Cellulite

PATHOPHYSIOLOGY AND TREATMENT
Second edition

Basic and Clinical Dermatology

Series Editor
Alan R. Shalita, M.D.
Distinguished Teaching Professor and Chairman
Department of Dermatology
SUNY Downstate Medical Center
Brooklyn, New York

Most recent titles

1. Cutaneous Investigation in Health and Disease: Noninvasive Methods and Instrumentation, edited by Jean-Luc Lévêque
2. Irritant Contact Dermatitis, edited by Edward M. Jackson and Ronald Goldner
3. Fundamentals of Dermatology: A Study Guide, edited by Franklin S. Glickman and Alan R. Shalita
4. Aging Skin: Properties and Functional Changes, edited by Jean-Luc Lévêque and Pierre G. Agache
5. Retinoids: Progress in Research and Clinical Applications, edited by Maria A. Livrea and Lester Packer
6. Clinical Photomedicine, edited by Henry W. Lim and Nicholas A. Soter
7. Cutaneous Antifungal Agents: Selected Compounds in Clinical Practice and Development, edited by John W. Rippon and Robert A. Fromtling
8. Oxidative Stress in Dermatology, edited by Jürgen Fuchs and Lester Packer
9. Connective Tissue Diseases of the Skin, edited by Charles M. Lapière and Thomas Krieg
10. Epidermal Growth Factors and Cytokines, edited by Thomas A. Luger and Thomas Schwarz
11. Skin Changes and Diseases in Pregnancy, edited by Marwali Harahap and Robert C. Wallach
12. Fungal Disease: Biology, Immunology, and Diagnosis, edited by Paul H. Jacobs and Lexie Nall
13. Immunomodulatory and Cytotoxic Agents in Dermatology, edited by Charles J. McDonald
14. Cutaneous Infection and Therapy, edited by Raza Aly, Karl R. Beutner, and Howard I. Maibach
15. Tissue Augmentation in Clinical Practice: Procedures and Techniques, edited by Arnold William Klein
16. Psoriasis: Third Edition, Revised and Expanded, edited by Henry H. Roenigk, Jr., and Howard I. Maibach
17. Surgical Techniques for Cutaneous Scar Revision, edited by Marwali Harahap
18. Drug Therapy in Dermatology, edited by Larry E. Millikan
19. Scarless Wound Healing, edited by Hari G. Garg and Michael T. Longaker
20. Cosmetic Surgery: An Interdisciplinary Approach, edited by Rhoda S. Narins
21. Topical Absorption of Dermatological Products, edited by Robert L. Bronaugh and Howard I. Maibach
22. Glycolic Acid Peels, edited by Ronald Moy, Debra Luftman, and Lenore S. Kakita
23. Innovative Techniques in Skin Surgery, edited by Marwali Harahap
24. Safe Liposuction and Fat Transfer, edited by Rhoda S. Narins
25. Pyschocutaneous Medicine, edited by John Y. M. Koo and Chai Sue Lee
26. Skin, Hair, and Nails: Structure and Function, edited by Bo Forslind and Magnus Lindberg
27. Itch: Basic Mechanisms and Therapy, edited by Gil Yosipovitch, Malcolm W. Greaves, Alan B. Fleischer, and Francis McGlone
28. Photoaging, edited by Darrell S. Rigel, Robert A. Weiss, Henry W. Lim, and Jeffrey S. Dover
29. Vitiligo: Problems and Solutions, edited by Torello Lotti and Jana Hercogova
30. Photodamaged Skin, edited by David J. Goldberg
31. Ambulatory Phlebectomy, Second Edition, edited by Mitchel P. Goldman, Mihael Georgiev, and Stefano Ricci
32. Cutaneous Lymphomas, edited by Gunter Burg and Werner Kempf
33. Wound Healing, edited by Anna Falabella and Robert Kirsner
34. Phototherapy and Photochemotherapy for Skin Disease, Third Edition, edited by Warwick L. Morison
35. Advanced Techniques in Dermatologic Surgery, edited by Mitchel P. Goldman and Robert A. Weiss
36. Tissue Augmentation in Clinical Practice, Second Edition, edited by Arnold W. Klein
37. Cellulite: Pathophysiology and Treatment, edited by Mitchel P. Goldman, Pier Antonio Bacci, Gustavo Leibaschoff, Doris Hexsel, and Fabrizio Angelini
38. Photodermatology, edited by Henry W. Lim, Herbert Hönigsmann, and John L. M. Hawk
39. Retinoids and Carotenoids in Dermatology, edited by Anders Vahlquist and Madeleine Duvic
40. Acne and Its Therapy, edited by Guy F. Webster and Anthony V. Rawlings
41. Hair and Scalp Diseases: Medical, Surgical, and Cosmetic Treatments, edited by Amy J. McMichael and Maria K. Hordinsky
42. Anesthesia and Analgesia in Dermatologic Surgery, edited by Marwali Harahap and Adel R. Abadir
43. Clinical Guide to Sunscreens and Photoprotection, edited by Henry W. Lim and Zoe Diana Draelos
44. Skin Moisturization, Second Edition, edited by Anthony V. Rawlings and James J. Leyden
45. Cellulite, Second Edition, edited by Mitchel P. Goldman and Doris Hexsel

Cellulite

PATHOPHYSIOLOGY AND TREATMENT
Second edition

edited by

Mitchel P Goldman, MD

Volunteer Clinical Professor of Medicine/Dermatology
University of California
San Diego, California
USA

Doris Hexsel, MD

Preceptor and Coordinator, Cosmetic Dermatology
Department of Dermatology
Pontifícia Universidade Católica do Rio Grande do Sul
Porto Alegre, Rio Grande do Sul
Brazil

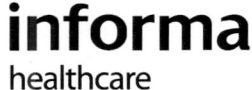

First published in 2006 by Taylor & Francis Group.

This edition published in 2010 by Informa Healthcare, Telephone House, 69-77 Paul Street, London EC2A 4LQ, UK.
Simultaneously published in the USA by Informa Healthcare, 52 Vanderbilt Avenue, 7th floor, New York, NY 10017, USA.

© 2010 Informa UK Ltd, except as otherwise indicated.

No claim to original U.S. Government works.

A CIP record for this book is available from the British Library.

ISBN-13: 9781439802717

Orders may be sent to: Informa Healthcare, Sheepen Place, Colchester, Essex CO3 3LP, UK
Telephone: +44 (0)20 7017 5540
Email: CSDhealthcarebooks@informa.com
Website: http://informahealthcarebooks.com/

For corporate sales please contact: CorporateBooksIHC@informa.com
For foreign rights please contact: RightsIHC@informa.com
For reprint permissions please contact: PermissionsIHC@informa.com

Typeset by Amnet Systems Private Limited
Printed and bound in the United Kingdom

Table of contents

Series introduction

Over the past twenty-one years we have edited a series of forty-five volumes relating to the art and science of dermatology. The series has been purposefully broad in content to attract the interest of a large variety of readers, from clinicians to basic scientists, affiliated with universities, industry, and in private practice.

The past decade has seen an explosion in interest in aesthetic dermatology. Significant advances have been made in cosmetic science and in new instrumentation for the treatment of aesthetic problems. Thus, a new focus has developed on the science of skin care both from the point of view of the practitioner as well as industry.

The latest addition to this series, *Cellulite: Pathophysiology and Treatment*, is the second edition of this popular work and demonstrates that the need for new information is compelling. The authors, Drs Mitchel Goldman and Doris Hexsel, not only are distinguished authorities in the field in their own right, but also have assembled a coterie of other distinguished contributors. We trust that this volume will again be of broad interest to scientists and clinicians alike.

ALAN R. SHALITA, M.D., Sc.D(hon)
Distinguished Teaching Professor and Chairman
Department of Dermatology
SUNY Downstate Medical Center
Brooklyn, NY, U.S.A.

Preface

Artists in painting and sculpture over the last two millennia have perceived beauty in a woman's figure as consisting in few muscles and a thick layer of subcutaneous fat. However, within the last four decades, there has been a radical change in perception, with today's society defining the ideal female body as youthful and almost pre-pubertal; well-defined musculature with very little body fat is now the ideal. This recent definition of beauty has led to the development of a new medical "disease," cellulite.

Cellulite can best be described as a normal physiologic state in post-adolescent women whose purpose is to maximize adipose retention to ensure adequate caloric availability for pregnancy and lactation. Almost all women who are not cachectic have cellulite.

The topic of cellulite appears every month on multiple television medical and talk shows, as well as in the lay public women's health magazines (which often show the cellulite in various female celebrities caught wearing a bathing suit, without the benefit of the air brushing that their publicity photographs undergo). Demand for the treatment of cellulite has become extremely popular: "90% of women have cellulite and the other 10% think they do." Sales of various topical therapies constitute a multimillion-dollar business; it is estimated that the sales of cellulite equipment is over 30 million dollars each year.

It is therefore time for a comprehensive textbook on the pathophysiology and treatment of cellulite. This subject is not taught in medical schools nor in residency training programs and there are few medical publications in the English language on this subject. As patients go to their physicians (mostly cosmetic and plastic surgeons and dermatologists) to seek advice on the pathophysiology and treatment of cellulite, physicians will need to educate themselves on this subject.

To this end, we have enlisted the enthusiastic support of some of the world's leaders in cellulite research. These respected professors and clinicians from the USA, Brazil, France, Italy, Argentina, Canada, Thailand and El Salvador are recognized as leaders on this subject. They have published numerous scientific papers on this subject in both their native languages and English. Our role as editors of this work, in addition to contributing separate chapters on our own unique research, is to ensure that this second edition of *Cellulite* is complete and up to date. We look forward to this textbook stimulating further research eventuating improved treatment of this cosmetically important condition.

Mitchel P Goldman
Doris Hexsel

List of contributors

Marie-Laurence Abella L'Oréal Recherche, Chevilly-Larue, France

Fabrizio Angelini Department of Endocrinology, University of Parma, Parma, Italy

Mathew Avram Department of Dermatology, Massachusetts General Hospital, Harvard Medical School, Boston, Massachusetts, USA

Pier Antonio Bacci University of Siena, and Cosmetic Pathologies Center, Arezzo, Italy

Marie Bazan Candela Corporation, Wayland, Massachusetts, USA

Christiane Bertin Johnson & Johnson Group of Consumer Companies, Paris, France

Régine Bousquet-Rouaud Dermatological Laser Unit, Millennium Clinic, Montpellier, France

Martin Braun Vancouver Laser and Skin Care Centre, Vancouver, British Columbia, Canada

Cristiano Brum Brazilian Center for Studies in Dermatology and Santa Casa Hospital Complex, Porto Alegre, Rio Grande do Sul, Brazil

Jean Chaintreuil Candela Corporation, Wayland, Massachusetts, USA

Taciana de Oliveira Dal'Forno Brazilian Center for Studies in Dermatology, Porto Alegre, Rio Grande do Sul, Brazil

Zoe Diana Draelos Department of Dermatology, Wake Forest University School of Medicine, Winston-Salem, North Carolina and Dermatology Consulting Services, High Point, North Carolina, USA

Agustina Vila Echague Candela Corporation, Wayland, Massachusetts, USA

Pietro Di Fiore Sports Medicine and Nutrition, Center for Prevention and Cure of Obesity, Palermo, Italy

Luca Gatteschi Sports Medicine Clinic, Florence, Italy

David J Goldberg Skin Laser Specialists of NY/NJ, and Mount Sinai School of Medicine, New York, New York, USA

Mitchel P Goldman Department of Dermatology, University of California, San Diego, California, USA

Mirko Guerra La Cittadella Socio Sanitaria di Cavarzere, Cavarzere, Italy

Enrique Hernández-Pérez Center for Dermatology and Cosmetic Surgery, San Salvador, El Salvador

José Enrique Hernández-Pérez Center for Dermatology and Cosmetic Surgery, San Salvador, El Salvador

Mauricio Hernández-Pérez Center for Dermatology and Cosmetic Surgery, San Salvador, El Salvador

Camile Luisa Hexsel Department of Dermatology, Henry Ford Hospital, Detroit, Michigan, USA

Doris Hexsel Department of Dermatology, Pontificia Universidade Católica do Rio Grande do Sul, Porto Alegre, Rio Grande do Sul, Brazil

Gustavo Leibaschoff University of Buenos Aires School of Medicine, and International Union of Lipolasty, Buenos Aires, Argentina

Woraphong Manuskiatti Department of Dermatology, Siriraj Hospital, Mahidol University, Bangkok, Thailand

Fulvio Marzatico Laboratory of Pharmacobiochemistry, Health Nutriceutical and Nutrition Research, University of Pavia, Pavia, Italy

Rosemarie Mazzuco Brazilian Center for Studies in Dermatology, Porto Alegre, Rio Grande do Sul, Brazil

Serge Mordon INSERM, Lille University Hospital, Lille, France

Alex Nkengne Johnson & Johnson Group of Consumer Companies, Paris, France

Carmine Orlandi Istituto di Ricerche Cliniche Ecomedica, Empoli, Italy

Michail M Pankratov Eleme Medical, Inc., Merrimack, New Hampshire, USA

Débora Zechmeister do Prado Brazilian Center for Studies in Dermatology, Porto Alegre, Rio Grande do Sul, Brazil

Massimo Rapetti   Istituto di Ricerche Cliniche Ecomedica, Empoli, Italy

Ana Beatris Rossi   Research and Development, Johnson & Johnson Group of Consumer Companies, Paris, France

Neil S Sadick   Department of Dermatology, Weill Medical College of Cornell University and Sadick Dermatology, New York, New York, USA

Gordon H Sasaki   Sasaki Advanced Aesthetic Medical Center, Pasadena, California and Linda Loma University Medical Center, Linda Loma, California, USA

Mariana Soirefmann   Brazilian Center for Studies in Dermatology, Porto Alegre, Rio Grande do Sul, Brazil

Attilio Speciani   Eurosalus, Milan, Italy

Amanda Stapenhorst   Brazilian Center for Studies in Dermatology, Porto Alegre, Rio Grande do Sul, Brazil

Jane Unaeze   Albert Einstein College of Medicine, New York, New York, USA

Molly Wanner   Department of Dermatology, Massachusetts General Hospital, Harvard Medical School, Boston, Massachusetts, USA

Magda B Weber   Department of Dermatology, Federal University of Health Science, Porto Alegre, Rio Grande do Sul, Brazil

1   Social Impact of Cellulite and Its Impact on Quality of Life
Doris Hexsel, Camile Luisa Hexsel, and Magda B Weber

Introduction

Almost all women have or believe they have cellulite. As it is more common to expose the body in certain cultures and in sunny countries such as Brazil, cellulite is of great concern to many women and also represents a problem of great social impact.

In today's globalized culture, physical well-being, including care taken with appearance, is highly valued. From this perspective, it is very important to evaluate the impact on quality of life (QoL) of such cosmetic problems as cellulite, wrinkles and aging. The fact that these have an impact on the QoL is indirectly shown by the growing interest in the investigation and treatment of these problems, which until recently were considered to be of minor significance. New studies involving QoL will benefit all those who suffer to a greater or lesser degree from these problems, and will be of great value in assessing the need for new scientific research into the treatment of these problems.

Medical treatments traditionally focused on quantitative factors, such as the reduction of morbidity and mortality and the assessment of treatment safety and social markers of health. Qualitative factors, such as patients' perceptions of well-being and capacity to perform activities of daily life were not a primary aim. In recent decades, however, the measurement of patient's quality of life and the evaluation of different treatments have been the focus of growing attention.

Sarwer et al. published a review of the literature that focused on psychological and social-cultural aspects, their relation to physical appearance, and their influence on the decision to undergo cosmetic treatments [1]. Their study revealed that in the 37 different cultures studied, men and women gave greater priority to sexual attraction in the choice of partners than to aspects of personality such as independence, emotional stability and maturity [1]. Dermatological diseases and cosmetic problems significantly affect self-esteem. As the symptoms are visible, the discomfort and psycho-emotional effects are frequently more serious than the physical alterations caused by the disease. Thus, it becomes very important to assess and quantify the emotional and social parameters in these patients, in order to understand the disruption that the problem causes in various daily activities. This will facilitate the follow-up and treatment evaluation, and consequently allow for improvements in the QoL of the patients.

The great importance given to QoL evaluation in clinical investigation and patient care has led to the development of questionnaires designed for the collection of information from the patients on the impact of the disease on their everyday lives. This knowledge allows the medical professional to better observe how the disease affects the patients physically, psychologically, and socially, and facilitates the evaluation of the effects on the lives of the patients.

In the case of cellulite, the reasons that lead the patient to seek treatment are generally social and, sometimes, also emotional. These may include the embarrassment caused by cellulite in social, affective, and sexual relations as well as the avoidance of normal everyday activities such as visiting a swimming pool or beach, practicing sports or exposing the body during intimacy.

A number of studies have been published that deal with QoL and recognize the value of specific questionnaires for dermatological diseases such as psoriasis, acne, melasma, atopic dermatitis, hyperhidrosis, and alopecia among others [2–9]. These studies have revealed the existence of similar facets related to QoL in patients from various countries [10] and point to the discomfort and the psycho-emotional effect on the patients. However, in general, little research has been done on the psychological, environmental, and social aspects of dermatological diseases. Moreover, to date, no study on the QoL of those afflicted by cellulite has been published.

Patients suffering from skin diseases should not be treated merely for the physical harm caused by the disease [10]. The skin is the most external and apparent organ, and skin contact contributes to the formation and structure of the personality.

Aspects of Cellulite Related to Qol

Cellulite is a clinical and aesthetic condition affecting most women. It may appear in preadolescence, adolescence, or adulthood. With cellulite, the connective tissue and adipose tissue undergo alterations, resulting in blood and lymphatic alterations [11]. Clinically, cellulite is characterized by alterations to the cutaneous surface, especially on the buttocks and thighs, giving the skin an orange peel or mattress appearance [12,13]. Clinically, cellulite is classified into degrees that range from 0 to III according to the clinical characteristics [14]. As well as classifying the cellulite, it is suggested that associated factors such as obesity [measured by the body mass index (BMI)] and degree of flaccidity (classified as light, moderate, or severe) be characterized.

Our clinical experience has shown that cellulite is a problem that has an impact on the QoL of both younger and more mature women, though the impact is greater in younger women. It also seems that cellulite is more frequent nowadays than many years ago.

We report here on a clinical study carried out in 62 female patients, aged between 18 and 45 years (average age 32) with BMIs between 18 and 25 (average 21.8), having various degrees of cellulite on the buttocks and thighs. Over a period of two months, these patients received mechanical treatment in both legs and topical treatment in only one randomly chosen leg. The degree of cellulite in each patient was evaluated before and at the end of the treatment and attributed a classification between 0 and III, according to the clinical appearance of the cellulite. No patients included in this study had a cellulite classification of 0.

These patients also answered a non-validated questionnaire created by the authors at the beginning and end of the treatment. This questionnaire evaluated patients' self-esteem and highlighted changes in the behavior of patients with cellulite such as avoiding wearing tight or small clothing; feeling embarrassed when frequenting swimming pools or at the beach, etc. The impact of cellulite in relation to age group was also evaluated, together with factors that patients believe may influence the cellulite, such as inheritance, diet, and physical activity, as well as the treatment performed and self-perception of the severity of their cellulite. A survey of the answers given to the questions permitted an assessment of:

1. patients' impressions of the problem of cellulite;
2. the everyday situations that result in restrictions or embarrassment for patients with cellulite; and
3. the impact of treatment on patients' QoL.

Some factors, in the opinion of the patient, may influence cellulite. When questioned regarding diet, 65% of patients believed that there is a relationship between cellulite and diet. For 60% of the patients interviewed, a specific diet can help with cellulite. Along the same lines, 90% of patients believed that practicing physical exercise is an efficient treatment for cellulite and may, in isolation, moderately reduce cellulite.

Cellulite was perceived before 20 years of age by 65% of patients. With regard to family inheritance, 80% of patients reported having first- or second-degree relatives with cellulite. Because it is a clinically diagnosed and easily recognizable problem, this information is highly indicative of the presence of positive family cases, bearing in mind that the great majority of patients reported a family member of the first degree, mother or daughter, as having the same problem.

Regarding the restrictions caused by cellulite, when questioned in a generalized way about the degree to which cellulite hampered their lives with the options of "not at all (1)," "a little (2)," "moderately (3)," or "greatly (4)," it was found that 70% of the interviewed patients considered that cellulite hampered their lives greatly. Regarding specific daily situations, it was noted that those suffering from cellulite experience some day-to-day restrictions. Each situation was evaluated by the patient and attributed a value from 1 to 5, in which "1" was given to situations in which having cellulite had no effect, "2" to little effect, "3" to a moderate effect, "4" to a significant effect, and "5" to a very significant effect.

The situations included wearing a bikini and tight clothing, sexual activity, practicing sports, and crossing the legs and sitting, which indicate the great social impact caused by cellulite. Keep in mind that, in all the situations presented and even after treatment, having cellulite influences to a moderate or significant degree the daily lives of the patients. We notice that the treatment, even though it might not be 100% effective for the problem, may modify the behavior of cellulite patients. The results obtained from the studied sample reveal that the presence of cellulite after treatment interferes less in certain activities when the responses from before and after treatment are compared. This reduction is most evident in the item "sexual life" when the total sample is examined: 21.9% of the patients mentioned that cellulite had great or very significant influence on their sexual life before treatment and, although the treatment may not have led to a marked improvement in the cellulite, only 8.3% of the patients gave the same response following treatment. The sitting position, a position that

supposedly makes the cellulite more apparent, reveals that before treatment, 48.9% of the patients interviewed considered the influence very significant, while after treatment this percentage fell to 15.1%. With regard to the embarrassment caused by the presence of cellulite in the practice of sports, the answers both before and after treatment were very similar. The results suggest that, for women, exposing the body during sport is not as embarrassing as in other situations, as for example during sexual relations.

According to Jorge [10], the psychological impact and in interpersonal relations, respectively, is more prejudicial for women than for men. Studies that evaluated patients with dermatosis, carried out in Sweden and Norway, suggest that those at risk of the greatest harm are females who are young and in whom that disease exists over an extended period of time [10]. As cellulite appears basically in women, this condition should be investigated in terms of its impact in QoL.

A study by Harlow et al, that evaluated the impact on quality of life of dermatological diseases during primary attention, noted the differences between men and women in relation to the various forms of constraints caused by the diseases from which they suffered [15]. Ten (10) attributes were evaluated: physical symptoms, feelings, daily routine, clothing, social and leisure, sport and exercise, work and study, personal relations, sexual relations and treatment. Of these, only in the question related to the degree to which the condition affected the practice of sports and exercise was the score given by males higher than that given by women [15]. This shows that the practice of sport may have greater significance in the male group than in the female.

We also checked the impact of treatment on the QoL of patients with cellulite. Each patient attributed a value from 0 to 9, with 0 representing very low self-esteem in relation to the fact of having cellulite, and 9 representing very high self-esteem. The clinical evaluation considered the improvement on the left and right sides, which were treated differently. Even without any improvement in the degree of cellulite noted by the examiner, there was an increase in self-esteem (evaluated from 0 to 9) after treatment. This improvement can be seen in the difference in the percentage of scores found from before and after treatment. This shows that the treatment did have a positive effect on the self-esteem of the patients, indicating that the simple fact of treating the cellulite and caring for themselves, even in the absence of any clinical improvement, influenced the well-being of the patients, who described themselves as better and more confident following the treatment. It may suggest that treatments should be tried, even if there is no cure for this condition.

In 2008, the authors conducted a new clinical trial with the aim to build a specific questionnaire on the QoL for cellulite patients. Fifty patients were included responding to a qualitative survey to evaluate the main spontaneous complaints of patients seen because of cellulite and the effect of cellulite on their quality of life. An open question was asked about the main complaint: "*We are trying to find out how much the fact of having cellulite affects the life of female patients. We would appreciate your cooperation, but your participation is totally voluntary and not compulsory. Could you please describe in what ways having cellulite has affected your life? You may include aspects of your professional and social life, personal relationships, leisure activities,*

Table 1.1 Summarized version of CelluQOL® questionnaire

	Not bothered at all	Bothered most of the time	No feelings either way	Bothered most of the time	Bothered all the time
Skin apperance	1	2	3	4	5
Clothing manners	1	2	3	4	5
Feeding habits	1	2	3	4	5
Physical and leisure activities involving exposure of the body in public	1	2	3	4	5
Physical or recreational activities involving the restricted exposure of the body	1	2	3	4	5
Sexual life	1	2	3	4	5
Negative feelings	1	2	3	4	5
Disbelief about results of treatments	1	2	3	4	5

or any other situation. Although we need to know how old you are, no further personal identification is necessary." The preliminary analysis of the questions answered by the volunteers showed factors and situations which are influenced by the presence of cellulite [16]. These patients mentioned that they usually avoid wearing white colored and beach clothing and prefer to wear black (90%); dislike walking on the beach without wearing beach jackets (56%), this is because they prefer to hide their cellulite; they also feel bothered and constrained by the presence of cellulite (38%); they are afraid about their partners noticing their condition (36%) and also have feelings of low self-esteem (20%). From the preliminary answers, it was possible to establish the main domains that affect the QoL due to the presence of cellulite: clothing choices, leisure habits, physical activities, relationships with partners, personal feelings about themselves, and daily habits [16].

The second part of the same study mentioned above involved 100 patients and aimed to create and validate a new instrument of Quality of Life on Celluite, called CelluQOL®. The authors created two versions of CelluQOL®, based on the domains revealed in the first part of the study, one complete and the other summarized (Table 1.1). All patients responded to both questionnaires which were compared and validated. The complete data of this study are in process of statistical evaluation and will be published soon. However, the data collected and pre-analyzed from this study suggests that a QoL questionnaire for patients presenting cellulite may be useful in clinical practice [16].

Conclusion
Thorough QoL evaluations will be necessary to evaluate not only the importance given to the problem of "cellulite", but also the need to develop new treatments for cellulite [17].

It is interesting to note that, even without techniques that can guarantee significant improvement of cellulite in its different degrees, cosmetic patients want alternatives and their emotional improvement is not directly related to the clinical improvement. Care and attention to cosmetic problems can lead to improvement in the emotional state of the patients.

Cellulite has a real impact on the QoL of patients, as it restricts those that suffer from the condition in everyday situations and activities. This causes damage in the psychological area in interpersonal relationships, as also occurs with other conditions that afflict the skin.

Patient complaints should be evaluated objectively regardless of whether defects are visible and pertinent or just imaginary, or even if the patient's concerns seem to be out of proportion with reality. As it is a very sensitive issue, techniques used for esthetic procedures should be improved, and their performance should lead to minimal side effects, faster recovery and greater safety. However, esthetic procedures may not be enough to deal with complaints that may in fact mask fears, anxiety and fantasies, and a full evaluation may be necessary to improve and preserve the doctor-patient relationship.

Finding out what aspects in each domain concern patients and measuring their possible impact may help to make decisions about what type of treatment should be prescribed for any specific patient. Also, the development of instruments to measure the QoL of patients presenting aesthetic complaints is an innovative and challenging area to be studied. The measurement of the aspects in each domain that concern patients may help to make decisions about more effective ways to treat specific patients.

REFERENCES

1. DB Sarwer, L Magge, V Clark. Physical appearance and cosmetic medical treatments: physiological and socio-cultural influences. Journal of Cosmetic Dermatology 2:29–39, 2003.
2. R Balkrishan, AJ McMichael, FT Camacho, F Saltzberg et al. Development and validation of a health-releated quality of life with for women with melasma. Br J Dermatol 149(3):572–7, 2003.
3. SP McKenna, AS Cook, D Whalley, LC Doward et al. Development of the PSORIQoL, a psoriasis-specific measure of quality of life designed for use in clinical practice and trials. Dr J Dermatol 149(2):323–31, 2003.
4. R Skoet, R Zachariae, T Agner. Contact dermatitis and quality of life: a structured review of the literature. Br J Dermatol 149:452–56, 2003.
5. LHF Arruda, S Ypiranga. Qualidade de vida em hiperidrose. In: AT Almeida, D Hexsel. Hiperidrose e Qualidade de Vida. Edição das autoras. São Paulo; 2003: 73–76.
6. AY Finalay, GK Khan. Dermatology life quality index (DLQI) – a simple pratical measure for routine clinical use. Clin Exp Dermatol 19:210–16, 1994.
7. S Shimidt, TW Fischer, MM Chren et al. Stratategies of coping and quality of life in women with alopecia. Br J Dermatol 144:1038–43, 2001.

8. C Swartling, H Naver, M Lindberg. Botulinum A toxin improves life quality in severe primancy focal hiperhidrosis. European Journal of Neurology 8:247–52, 2001.

9. E Mallon, JN Newton, A Klassen et al. The quality of life in acne: a comparison with general medical conditions using generic questionnaires. Br J Dermatol 140:672–76, 1999.

10. HZ Jorge. Avaliação de Qualidade de Vida em Pacientes com Dermatoses: Estudo De Adaptação e Validação da Dermatology Life Quality Index: (DLQI) para uma amostra Sul-Brasileira. Tese de Mestrado, Faculdade de Psicologia, Pontifícia Universidade Católica do Rio Grande do Sul 2004.

11. GW Lucasse, WLM Van-der-Sluys et al. The effectiveness of massage treatment on cellulite as monitored by ultrasound imaging. Skin Re Technol 3:154–60, 1997.

12. AM Segers, J Abulafia et al. Celulitis. Estudo histopatológico e histoquímico de 100 casos. Med Cut ILA 12:167–72, 1984.

13. C Scherwitz, O Braun-Falco. So-called cellulite. J Dermatol Surg Oncol 4(3):230–34, 1978.

14. D Hexsel, R Mazzuco. Subcision: a treatment for cellulite. Int J Dermatol 39:539–44, 2000.

15. D Harlow, T Poyner, AY Finlay, PJ Dykes. Impaired quality of adults with skin disease in primary care. Br J Dermatol 143:979–82, 2000.

16. D Hexsel, M Weber, ML Taborda, JF Souza. Preliminary results of the elaboration of a new instrument to evaluate quality of life in patients with cellulite: CelluQOL. JAAD Poster Abstracts 3(60):P1192, 2009.

17. KG Bergstrom, K Arambula, AB Kimball. Medication formulation affects quality of life: a randomized single-blind study of clobetasol propionate foam 0.05% compared with a combined program of clobetasol cream 0.05% and solution 0.05% for the treatment of psoriasis. Cutis 72(5):407–11, 2003.

2 Psychological Impact of Cellulite on the Affected Patients
Cristiano Brum

New cellulite research is appearing in literature every day, including a new classification [1] system, new techniques and tools [2,3,4], with the aim of achieving better results and greater patient satisfaction. This process is a response to the explosion in popularity of other aesthetic treatments and it is mainly due to the safety of less-invasive procedures developed over the last two decades. As a result, these procedures received increased media attention and therefore more individuals were willing to undergo cosmetic treatments with the goal of enhancing their physical appearance [5] as well as increasing aspects of their quality of life, especially regarding body satisfaction and health [6].

Beauty is an attribute that has been desired by mankind since ancient times. Plato understood that beauty, good health and wealth acquired by honest means, are the most important wishes of every man [7]. Beauty inspired poets, painters, writers, and wars, as depicted in the *Iliad*, in which Homer describes the epic battles of the Trojan War caused by Paris's abduction of Helen – said to be the most beautiful woman who ever lived – from her husband, King Menelaus. Beauty was also correlated to Darwin's theory of evolution, in which physical signs of youth and health are the most reliable physical markers of fertility [8].

Beauty plays an important role in human relationships in a social setting. Koblenzer [9] mentions some studies that demonstrate real benefits from maintaining an appearance of youthfulness and beauty during all stages of life. For example, "cute" babies receive more care-taking attention, nice-looking children are assumed by their teachers to be more intelligent, attractive adolescents are preferred as friends or dates, employers are more likely to hire applicants with nicer appearances, at higher salaries, whom they promote rapidly.

Nowadays, one of the reasons for women's dissatisfaction with their appearance is cellulite – a clinical condition that affects a significant number of women worldwide. It was noted that those suffering from cellulite, experience some day-to-day restrictions, including clothing choices, physical and sexual activity, among others. These problems suggest a great social impact of this condition on their lives [10]. There are no references in medical literature about the psychological aspects of women that undergo cosmetic treatments for cellulite, except for the incipient studies regarding quality of life in this population [11].

To fill in this gap, the research group from the Brazilian Center for Studies in Dermatology (Porto Alegre, Brazil) collected new data from 30 healthy female volunteers, ranging in age from 20 to 45 years old. They answered a questionnaire focusing on the psychological aspects, symptoms of eating disorders, body image concerns, social functioning, previous psychotherapy and psychiatric problems, feelings related to their cellulite, social embarrassment, and cellulite treatment expectations [12].

Regarding the onset of cellulite, most of the patients (40%) mentioned the adolescent period, 33% their 20s, and the others varied situations, during weight loss and gain, after pregnancy,

and after 40s were mentioned by 16.5%. It seems that early in life cellulite becomes a great concern for women [12].

Eighty-six percent of patients presenting cellulite stated that they notice cellulite in others. According to the patients' opinions, they pay attention to the cellulite in other women to compare the severity (19%), to help them feel better about themselves because of the fact that they share the same condition with other women (15%), for both cited reasons (54%) and 12% for other reasons. When asked whether they thought men paid attention to their cellulite, 50% of women said yes, and the others said no [12].

When these patients stare in the mirror and see their cellulite, they experience diverse negative feelings, like anger, guilt, sadness, impotency, shame, discomfort and the desire to cover themselves. Among these feelings, the most frequently mentioned by this sample was frustration (26%). The volunteers also reported that they feel ashamed of their cellulite. For 67%, the feeling of shame is presented in only certain situations. In 30% of these patients, this feeling occurred more frequently, whereas only one woman denied feeling ashamed of her cellulite. Interestingly, the majority of patients (63.3%) mentioned that these negative feelings do not interfere in their daily activities. In 23.3%, these feelings have a positive impact on their self-care (health and appearance), and only 13.3% reported low self-esteem and isolation [12].

The leading cause for seeking cellulite treatments was personal motivation, reported by 63.3% of the patients. The second most common was media, responsible for 20%. Recommendations from partners, friends, or family also played an important role accounting for 13%. Overall, the volunteers believe that treating their cellulite will improve certain aspects of their lives, such as self-esteem and sociability [10].

Personal motivation is directly related to the inner world of each individual, their life story, parental support, self-esteem, formation process of their body image, and their personality traits. However, external influences are an important factor in the pursuit of a perfect and attractive cellulite-free body. Some research shows that media significantly contributes to the creation of the thin body ideal, eating habits, altering moods, and satisfaction with their own body.

Pinhas et al. [13] and colleagues examined changes in female university students' mood states resulting from viewing pictures in fashion magazines of models who represent the thin ideal. The authors observed that viewing images of female fashion models had an immediate negative effect on women's moods, represented by more depressed and angry states. Hawkins et al. [14] showed further aspects related to the exposure of women to thin-ideal magazine images, such as an increase in body dissatisfaction, negative mood states, eating disorder symptoms, and lowered self-esteem.

In a recent study, participants were randomly divided in two groups, one of which watched a reality TV cosmetic surgery program, while the other watched a reality TV home improvement program. The authors concluded that among the participants, particularly those who had internalized the thin body-ideal and watched the cosmetic surgery program, reported greater perceptions of media pressure to be thin [15].

Using functional neuroimaging in 18 healthy young women, Friederich et al. examined brain responses and levels of anxiety from images of slim-idealized bodies (active condition) and interior designs (control condition) were measured. In active condition, participants initiated their body shape processing network. The authors believe that brain networks associated with anxiety induced by self-comparison to slim images may be involved in the genesis of body dissatisfaction and hence with vulnerability to eating disorders [16].

In our study, bulimic symptoms were found in three patients, 10% of the sample. One volunteer reported she had a diagnosis of bulimia and was being treated by a psychiatrist [12]. The same proportion was described by Alagöz et al. [17] in research that investigated self-esteem, body imaging scale, and applied eating attitude scale tests in patients who had undergone cosmetic surgery.

Another important finding from this study was the fact that twenty-one patients (70%) reported using weight-loss drugs, many volunteers taking more than one medication for this reason. Amphetamines were cited by four patients, eight volunteers took laxatives, three used diuretics, and eight received a prescription of sibutramine from their doctors [12]. This data suggests that many patients look for magic formulas to lose weight instead of adopting healthier lifestyles.

Because these patients might be using such medications without knowing their possible side effects and the health threats, doctors should advise their patients about amphetamines' adverse effects, such as paranoid delusions, hallucinations, anxiety disorders, mania, insomnia, irritability, chemical dependence and physical symptoms (hypertension, tachycardia, palpitation, mydrasis, bruxism, tremor and headache) [18].

The purchase and use of prescribed medications, without a prescription, is a very common practice in many countries worldwide, including Brazil. This is a major problem because the misuse of these medications can cause adverse effects, such as diuretics, resulting in hyponatremia, hyperkalemia, hypokalemia, increased levels of blood sugar and cholesterol, rash, joint disorders (gout), and menstrual irregularities. It is important to advise patients about misconceptions, as many women think diuretics help lose weight [19]. Laxatives are sometimes used by normal and bulimic women. This medication can cause fluid and electrolyte imbalances, steatorrhea, osteomalacia, diarrhea, and, cathartic colon. Although there is no evidence on the structural or functional impairment of enteric nerves or intestinal smooth muscle, nor colorectal cancer and other tumors, laxatives should be taken with caution [20].

When sibutramine is prescribed by doctors, patients should be aware of the side effects, which include drug intolerance, headache, insomnia, nausea, dry mouth, constipation, tachycardia, and hypertension-related events [21], as well as the case of patients with bipolar disorder, which could result in mania or mixed mood states [22].

Many patients want an "easy way" to lose weight. These patients also expect magic results from cellulite treatments. In our preliminary research, 11 patients (37%) expect their cellulite to disappear with the treatment, another 37% are more realistic and expect some improvement after the procedure, 16% have never done any treatment and 3% believe that there is no effective treatment for cellulite [12].

Crockett et al. [23] mentioned that patients who regularly watched one or more reality television show reported the following: a greater influence from television and media to pursue cosmetic surgery; felt more knowledgeable about cosmetic surgery in general; and felt that plastic surgery reality television was more similar to real life than did non-frequent viewers. The results of this study suggest that many patients come to offices with unrealistic ideas and expectations regarding cosmetic procedures. The evaluation of the psychological profile, expectations and knowledge about the technique may be helpful to improve the relationship between physicians and patients, especially when undergoing cosmetic procedures. Moreover, it is also important to manage their expectations, advise them about contraindications, possible side effects and complications, including limitations of each indicated procedure.

Considering that patients usually do not inform doctors about their psychiatric problems if not asked, and that some psychiatric conditions do interfere with patient's satisfaction, the psychological history should be carefully evaluated. Certain psychiatric disorders, especially those interfering with the body image, seem to be more prevalent in cosmetic patients, and they may be considered a contraindication to perform some cosmetic procedures [24]. Attention should be given to psychosis, eating disorders, body dimorphic disorder, depression, and anxiety [24,25]. In our research, 30% of the patients had a history of psychiatric disorders and previous psychotherapy. The main causes were depression, bulimia, anxiety, panic disorder, and psychological conflicts. None were diagnosed with body dimorphic disorder.

It is important to mention that we learned that 77% of the patients would like to better evaluate their emotional symptoms and were open to this conversation. This emphasizes the importance of the medical and psychological approach to cosmetic patients, especially those undergoing surgical procedures, to avoid patient and surgeon frustration and unexpected, negative outcomes.

REFERENCES

1. D Hexsel, T Dal'Forno, CL Hexsel. A validated photonumeric cellulite severity scale. J Eur Acad Dermatol Venereol (5):523–8, 2009.
2. K Altabas, V Altabas, MC Berković, VZ Rotkvić. From Cellulite to smooth skin: Is Viagra the new dream cream? Med Hypotheses 73(1):118–9, 2009.
3. S Bielfeldt, P Buttgereit, M Brandt et al. Non-invasive evaluation techniques to quantify the efficacy of cosmetic anti-cellulite products. Skin Res Technol 14(3):336–46, Aug 2008.
4. A Goldman, RH Gotkin, DS Sarnoff et al. Cellulite: a new treatment approach combining subdermal Nd: YAG laser lipolysis and autologous fat transplantation. Aesthet Surg J 28(6):656–62, Nov-Dec 2008.
5. DB Sarwer, CE Crerand. Body image and cosmetic medical treatments. Body Image 1(1):99–111, 2004.
6. NA Papadopulos, L Kovacs, S Krammer et al. Quality of life following aesthetic plastic surgery: a prospective study. J Plast Reconstr Aesthet Surg 60(8):915–21, 2007.

7. M Alam, JS Dover. On beauty: evolution, psychosocial considerations, and surgical enhancement. Arch Dermatol 137(6):795–807, 2001.

8. DB Sarwer, TA Grossbart, ER Didie. Beauty and society. Semin Cutan Med Surg 22(2):79–92, 2003.

9. CS Koblenzer. Psychosocial aspects of beauty: how and why to look good. Clin Dermatol 21(6):473–75, 2003.

10. D Hexsel, C Hexsel. Social impact of cellulite and its impact on quality of life. In: MP Goldman, PA Bacci, G Leibaschoff et al (eds). Cellulite: pathophysiology and treatment. New York: Taylor & Francis; 2006: pp1–5.

11. D Hexsel, JF Souza, M Weber, ML Taboreda. Preliminary results of the elaboration of a new instrument to evaluate quality of life in patients with cellulite: CELLUQOL. J Am Acad Dermatol 60(3) (Suppl 1):62, 2009.

12. D Hexsel, C Brum, R Mazzuco, T Rodrigues. Psychologic aspects of women who underwent celulite treatments: Piolot study. Poster presented at 67th Annual Meeting of American Academy of Dermatology, March 6–10th, 2009. San Francisco, California- PP1131.

13. L Pinhas, BB Toner, A Ali et al. The effects of the ideal of female beauty on mood and body satisfaction. Int J Eat Disord 25(2):223–26, 1999.

14. N Hawkins, PS Richards, HM Granley, DM Stein. The impact of exposure to the thin-ideal media image on women. Eat Disord. 12(1):35–50, 2004.

15. SE Mazzeo, SE Trace, KS Mitchell, RW Gow. Effects of a reality TV cosmetic surgery makeover program on eating disordered attitudes and behaviors. Eat Behav 8(3):390–97, 2007.

16. HC Friederich, R Uher, S Brooks et al. I'm not as slim as that girl: neural bases of body shape self-comparison to media images. Neuroimage 15;37(2):674–81, 2007.

17. MS Alagöz, AD Başterzi, AC Uysal et al. The psychiatric view of patients of aesthetic surgery: self-esteem, body image, and eating attitude. Aesthetic Plast Surg 27(5):345–48, 2003.

18. BJ Sadock, VA Sadock. Kaplan and Sadock's Synopsis of Psychiatry: Behavioral Sciences/Clinical Psychiatry; 2007.

19. C Brater. Diuretic Therapy. NEJM 339(6):387–95, 1998.

20. A Wald. Is chronic use of stimulant laxatives harmful to the colon? J Clin Gastroenterol 36(5):386–89, 2003.

21. AP Maggioni, I Caterson, W Coutinho et al. SCOUT Investigators Tolerability of sibutramine during a 6-week treatment period in high-risk patients with cardiovascular disease and/or diabetes: a preliminary analysis of the Sibutramine Cardiovascular Outcomes (SCOUT) Trial. J Cardiovasc Pharmacol 52(5):393–402, 2008.

22. Q Cordeiro, H Vallada. Sibutramine-induced mania episode in a bipolar patient. Int J Neuropsychopharmacol 5(3):283–84, 2002.

23. RJ Crockett, T Pruzinsky, JA Persing. The influence of plastic surgery "reality TV" on cosmetic surgery patient expectations and decision making. Plast Reconstr Surg 120(1): 316–24, 2007.

24. TA Grossbart, DB Sarwer. Psychosocial issues and their relevance to the cosmetic surgery patient. Semin Cutan Med Surg 22(2):136–47, 2003.

25. D Veale. Psychological aspects of a cosmetic procedure. Psychiatry and Medicine 5(3):93–95, 2006.

3   Anatomy of Cellulite and the Interstitial Matrix
Pier Antonio Bacci

Introduction

The understanding of the structure and function of the interstitial (or extracellular) matrix constitutes a relatively recent conceptual revolution. Prof. Francesco Albergati of Milan, student of Prof. Sergio Curri, was the first to study and describe the clinical relevance of this microvascular tissue unit [1]. A brief overview is given here.

Cellulite

The body's silhouette is characterized by a particular localization of the subcutaneous adipose tissue over the osteomuscular structure. The human body is characterized by the presence of rigid fasciae and especially deep muscular fasciae that start from the base of the cranium and continue to the ankles and metatarsus promoting various physiological functions: vascular, neurophysiologic, and orthopedic. Cellulite is a degenerative and evolutional affect on subcutaneous tissue. The authors describe cellulite from a histomorphologically point of view, defining it as a PEFS: "panniculopatia edematofibrosclerotica (edematofibrosclerotic dermo-lipodermic pathology)" [2].

Cellulite is considered as a series of events characterized by interstitial edema, secondary connective tissue fibrosis, and consequent sclerotic evolution. Recent clinical observations demonstrated that if PEFS is a true part of cellulite, it does not represent all the various clinical aspects of cellulite. In fact there are often particular forms of connective and interstitial damage or diffuse syndromes characterized by a lipedema associated with a lymphedema and/or lipodystrophy. Such pathologies are mainly observed on the gluteal muscle and on the lower limbs of women.

Fundamental here is acceptance that cellulite is not a female whim or something considered unsightly, but a real disorder, or rather, different disorders that represent aesthetic pathologies that must be cared for from a medical and cosmetic point of view.

- The cellulite disorder normally is an expression of lipolymphedema, or more precisely a typical expression of mesenchimopathy with microvessel alterations.
- It is, above all, an endocrine-metabolic disorder that may or may not be associated with lipolymphedema, localized adiposity, and lipodystrophy with an alteration of the interstitial matrix and connective tissue. It, therefore, presents various aspects that call for different therapies.
- First and foremost, it displays alterations of the purifying organs that must be controlled and brought back into balance. There are also alterations of the basic regulation of temperature, pH, and the oxidation–reduction systems.
- Such alterations can be discovered with tests to assay free radicals and heavy metals, and by video capillaroscopy. These dismetabolic situations can be corrected through diet (especially protein therapy in two-week cycles), physical activity, and polyvitaminic, alkalinizing, and orthomolecular therapy [3–10].

- Cellulite is often also associated with venous lymphatic insufficiency; however, cellulite formation occurs before, not after, the venous disease. It is the cause, not the effect.
- Lipolymphedema and cellulite are the greatest expressions of an alteration of the functionality of the cleansing organs. We also know that unnecessary nongraduated elastic stockings are one of the causes of superficial cellulite due to compression and the slowing of microcirculation [11].

We know that three forms of edema can be associated with cellulite disorder: venous edema, lymphatic edema, and lipedema.

1. *What is venous edema?*
   Venous edema is basically characterized by a release of kinins, toxic substances, and iron that carries calcium with it. It is an edema associated with phlogosis of the tissues and deposition of hemosiderin.
2. *What is lymphedema?*
   Lymphedema is a pathological condition characterized by a state of tumescence of the soft tissues, usually superficial, due to accumulation by stasis of high protein–content lymph caused by primary and/or secondary alterations of the lymphatic vessels. Lymphatic edema is linked to alterations of the lymphatic vessels, and is characterized by free water in the interstices that has bonded with proteins and solutes, forming an edema of lymph with interstitial hyperpressure [12].
3. *What is lipedema?*
   Lipedema is a particular syndrome characterized by subcutaneous deposition of fatty tissue and water, especially in the buttocks and lower limbs, which may or may not be associated with lymphedema and/or lipodystrophy [13,14]. It is an edema characterized by an increase of free water in the interstices; it is not lymph—it is free water and fatty tissue.

Lymphedema

Lymphedema is a chronic and progressive affliction that is very difficult to cure. The aim of treatment is to keep the disease stable in order for the patient to live normally. In this type of pathology, the first component is edema and the second is fibrosis. The increase of protein levels in the tissues contributes to the development of edema and probably causes chronic inflammation and subsequently the fibrosis.

The basic clinical sign of lymphatic problems, either mechanical or dynamic, is a cold and pale swelling, which is initially viscous and later hardens but is not painful in most cases. With the increase in severity of edema, there is an increase in limb volume. At this point, it is not sufficient to hold the limb in an elevated position in order to reduce edema; fibrosis is already present.

Lipedema and Lipolymphedema

Lymphedema is described as a pathology characterized by a tumescent state of soft tissues, usually superficial [15], and is related to an accumulation of lymph with high protein content due to stasis in the interstitial space. It is determined by primary and/or secondary damage of the transport vessels. In contrast, lipedema is a particular syndrome with a poorly understood etiology characterized by fat and water deposits in the subcutaneous tissue (particularly in lower limbs and gluteal muscle), and associated with lymphedema and/or lipodystrophy.

Lipedema was described for the first time as an accumulation of subcutaneous fat with hard leg edema excepting the feet. In various descriptions [16], the following observation has always been underlined: foot hypothermia with a localized gradient of temperature. Such pathology, often superficially defined as a lymphedema or venous insufficiency or cellulite, is observed in more than 65% of women between the ages of 14 and 35 years, becoming lipodystrophic lipolymphedema after the age of 40. The common characteristics of a lipolymphedema are the absence of venous insufficiency (eventually secondary) and the close relation with the fat tissue metabolism.

Lipolymphedema is a syndrome of unknown etiology, characterized with fat deposition in the subcutaneous tissue and associated with orthostatic and recurrent edema in the legs and gluteal muscle that induces the impression of an increased volume in the limbs. Lipedema always begins in the legs, excluding the ankle and foot, which makes it different from lipolymphedema. It can be related to weight increase but is often independent of it. It is often related to familial factors. The characteristic of this extremely frequent disease is that edema always succeeds fat deposition. The latter is subsequent to endocrinometabolic disorder of the interstitial matrix and is not accompanied with obesity.

The edema here is not caused by structural changes of venolymphatic vessels, but by the modified ratio of the distance from the adiposity and connective structure with a loss of support. It is an edema that worsens with walking and standing, in contrast to phlebolymphedema. Another difference from lymphedema is its softness and the possibility of its making a skin fold that is not obstructed by the viscosity. Thus it is different from lipolymphedema, phlebolymphedema, Barraquer–Simmond disease (characterized by upper body thinness), and Dercum syndrome; the latter, which is clinically similar, has an etiology related to toxicities of the autonomous nervous system linked to an intestinal dysbiosis.

Dercum Syndrome

The word "lipodystrophy" means a pathology characterized by structural and functional damage of adipose tissue. Lipodystrophy can be associated with some form of lipolymphedema, the more typical being Dercum lipodystrophy or painful lipodystrophy. Women are affected early with recurrent lipedema. Typically painful fat nodules are often preceded by the appearance of lipedema and are often associated with asthenia, neuropsychic and adynamical troubles (depression or anxiety), and intestinal dysbiosis. Limb pain is different from the pain of lipolymphedema or from superficial hypoxia, where pain is induced by pinching the subcutaneous tissue and is associated with tissue viscosity due to interstitial hyperpressure of toxic lymph.

Pathogenesis of the Dercum syndrome is not endocrine or metabolic (as in recurrent lipedema), but from nerve damage of the neurovegetative—either the hypothalamic or the peripheral—system. Interstitial inflammation phenomena have been demonstrated to be related to the nervous network linked to the adipose tissue in the environment of the extracellular matrix.

In this context, bacteria from intestinal origin have also been found. This disease is certainly attributable to a suffering of interstitial mesenchyma with exaltation of the lipogenesis (slowdown of the microcirculatory flux and damage of the α-2-fibers) due to the damage to the peripheral neurovegetative regulatory system.

"Big Leg"

For Robert Stemmer [16], famous French phlebologist and memorable president of the International Union of Phlebology, "big leg" means a lower limb in which volume increase is measurable and palpable. A total or partial big leg can be observed, but there are also different kinds of big leg such as venous, post-phlebitis syndrome, posttraumatic, angiodisplasic, lymphatic, adipose, or cellulitic big leg. The main characteristic of big leg is edema—systemic, lymphatic, venous, or interstitial edema. Considering that lymphatics run in the interstitial subcutaneous tissue, it is easy to assume that the increase of lymphatic edema or of adipose tissue could induce a lymph slowdown. We know that there is a neoangiogenesis, stimulated by collagen production, obtained after adipocyte rupture. Such collagen production also stimulates fibrinogenesis and vascular formation. The difference between localized adiposity and lipodystrophy or angiolipodystrophy is this: Localized adiposity means physiological or pathological accumulation of fat tissue in determined body areas, without a dystrophic process. Lipodystrophy means a pathologic affection of both supporting tissue and subcutaneous adipose tissue, characterized by various circulatory and metabolic damages. For this type of pathology, we now essentially use liposculpture.

Interstitial Matrix

These cells represent the functional units of all living organisms by virtue of their specific structural organization. They possess complicated biochemical and molecular systems, complexly organized and highly sophisticated. Such systems not only guarantee the survival of the cell, but they also (above all) allow numerous fundamental activities to take place for the biological life of the cell. This affirmation could appear banal at first: In reality the cell and its functional organization represent an extraordinary example of "natural functionality," as the natures of both are able not only to organize the constitutive elements of the tissues but also to predispose them, in the functional sense, to their precise and mutable adaptation in answer to the different biological changes that happen every second in the living organism.

An example of the importance of such sophisticated mechanisms is that some cellular passages are open only to sodium but not to potassium ions, while others are open only to glucose but not to amino acids. The protein in the transport membrane functions as a real "organ" to a degree that allows, through specific sites of recognition, the selective entry of substances into cells, determined by some precise passages. The ionic transport has extreme importance in biology. Perfect operation of the ionic pumps is vital for cellular life. The ionic movement through the membrane is also at the base of the production of adenosine triphosphate (ATP) in all cells, and particularly for the nervous system [17].

The ionic concentrations in the intra- and extracellular environments are shown in Fig. 3.1 [18].

As is known, the large concentration of Na^+ outside of the cell is compensated by the concentration of Cl^- while the strong

Component	Intracellular (nM)	Extracellular (nM)
Na^+	5–15	145
K^+	140	5
Mg^{2+} (citosol)	0.5	1–2
Ca^{2+} (citosol)	1/100000	1–2
H^+	7 x 1/100000	4 x 1/100000
Cl^-	5–15	110
Fixed anions	Tall	0

Figure 3.1 The ionic concentrations in the intra- and extracellular environments.

concentration of K^+ is counterbalanced by a series of negative intracellular ions. For example, this narrow joining ensures the activity of the pump only when there are proper ions to transport, so that there is no wastage of ATP (Fig. 3.2).

Every cell, as a separate living cellular mechanism, has the vital necessity "to feel" its environment and "to interact" with it, to be able to survive dispatching its vital functions.

We could say that every cell necessarily has to have a "social life," and it therefore must develop "senses" that allow it to communicate with other cells and with the whole extracellular environment, or rather with the "extracellular matrix."

In a multicellular organism, cells have to coordinate their behavior in many different ways, exactly as happens in a community of human beings; here, in fact, communication is constant and fervent: Nearby individuals are spoken to and discussions are held with them; public announcements are transferred to whole populations; urgent messages are delivered from near or far to precise individuals; and precise alarms are sounded when dangers or threats draw near. What would seem difficult to humans is in reality even more difficult (but not impossible) for the individual constituents of our body, firmly created to be gathered in "organs" and "apparatuses" developing precise and defined functions.

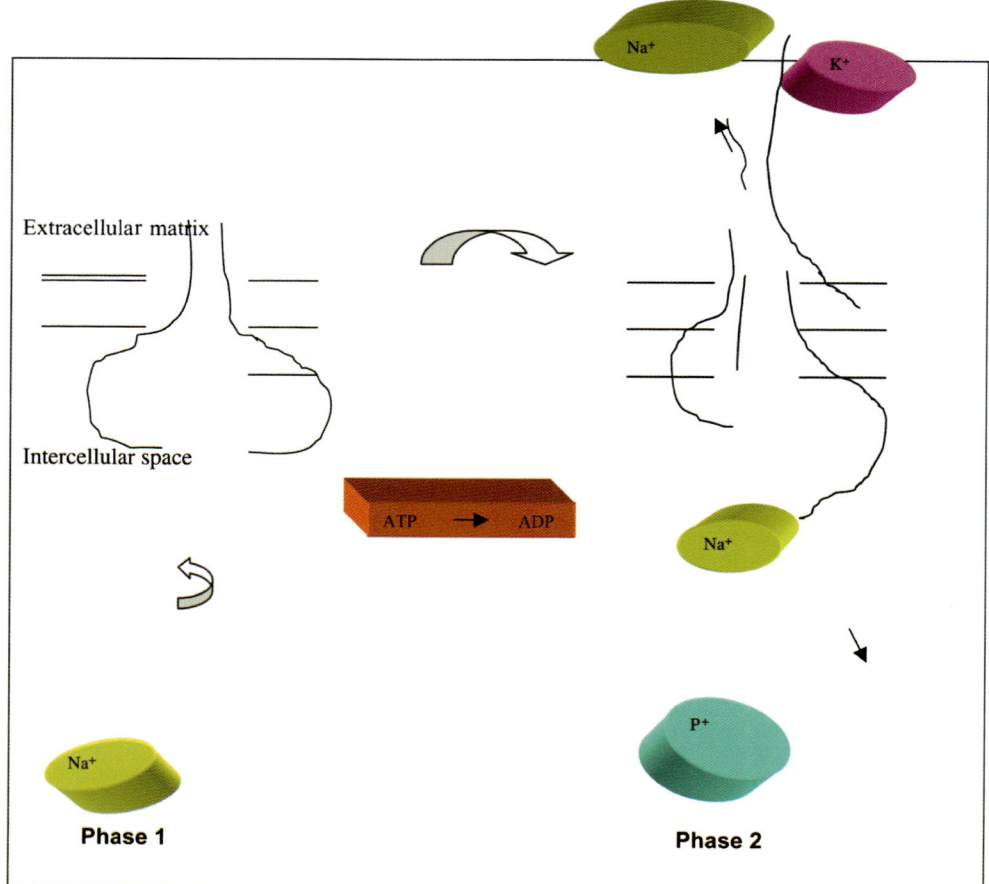

Figure 3.2 The ionic pumps.

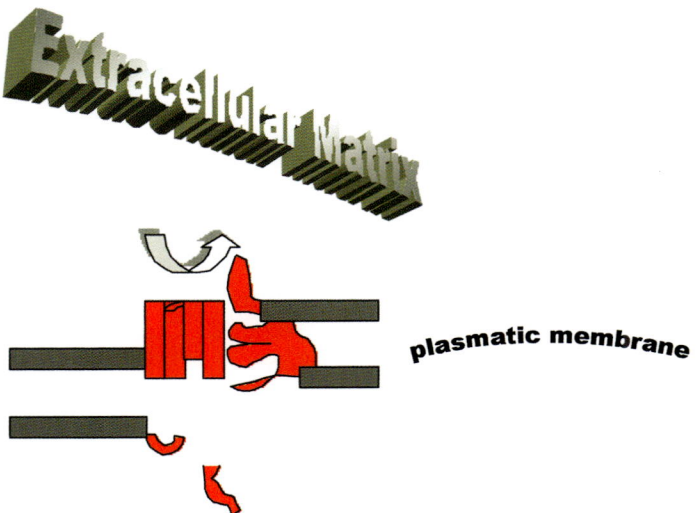

plasmatic membrane

Cells come into contact with the complicated extracellular world through their surface, constituted by lipid and protein molecules composing the plasma membrane. Additionally, they come into contact with the specific areas of these molecules that are found, because of their steric and biochemical encumbrance and their conformation, in the extracellular environment, forming intimate and complex biochemical-functional relationships with the extracellular matrix. Thanks to the continuous activity of this real interface of cellular contact, the cells are able to recognize other cells, near or distant, as real functional entities of a similar subject, or as structures extraneous to them; to send and to continually receive chemical and physical signals; and to stick to other cells or other substances present in the interstitial spaces of the extracellular matrix. For example, cellular receptors have great importance, especially the receptors that tie the molecular protein conducting the signal to the extracellular matrix, where the union happens with the membrane (Fig. 3.3).

Figure 3.3 Schematic representation of a G protein coupled receptor. The receptors that tie the protein molecules (signal protein) ask for a site at the extracellular matrix level, formed by the polypeptidical substance identified on the figure. Smaller molecules (signal protein), such as adrenaline, ask for a small extracellular site.

To transmit a message "person to person," we can write it on paper, then repeat it by voice, sending it in the form of "sensorial" impulses, for example by telephone. This sensorial impulse will come to another individual that will turn it into nervous impulses.

In the various phases of this simple communicative run, the same message is represented with different forms of signals: The real critical points of the transmission meet when information is converted from one form into another. This process of conversion is known as "translation of the signal."

The cellular membranes are responsible for the internal organization of cells as well as for interaction with external stimuli and for "structural integrity." The plasma membrane prevents a mixing of cellular contents with extracellular molecules and acts as the first element of "contact" between the cells and the extracellular environment. The composition and the maintenance of this structure is essential for the generation and regulation of different functional signals and biochemicals, both in the normal and in the pathologic cells [19,20].

The extracellular matrix is represented by a complex structural entity that surrounds, nourishes, and furnishes support to all the cells. The extracellular matrix is generally described as being composed of three biomolecular classes of substances:

1. structural proteins (collagens and elastin)
2. specialized proteins (fibrillates, fibronectin, laminin, etc.)

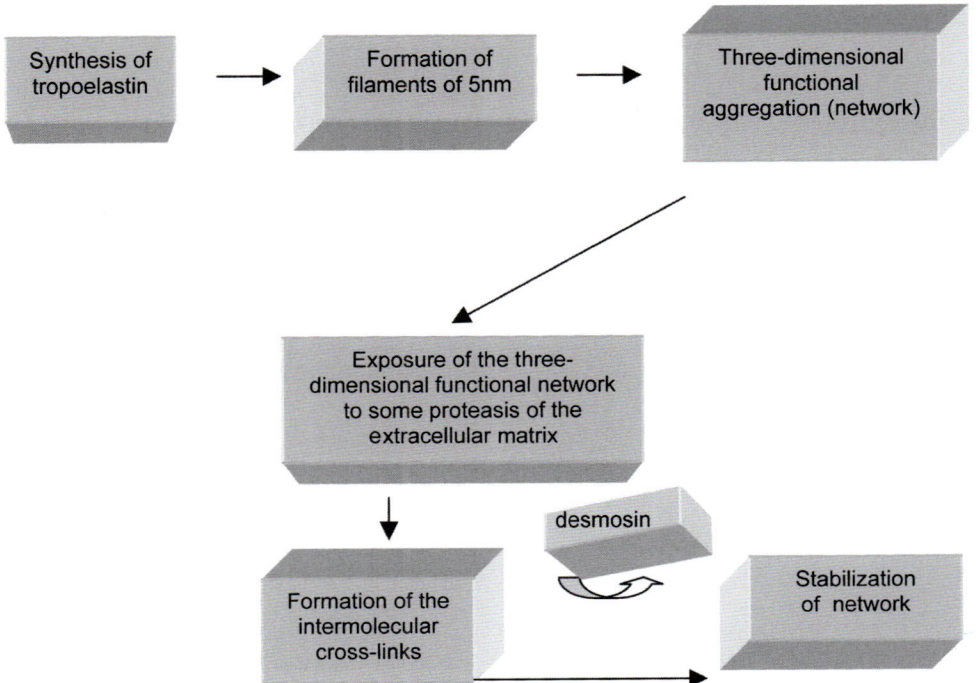

Figure 3.4 Interpretative scheme of the formation of the elastin from the tropoelastin.

3. proteoglycans (composed of a "core" of protein with long chains of two saccharides of glycosaminoglycan forming, in such a way, complexes of high molecular weight that represent a cardinal part of the extracellular matrix)

The connective system has great importance in the interstitial matrix. Many trials could be represented by the scheme in Fig. 3.4, reported to be the interpretative scheme of the formation of elastin by tropoelastin.

Therefore, it appears fundamental to begin to consider cellular homeostasis, both in a molecular and in an anatomic-functional biological sense, as a complex interaction of mechanisms and reactions that can begin and also evolve from the outside of the cell in the extracellular matrix [21]. The cellular matrix, the fundamental substance for life, is found as a rule as a solution. Some alterations can make it vary into a gel. These variations play a role in physical, chemical, and metabolic changes, among which are the alterations typical of cellulite [22]. In the dermal site and in the superficial subcutaneous site, we can have an activation of "metalloproteases-2" directly connected with the evolution of lymphedema, lipolymphedema, and mesenchymopathies [23–28].

REFERENCES

1. S Curri. Inquadramento nosologico e classificazione delle 1. panniculopatie da stasi (Classification of panniculopathy by venous lymphatic stasis). In: Flebologia. Torino, Italy: Minerva Medica; 1990: 1:15–19.
2. PA Bacci, C Allegra, S Mancini et al. Randomized, placebo controlled double blind clinical study on efficacy of a multifunctional plant complex in the treatment of the so called cellulites. J Aesthet Surg Dermatol Surg 5(1), 2003.
3. PA Bacci. Valutazione clinica controllata in doppio cieco di prodotti fitocomposti nel trattamento della cosiddetta cellulite (Double blind clinical study of a multifunctional plant complex in the treatment of the cellulitis). In: PA Bacci, S Mariani (eds). La Flebologia in Pratica. Arezzo, Italy: Alberti; 2003: 92–111.
4. U Cornelli, M Cornelli, R Terranova et al. Invecchiamento e radicali liberi (Aging and free radicals). Prog Nutr 3:37–50, 2000.
5. C Vassalle, V Lubrano, C Boni et al. Valutazione dei livelli di Stress ossidativo in vivo mediante metodo colorimetrico ed immunoenzimatico (Valuation of oxydative stress by immunological methodology). Report of CNR (recherche national center), Istituto di Fisiologia Clinica, Pisa, Italy; 2001.
6. KH Cheeseman, TF Slater, S Vaisman. Radicais livres em medicina. Interlivros, Rio de Janeiro 1996.
7. F Terranova. Apoptosi e senescenza cellulare nella cute (Apoptosis and cellular skin aging). In: Atti 2° Congresso Nazionale. Milano, Italy: Medicina Estetica; 2000: 45–46.
8. M Carratelli, R Porcaro, M Ruscica et al. Reactive oxygen metabolites (ROMs) and prooxidant status in children with Down's syndrome. Int J Clin Pharmacol Res 21(2):79–84, 2001.
9. G Belcaro, M Caratelli, R Terranova et al. A simple test to monitor oxidative stress. Int Angiol 18(2):127–30, 1999.
10. PA Bacci. Le Celluliti. Arezzo, Italy: Alberti Editori; 2000: 175–85.
11. C Campisi. Il linfedema. In: Flebologia Oggi. Torino, Italy: Minerva Medica; 1997: 23–29.
12. M Lucchi, S Bilancini. Il lipoedema. In: PA Bacci (ed.) Le Celluliti. Arezzo, Italy: Alberti Editori; 2000: 80–85.
13. PA Bacci, G Leisbashoff. Las celulitis y el protocollo BIMED. Buenos Aires: Medical Books; 2000: 93–103.
14. J Casley-Smith. Fine structure properties and permeabilities of the lymphatic endothelium. New trends in basic lymphology. Experentia (Birkhauser) (suppl 14):19–40, 1981.
15. PA Bacci. Il cosiddetto Lipolinfedema. In: Flebologia Oggi. Torino, Italy: Atti Congresso Nazionale Collegio Italiano Flebologia; 1998: 2:27–32.
16. R. L'edema Stemmer. In: G Bassi (ed.) Terapia Flebologica. Torino: Minerva Medica; 1986: 164–81.
17. L Rosenberg, JE Scott et al. London, UK: Portland Press.
18. FG Albergati, PA Bacci. La Matrice Extracellulare. Arezzo, Italy: Minelli Editore; 2004.
19. Y Yamaguchi, DM Mann, E Ruoslahti. Negative regulation of transforming growth factor-beta by the proteoglycan decorin. Nature 346(6281):281–84, 1990.
20. HC Whinna, HU Choi, LC Rosenberg, FC Church. Interaction of heparin cofactor II with biglycan and decorin. J Biol Chem 268(6):3920–24, 1993.
21. F Albergati, PA Bacci et al. Valutazione degli effetti microcircolatori dopo terapia della matrice extracellulare in pazienti affette da flebolinfedema agli arti inferiori (Valuation of the microvascular effect in patient with limphedema). Atti 1° Congresso Nazionale Medicina Estetica SMIEM, Milano; 1999: 20.
22. PA Bacci. Le Celluliti nel 2004. Arezzo, Italy: Minelli Editore; 2004.
23. JF Bourgeois, B Guillot et al. – Montpellier University & Centre Regional de Lutte Contre le Cancer, Val d'Aurelle, Montpellier, France "A randomized, prospective study using the LPG Technique in treating radiation-induced skin fibrosis. Clinical and Profilometric analysis"; Skin Research and Technology; 2007: Vol.3:12–18.
24. A Couillandre, M-J Duque Ribeiro, P Thoumie, P Portero. – Université de Paris "Modification des paramétres d'équilibration et de force associés reconditionnement sur plateforme motorisée de rééducation: étude chez le sujet sain". Annales de Rèadaptation et de Médecine Physique; 2007 (in press).
25. C Monteux, M Lafontan. – LPG Systems, Valence France "Use of Microdialysis technique to assess lipolytic responsiveness of femoral adipose tissue after 12 sessions of mechanical massage technique". Journal of Cosmetic Dermatology; 2007 (in press).
26. D Innocenzi et al. – "Evidenza delle modificazioni cutanee indotte della tecnica LPG mediante analisi d'immagine"; DermoCosmetologia anno II numero 1- Gennaio- Marzo; 2003: p.9–15.
27. P Portero. "Delayed onset muscle soreness induced by eccentric muscle exercise: from the origin to the resolution". Kinésithérapie Scientifique n. 416, Novembre 2001.
28. JP Ortonne. – "Cellulite: evaluation and treatment"; International Master Course on Ageing Skin (IMCAS); January 6–8, 2006; Paris, France.

4 Definition, Clinical Aspects, Classifications, and Diagnostic Techniques
Doris Hexsel, Taciana de Oliveira Dal'Forno, and Rosemarie Mazzuco

Definition

Cellulite is a very common topographical alteration [1,2] in which the skin acquires an orange peel, mattress or cottage cheese appearance (Fig. 4.1) [3,4]. There are many theories to explain the physiopathology of this condition. The majority of the theories involve modifications that occur to the adipose tissue and microcirculation, resulting from blood and lymphatic disturbances, causing fibrosclerosis of the connective tissue [2]. It is generally considered a non-inflammatory, degenerative phenomenon that provokes alterations to the hypodermis [5] producing irregular undulations on the skin overlying affected areas.

Cellulite results from many complex events that involve the epidermis, dermis and subcutaneous tissue [1]. Cellulite can be divided into four stages:

1. alterations to the precapillary arteriolar sphincter, leading to changes in vascular permeability and capillarectasia resulting in pericapillary and interadipositary transudation, leading to edema;
2. edema, provoking metabolic changes that result in hyperplasia and hypertrophy of the reticular network, leading to the formation of pericapillary and interadiposity transudation, leading to edema;
3. organization of collagen fibers around groups of adypocytes forming micronodules; and
4. union of the micronodules to form the macronodules that cause sclerosis [6].

Anatomically, the cutaneous alterations found in cellulite are largely due to fibrosis of the connective tissues present in the dermis and/or in the subcutaneous tissue [7]. The connective tissue of the reticular dermis is connected to the deep fascia (SMAS), by means of the interlobular trabeculas (fibrous septa). Subcutaneous fat lobes are separated from one to another by these thin, usually rigid strands of connective tissue, which cross the fatty layers and connect the dermis to the underlying fascia. These septa stabilize the subcutis and divide the fat [8]. The shortening of these septum due to fibrosis provokes retraction at the insertion points of the trabeculas [9], causing the depressions that are characteristic of cellulite.

Nürnberger and Müller studied the anatomy and histology of fat and the connective tissue structure of the subcutaneous tissue in cellulite patients. They demonstrated the anatomical basis of the characteristic mattress aspect of cellulite and pointed out important differences in the organization of the subcutaneous between genders [10,11]. They also showed that in women the fibrous septa are usually orientated perpendicularly in relation to cutaneous surface, while in men they have a crisscross pattern [11]. Several studies have shown that the fat is divided into lobes, and in women these are larger and more rectangular when compared with those in men [4,11–15]. These anatomical and histological findings explain the greater frequency of cellulite in women.

Nomenclature

In France in 1920, Alquier and Paviot described cellulite as an unaesthetic condition [6,16]. In the same decade, Lagueze described cellulite as a disease of the hypodermis, characterized by interstitial edema and an increase in subcutaneous fat [17].

Initially Curri denominated cellulite as nodular liposclerosis [6,18] and, later, adopted the term "cellulitic dermohypodermosis" [19]. In 1958, Merlen defined cellulite as a histoangiopathy [20] and, in 1978, Benazzi and Curri, after a histopathological study, suggested the term "sclerotic-fibrous-edematous paniculopathy" [21,22]. Nurberguer and Müller used the name panniculosis of the dermis [16,23] to describe cellulite from the histopathological viewpoint. Bacci and Leibaschoff suggest the terms cellulitic hipodermosis [16].

In recent years, the term "gynoid lipodystrophy" (GLD) has been mentioned in some studies [2,9,24]. The terms hydrolipodystrophy or herniation of the fat with hypodermic tension bands are also used to describe cellulite [25,26].

The presence of the suffix "ite" in a medical term indicates inflammation, therefore, the term cellulite is more appropriately used to designate inflammation and/or infection of the subcutaneous tissue [27]. However, the term cellulite has become very popular, and its use has been consecrated [20,28], being accepted throughout the world. Other synonyms often used for cellulite are listed in Table 4.1.

Clinical Aspects

Although it is found in all age groups and in both sexes [10,29,30], cellulite occurs mainly in women [6,31], especially after puberty [32] and in obese people, being considered a normal manifestation of obesity by Burton and Cunliffe [12,29].

There is evidence to suggest that estrogen is the most probably involved element in the initial dysfunction, aggravation and persistence of cellulite [1,20,33]. The greater incidence of cellulite in females, post puberty onset, the worsening of the condition in relation to some conditions, such as pregnancy, menstrual cycle, use of contraceptives and hormonal replacement, are cited to support this hypothesis [1].

Cellulite normally manifests itself in areas of greatest fat accumulation, such as the buttocks, thighs [29] (Fig. 4.2), flanks, abdomen [6,29] and upper legs [26,29,32].

The lesions are essentially asymptomatic. However, in severe cases of cellulite, symptoms such as a sensation of weight and pain are reported by patients in the affected areas [10,20,29]. Some authors believe these probably occur as a result of compression of the nervous terminals or the presence of inflammatory reactions [16,19].

(a)

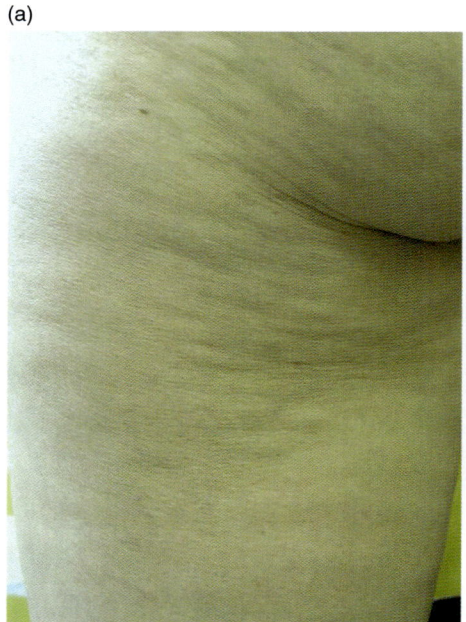

(b)

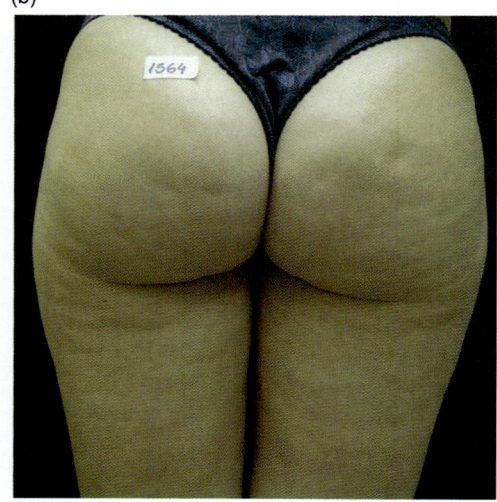

(c)

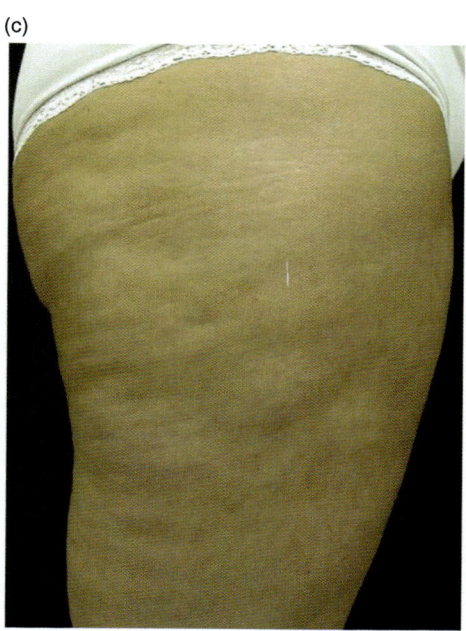

Figures 4.1a, 1b and 1c Clinical aspect of cellulite.

The main clinical manifestations of cellulite are:

1. flaccid "mattress-like" skin, with multiple depressions and some elevations, caused by irregular retraction of the skin, forming a surface where protuberances and depressed areas alternate (see Fig. 4.1) [6,16,34];
2. "orange peel" skin due to the tumefaction of the skin and the dilation of the follicular pores [6,16,34];
3. "cottage cheese" (1) appearance of the skin in the affected areas.

The cutaneous surface alterations that characterize cellulite are predominantly depressed, when compared to cutaneous surface of the affected area [29]. These depressions have the same color and consistency as normal skin, and the number of lesions may vary from one to many [29]. The shape of these lesions is varied [29]: rounded, oval or linear (Fig. 4.3). Most lesions are oval, as the longest axis of the lesions lies parallel to the relaxed skin tension lines (Figs. 4.4a-e). They are usually found in the lower portion of the buttocks and the upper thigh (see Figs. 4.4a-e), where just below the gluteus fold, the longest axis is in the horizontal direction, with the lateral extremities slightly elevated. In these locations cellulite may be more evident due to the flaccidity of the epidermis, which tends to become aggravated with age. This can be demonstrated by the diminishing or even the disappearance of the lesions when the buttocks are lifted to their original position. It is interesting to note that lesions not presenting this disposition in relation to the relaxed skin tension lines, in general, originate from secondary fibrosis of the subcutaneous tissue, such as injections trauma, etc.

Table 4.1 Classification of cellulite

Grade or stage 0 (zero)
There is no alteration to the skin surface
Grade or stage I
The skin of the affected area is smooth while a subject is standing or lying, but the alterations to the skin surface can be seen by pinching of the skin or with muscle contraction (Fig. 5).
Grade or stage II
The orange skin or mattress appearance is evident when standing, without the use of any manipulation (skin pinching or muscle contraction) (Fig. 6).
Grade or stage III
Presence of alterations described for grade or stage II plus raised areas and nodules (Fig. 7).

Classification

Several authors have classified cellulite into four clinical stages or grades (shown in Table 4.1), based on clinical alterations observed with the patient standing at rest and/or applying pinch test or muscular contraction [6,29,34], to make the lesions more evident.

While the current classification of cellulite (Table 4.1) describes different grades of this condition, which is very important, additional key morphological aspects affect the severity of cellulite and are useful in clinical evaluation and to define treatment options. For this reason, Hexsel, Dal'Forno and Hexsel created and validated a new method to measure and classify the severity of cellulite, called Hexsel, Dal´Forno & Hexsel Cellulite Severity Scale (CSS). This scale complements the current classification by suggesting the assessment of additional important clinical and morphological

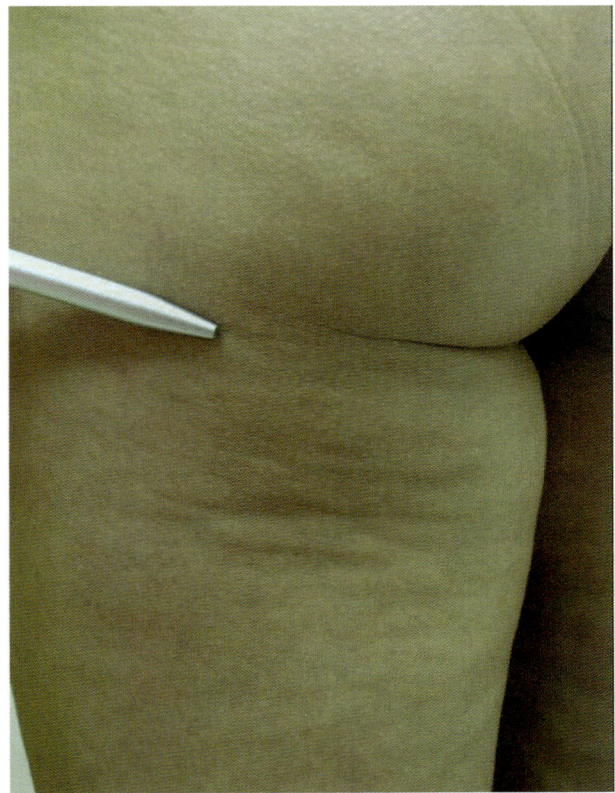

Figure 4.3 Oval and linear lesions of cellulite.

aspects [35] (Attachment 1 – Cellulite Assessment Protocol). The proposed new scale expands the current classification by adding four items, therefore allowing a comprehensive measurement of the intensity of the condition. It is an objective method that facilitates patient follow-up and allows a better measurement of treatment outcomes. In CSS, each morphological aspect of cellulite is graded from 0 to 3, allowing a final sum of scores which range numerically from 1 to 15. The scores of these five items of the new CSS facilitate the objective quantitative and qualitative classification of cellulite as mild, moderate or severe. Data analysis of CSS demonstrated that it is a consistent, comprehensive, reliable and reproducible tool for the complete assessment of cellulite severity and can therefore, be successfully used by dermatologists as a valuable instrument for research and clinical evaluation of patients with cellulite.

Cellulite is diagnosed based on clinical alterations to the skin surface, without specific histological or laboratorial findings. Based in its clinical concept, it can also be classified as either primary or secondary cellulite. In primary cellulite, lesions appeared spontaneously as a consequence of its anatomical bases; no aggravating factors or secondary causes, such as traumas, are involved. In secondary cellulite, lesions are related to secondary causes, such as increase in localized fat, important saggy, loose skin, previous traumas, including traumas from liposuction, lipoatrophy after injections of lipodissolve agents, subcutaneous fibrosis from any inflammatory/infectious process. These circumstances may be present accompanying or aggravating primary cellulite and should be detected and investigated through the medical history and physical examination. Treatment, in this case, implies the correction of the primary factor.

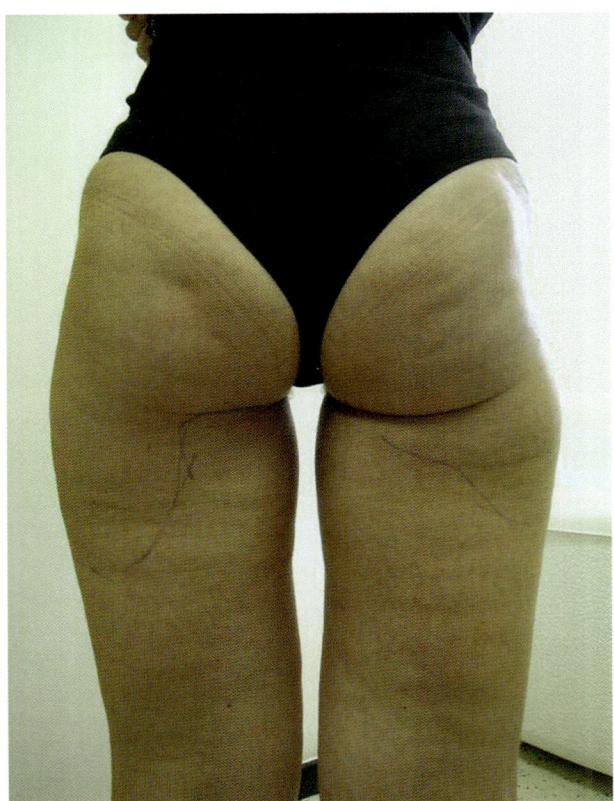

Figure 4.2 Areas commonly affected by cellulite: upper part of the thighs and buttocks.

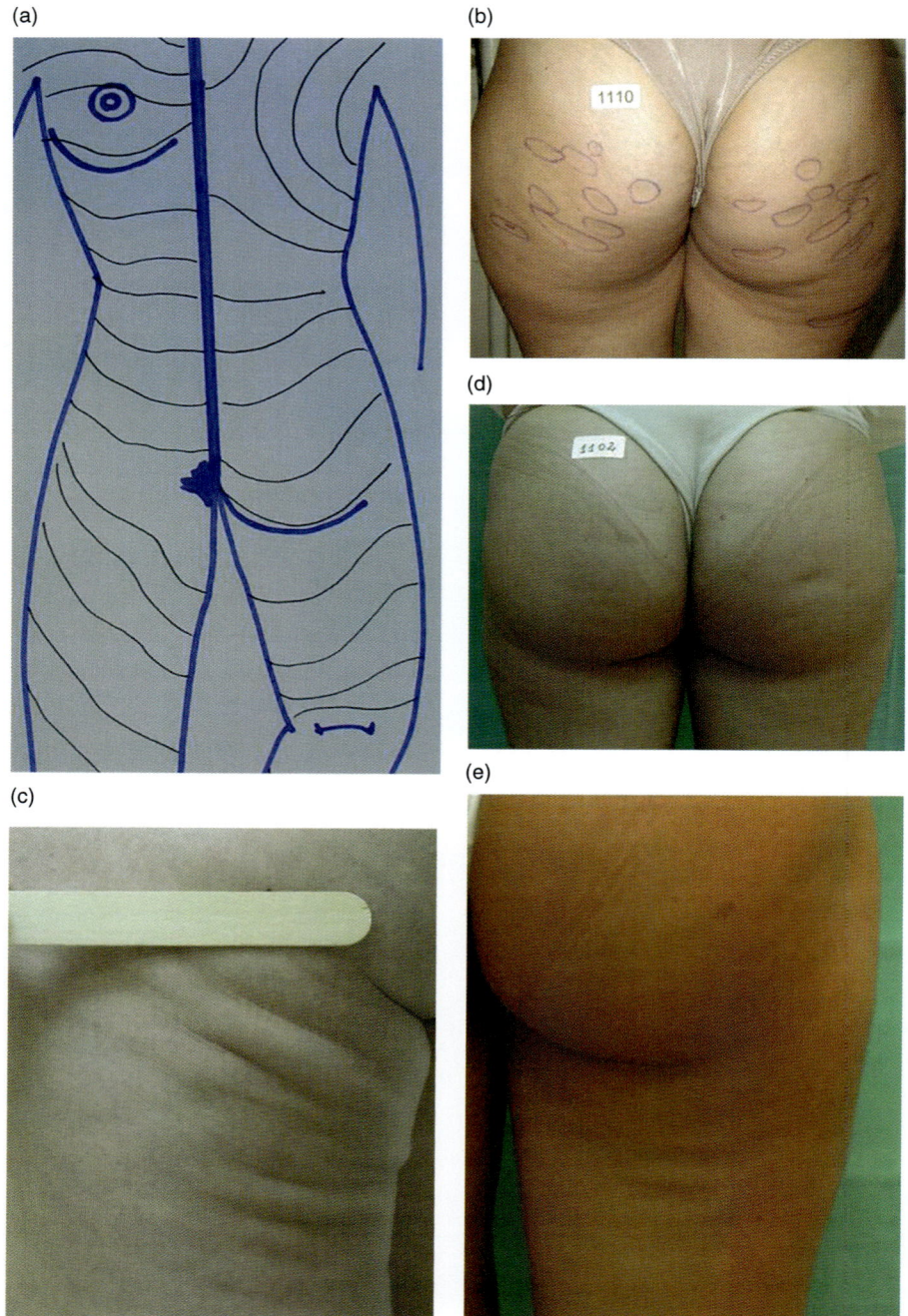

Figure 4.4 Relaxed skin tension lines mapped on body scheme. (a) The left half shows the frontal view and the right half, the back view. (b-e) Cellulite lesions follow the relaxed skin tension lines.

Clinical Evaluation of Cellulite Patients

As with other pathologies, the medical history should be detailed in the evaluation of cellulite. The patient should be questioned regarding the age of onset of cellulite, prior occurrence of trauma, liposuction or injections in the affected area, the history of prior disease or surgery, family history, the presence of chronic vascular or associated hormonal diseases, the occasional or regular use of medications and previous or current history of hormonal treatment or the use of any medicine that may contribute toward increasing the deposit of fat in the affected areas. Other aspects that should be researched with patients are: sedentary life, diet programs, psychosomatic factors, smoking habits, prior

pregnancies and the behavior of cellulite during pregnancy or other conditions.

Although smoking and circulatory problems are frequently cited as causative agents of cellulite, in the experience of the present authors, in a sample of 1500 patients with high degree cellulite, the vast majority were neither smokers (more than 85%) nor those having varicose veins or other circulatory problems.

The physical examination should be performed with the patient in standing position with muscles relaxed [9,10,29]. Cellulite can be better observed if the pinch test is applied in the affected areas. The pinch test is performed by pinching the skin between the thumb and index finger to form a fold by skinfold

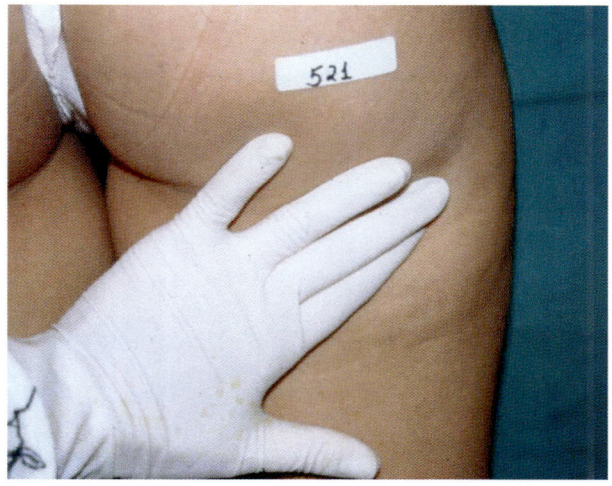

Figure 4.5 First degree cellulite, in which there are no alterations to the skin surface in standing position and relaxed gluteous muscles. Alterations are found under the pinch test applied to the skin of the affected area.

plicometry or through the contraction of the muscles in the area (Figs. 4.8 and 4.9) [9]. Overhead or tangential illumination of the patient facilitates the visualization of cellulite lesions [29]. There are significant differences in the appearance of cellulite, depending on the position and the method used for its classification. For this reason, the standing position is the most recommended for the examination of a patient with cellulite.

Palpation should always be performed to check the elasticity of the skin and subcutaneous tissue. However, at present, there are no exact parameters for the classification of skin elasticity.

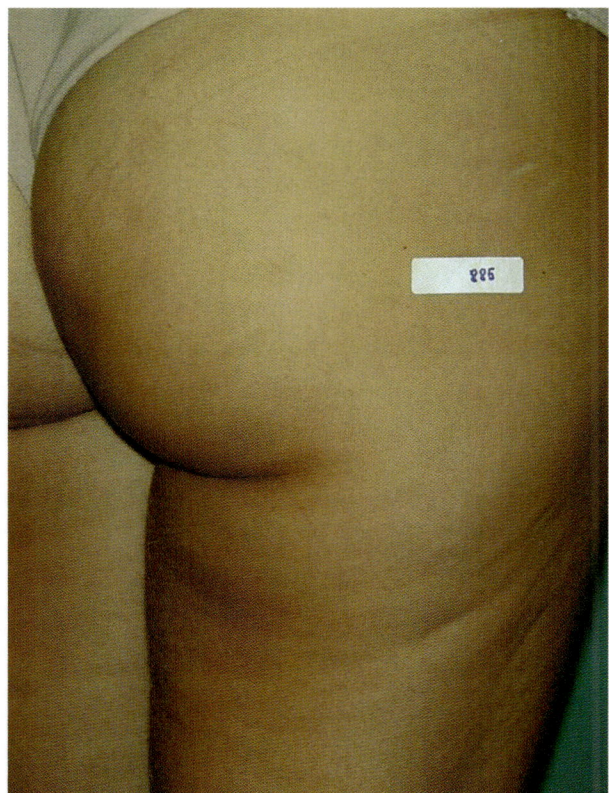

Figure 4.6 "Orange peel" or "mattress appearance" of second stage of cellulite.

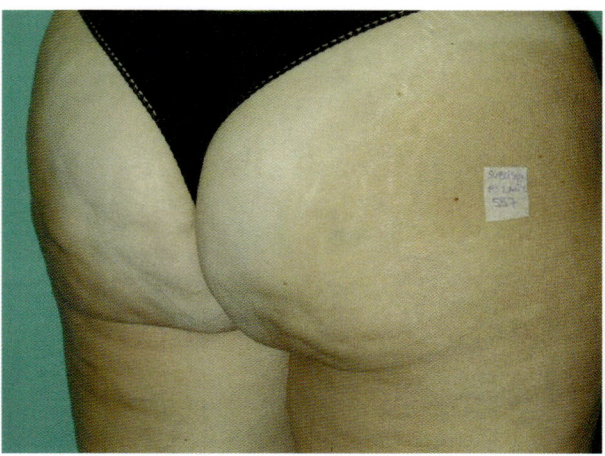

Figure 4.7 Third degree cellulite showing raised and depressed areas and modules plus orange peel or mattress appearance.

Venous or lymphatic insufficiency may, in theory, aggravate cellulite and should be checked during the physical examination [36].

One should make note of the presence of varicose and telangiectatic leg veins as well as any pitting edema or indurations of the skin. A Doppler or duplex ultrasound examination of the superficial venous system will also help to classify the significance of venous insufficiency and its efficient treatment.

Aggravating Factors
A number of clinical conditions are frequently found accompanying or aggravating cellulite, especially obesity, localized fatty deposits and flaccidity.

Obesity promotes a generalized increase in body weight (skeletal, muscular, interstitial fluid, organ hypertrophy, etc.). After a return to the original baseline weight, an increased accumulation of fat can be observed [37]. The clinical manifestation of localized adiposity is an increase in the ill-defined symmetrical and bilateral diffuse volume, owing to an increase in the adipose tissue [29]. The localized increase in adipose tissue in the subcutaneous tissue leads to the aggravation of cellulite lesions by contributing to a worsening of the irregular undulations of the skin. The increase in subcutaneous fat leads to the appearance of raised areas as well as to an augmentation of tension forces within the lobes, aggravating the depressions, causing an effect similar to that of a stuffed quilt [29]. These also contribute to the appearance of the mechanical and circulatory alterations in the fat lobes, that may occur in cellulite. Greater thickness of the subcutaneous fat in the affected areas may be seen by histopathological examination and can be measured by special instruments or by the pinch test (Fig. 4.9) [37].

Rosenbaum et al. described the exacerbation of cellulite with weight gain and the correlation with the Body Mass Index (BMI). This study demonstrates the protrusion of the adipose tissue into the dermis when the volume of subcutaneous fat is augmented, which explains the mattress-like appearance [31].

Flaccidity or loose skin is caused by physiological ptosis of the subcutaneous structures, making the skin permanently distended and loose. This condition frequently occurs in the buttocks, thighs, the region above the knee and the inner surface of the

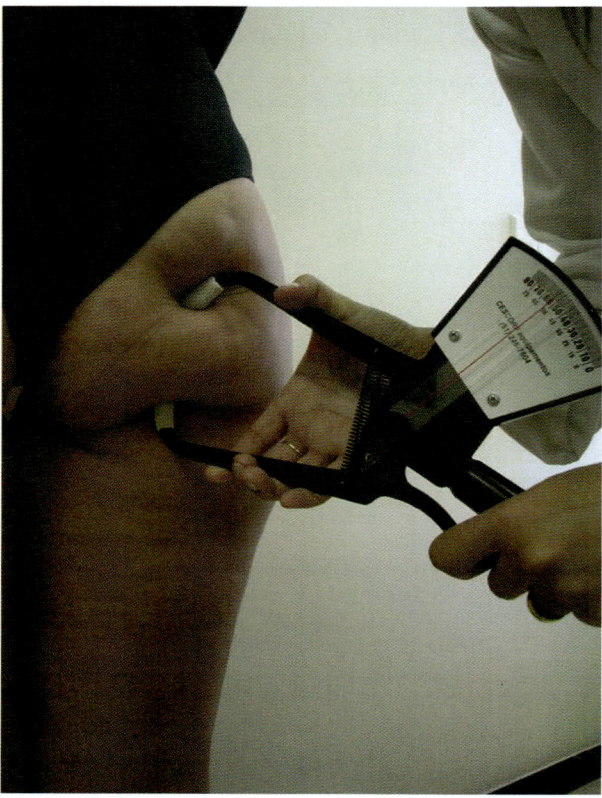

Figure 4.8 Pinch test using aial device, the skinfold plicometry.

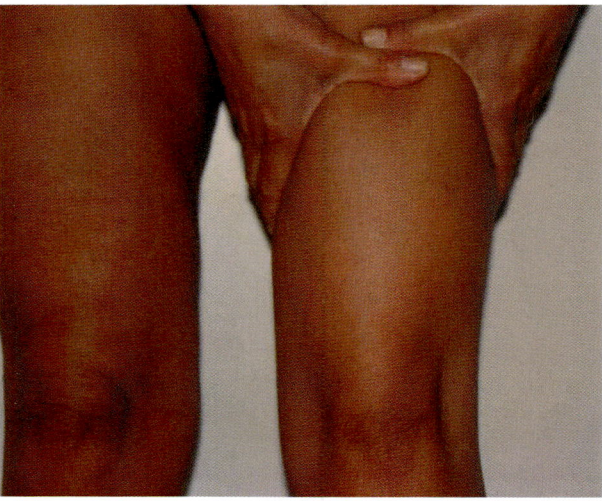

Figure 4.10 The patient shown in Fig. 9 showing improvement to the skin surface when stretching the skin in the direction opposite to forces of gravity.

arms, regions where the skin probably has less retentive capacity and suffers the mechanical action of weight exerted by the adipose tissue and by the other subcutaneous structures [29]. The weight of these structures also increases, the effects of gravity worsen the alterations to the skin surface, seen as laxity and looseness [29]. The reduced elasticity of the skin, sudden loss of weight [29] or subcutaneous fat due to liposuction [38] are conditions that can bring about or aggravate flaccidity.

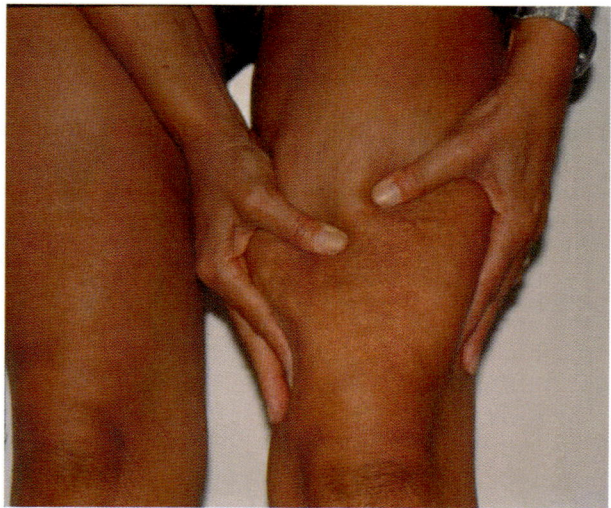

Figure 4.9 Patient with cellulite secondary to flaccidity or loose skin. Alterations to the skin surface became more evident pinching the skin.

Being of great importance, the presence of flaccidity or other aggravating conditions should be evaluated in patients with cellulite. In the absence of flaccidity, a distension test of the skin and subcutaneous tissue in the antigravity direction tends not to diminish the lesions. In the presence of flaccidity, however, such a test can lead to the reduction or even disappearance of cellulite lesions (Fig. 4.10). The pinch test causes an increase in tension inside the lobes, making cellulite more evident, as the lobes bulge and aggravate the traction of the septa in the pinched area (Fig. 4.11). Moreover, flaccidity has a similar effect to that of pinching by compressing the lobes and, thus, augmenting the tension within them. This situation is responsible for the emergence or worsening of cellulite lesions, especially after the fourth or fifth decade of life when the elastic properties of the skin diminish [39]. This, together with the weight of the subcutaneous fat, determines the worsening of distension of the skin.

Other notable conditions that cause secondary cellulite or that aggravates cellulite are subcutaneous fibrosis caused by previous surgery, mainly liposuction and the subcutaneous fibrosis and lipoatrophy originating from the trauma or caused by injections in the affected areas. Alterations to cutaneous surface resulting from liposuction usually appear late, from three months to one year after surgery. They may be slight, moderate or severe, and always emerge in previously treated areas, such as the lateral and posterior thighs, buttocks, abdomen (Fig. 4.12), flanks and the region above the knees. Like cellulite, the cutaneous sequelae from liposuction are predominantly depressions, but also raised and depressed areas may intercalate and vary in number and shape, as a reflection of the number and variety of liposuction cannula insertions, as well as the size and type of cannulas used in the procedure. Generally, they form larger depressions with bizarre shapes and do not necessarily follow the direction of the relaxed skin tension lines, as seen in primary cellulite lesions. Instead, they follow the direction of cannula insertion (Fig. 4.12).

The cutaneous surface alterations caused by previous injections (such as insulin injections in diabetics) occur in places where the injections are normally applied, that is, in the upper, outer quarter of the buttocks. They also vary in number and shape, and usually do not follow the skin tension lines.

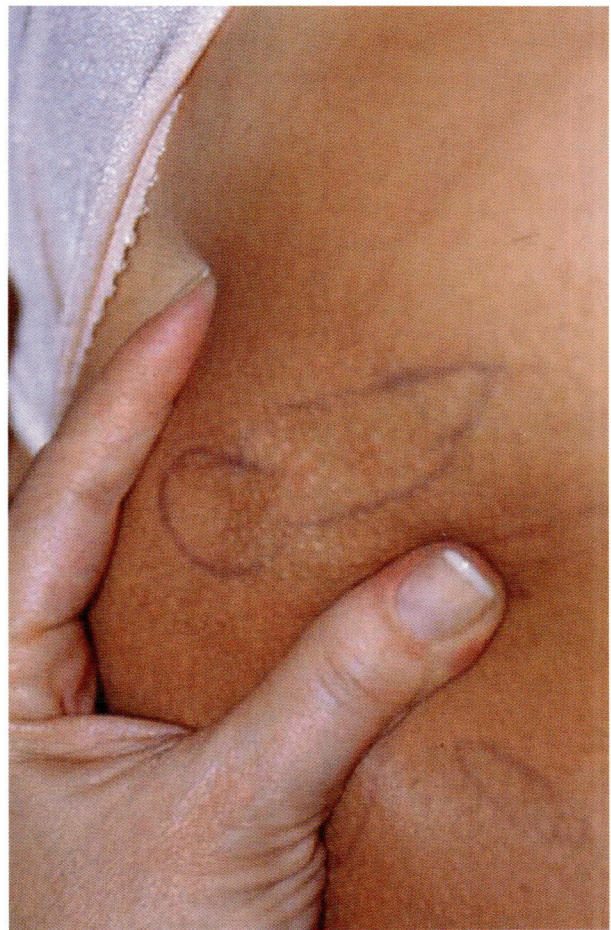

Figure 4.11 Pinch test, which makes the septa pulling the skin surface more evident.

Atrophic scars in the areas often affected by cellulite can also simulate or aggravate cellulite.

Other Diagnostic Techniques

The Body Mass Index (BMI) is widely used and cited by some authors, as a simple, low cost examination, considered

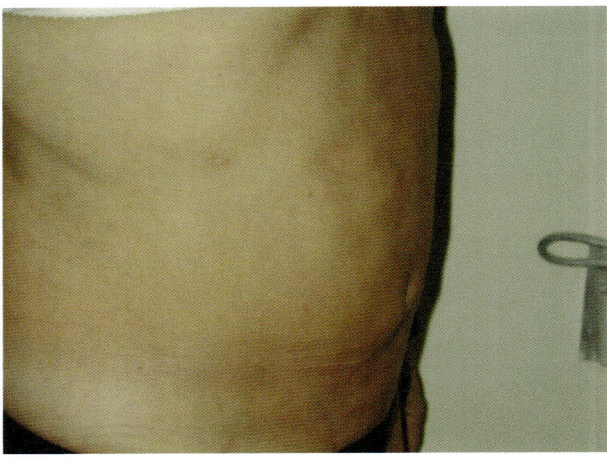

Figure 4.12 "Cellulite-like" liposuction sequelae on the abdomen, one year after the surgery.

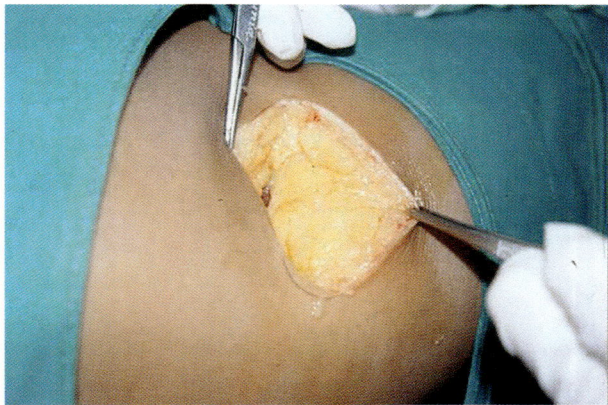

Figure 4.13 Macroscopic aspect of subcutaneous fat from a corpse.

fundamental for the evaluation of the clinical cellulite [6,40]. This is a quantitative method that measures weight and height in order to assess the degree of obesity [40]. By using this index, it is not possible to distinguish the percentage of body fat in the muscular mass. BMI is an uncertain diagnostic index of obesity [41]. Studies reveal that the estimation standard error of the percentage of body fat of BMI was approximately 5–6% [40].

The present authors evaluation of a small sample of 32 patients aged between 18 and 45 years old, by physical examination, BMI calculation, assessment of body fat percentage by skinfold plicometry [40], revealed that cellulite manifested even in patients with a low percentage of body fat and a normal BMI.

Two-dimensional ultrasound is a non-invasive method of evaluating variations [42,43] and alterations of the subcutaneous fatty tissue, and with the assistance of Doppler, it evaluates the local circulation [6]. This examination has been used in some studies for the evaluation of cellulite, and has demonstrated a diffuse pattern of extrusion of underlying adipose tissue into the reticular dermis in affected individuals, but not unaffected individuals [2,31].

Computerized tomography [44] and magnetic resonance imaging (MRI) [45,46] are examinations used for measuring the thickness of the adipose tissue, which do not allow evaluation of the dermis or microcirculation [6]. In one study, the MRI quantified deeper indentations of adipose tissue into the dermis and evidenced for the first time a great increase in the thickness of the inner fat layer in women with cellulite [47].

Mirrashed et al. successfully showed that *in vivo* MRI can visualize changes in skin architecture associated with cellulite. The structural alterations of the skin correlated with cellulite grade were measured by assessment of the hypodermis and dermis thickness, the percentage of hypodermic invaginations inside the dermis, and the percentage of adipose vs. connective tissue in a given volume of the hypodermis [48].

A study conducted by Hexsel et al. aimed to compare the subcutaneous tissue in the areas with and without cellulite on the buttocks of same subjects with MRI. This exam was used to measure the adipose volume according to body site and for the visualization of the subcutaneous structures. Thirty female patients participated in the study. An area with cellulite and another without cellulite on the contralateral buttock were selected to be evaluated by MRI. Two soft gelatin capsules of different sizes were used as skin markers. Thicker fibrous septa

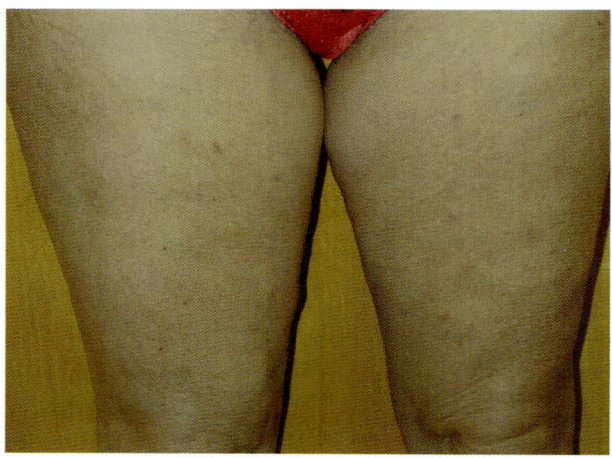

Figure 4.14 Lipomatosis from cellulite.

were visualized in 96.7% of the cellulite depressions, most of them were ramified, although in the areas without cellulite, MRI showed that only 16.7% fibrous septa. All fibrous septa found in the examined areas were perpendicular to the skin surface. This study showed that cellulite depressions were significantly associated to the presence of underlying fibrous septa [49].

Although invasive, histological examination may be useful as a method for evaluating cellulite [3,6,13], it is only rarely used. The stains used in this examination include hematoxylin-eosine for routine histological examination, Alcian blue for polysaccharides, periodic acid-Schiff for basement membranes, Weigert-Van Gieson (fuchsin-resorcin and acid fuchsin) for highlighting elastic, collagen and flat muscle fibers, and, Masson trichromic to demonstrate contrast between collagen and muscles fibers [6]. With this examination, it is also possible to observe the diffuse extrusion pattern of underlying adipose tissue distending the reticular dermis in people with cellulite [31]. The macroscopic aspect of subcutaneous fat from corpses is shown in Fig. 4.13.

Differential Diagnosis

As previously mentioned in this chapter, of particular importance in the differential diagnosis of cellulite are aggravating and

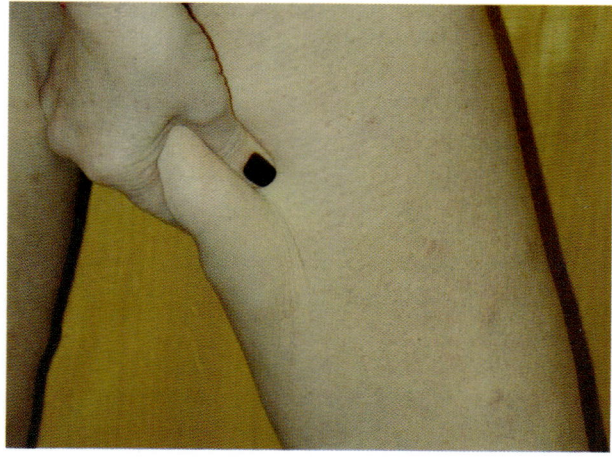

Figure 4.15 Lipomatosis from cellulite.

associated conditions, such as localized deposits of fat [13], flaccidity, liposuction surgical sequelae (Fig. 4.12) or from other traumas [50], presence of lipomas or lipomatosis (Figs. 4.14 and 4.15), and depressions caused by multiple atrophic scars, after furunculosis or other pathologies, in the affected areas. It is also necessary to differentiate from cellulite those cutaneous depressions that occur as a result of injections of medicines that cause fibrosis or atrophy of the subcutaneous tissue, for example, corticosteroid injections [51]. When unilateral, localized scleroderma or morphea should be part of the differential diagnosis [29]. In these cases, the treatment of these conditions is crucial and mandatory.

Conclusion

Cellulite is a common and challenging condition, currently affecting almost every woman from every culture and country. It can be considered an anatomical expression of normal structures of the affected area. This condition is easily diagnosed. Evaluation of the morphological clinical aspects and associated conditions are important to determine the degree and severity of cellulite and other factors involved in its origins as well as to indicate different treatment options.

REFERENCES

1. ZD Draelos. Cellulite. Etiology and purported treatment. Dermatol Surg 23:1177–81, 1997.
2. GW Lucassen, WLN Van-Der-Sluys et al. The effectiveness of massage treatment on cellulite as monitored by ultrasound imaging. Skin Res Technol 3:154–16, 1997.
3. AM Segers, J Abulafia et al. Celulitis. Estudo histopatológico e histoquímico de 100 casos. Med Cut ILA 12:167–72, 1984.
4. C Scherwitz, O Braun-Falco. So-called cellulite. J Dermatol Surg Oncol 4(3):230–34, 1978.
5. M Ronald, Di Salvo. Controlling the appearance of cellulite. Cosmetics and Toiletries 110:50–58, 1995.
6. ABR Rossi, AL Vergnanini. Cellulite: a review. J Eur. Acad Dermatol Vener 14:251–62, 2000.
7. DM Hexsel, D Gobbato, R Mazzuco, CL Hexsel. Lipodistrofia ginóide. In: MPV Kede, Sabatovich (eds). Dermatologia Estética. 1st ed. Atheneu: São Paulo; 2003: 350–59.
8. GF Murphy. Histopathology of the skin. In: DE Elder, R Elenitsas, C Jaworsky, BL Johnson Jr. (eds). Lever's histopathology of the skin. Lippincott-Raven: Philadelphia; 1997: 5–50.
9. D Hexsel, R Mazzuco. Subcision: Uma alternativa cirúrgica para a lipodistrofia ginóide ("celulite") e outras alterações do relevo corporal. An Bras Dermatol 72(1):27–32, 1997.
10. DM Hexsel, NIM De Oliveira. Tratamento da celulite pela subcisão. In: Horibe EK (eds). Estética Clínica e Cirúrgica. Revinter: Rio de Janeiro; 2000: 261–64.
11. F Nurnberger, G Muller. So-called cellulite: an invented disease. J Dermatol Surg Oncol 4:221–29, 1978.
12. JL Burton, WJ Cunliffe. Subcutaneous fat. In: RH Champion, JL Burton, FJG Ebling (eds). Textbook of Dermatology, 6th ed. Blackwell Science: Oxford; 1992: 2140.
13. O Braun-Falco, E Buddecke et al. Zellulitis. Round-Table-Gesprach. Med Klin 66:827–32, 1971.
14. SJ Salache, G Bernstein, M Senkarik. Superficial musculoaponeurotic system. In: SJ Salache, G Bernstein, M Senkarik (eds).

Surgical Anatomy of the Skin. Appleto e Lange: Norwalk; 1988: 89–97.

15. J Franchi, F Pellicur et al. The adipocyte in the history of slimming agents. Pathol Biol 51(5):244–47, 2003.

16. PA Bacci, G Leibaschoff. La Cellulite. Medical Books. Gasgón 19:196, 2000.

17. P Laguese. Sciatique et infiltration cellulalgique. These Méd. Lyon, 1929.

18. SB Curri. Las paniculopatias de estasis venosa: diagnóstico clínico e instrumental. Hausmann, Barcelona; 1991.

19. SB Curri. Aspects morphohistochimiques e bioquimiques du tissue adipeaux dans la dermo hypodermose cellulitique. J Med Esth 5:183, 1976.

20. LB Medeiros. Lipodistrofia ginóide. Abordagem Terapêutica. In: MP Kede, Sabatovich (eds). Dermatologia Estética, 1st ed Atheneu: Rio de Janeiro; 2003: 337–42.

21. RM Di Salvo. Controlling the appearance of cellulite: surveying the cellulite reduction effectiveness of xantines, silanes, Coa, 1-carnitina and herbal extracts. Cosm Toil 110:50–59, 1995.

22. M Binazzi, E Grilli-Cicioloni. A propósito della cosidetta cellulite e della dermato-paniculopatia edemato fibrosclerótica. Ann It Derm Clin Sper 31:121–25, 1977.

23. M Binazzi. Cellulite. Aspects cliniques et morpho-histologiques. J Med Esth Et Chir Derm 10(40):229–23, 1983.

24. H Ciporkin, LHC Paschoal. Clínica da L.D.G. In: Atualização terapêutica e fisiopatogênica da lipodistrofia ginóide (LDG) "celulite" São Paulo: Santos; 1992: 141–54.

25. RT Francischelli, MN Francischelli. Hidrolipodistrifia. Avaliação epidemiológica e uma proposta de classificação. SBME 12:27–36, 2001.

26. Ge Pierard, JL Nizet et al. Cellulite: from standing fat herniation to hypodermal stretch marks. Am J Dermatopathol 22(1):34–37, 2000.

27. RJ Hay, BM Adriaans. Bacterial Infections. In: RH Champion et al. Rook/Wilkinson/Ebling (eds). Textbook of Dermatology, 6th ed. Blackwell Science: Oxford; 1998: Vol 2:1112–6.

28. CF Sanches. Celulitis. 3rd ed. Celcius: Buenos Aires; 1992: 3–225.

29. DM Hexsel. Body repair. In: LC Parish et al. In: Women's dermatology: Parthenon Publishing: Nova Iorque; 2001: 586–95.

30. AS Garder. New insight on the etiology and treatment of cellulite according to Chinese medicine: More than skin deep. Am J Acupunct 23(4):339–46, 1995.

31. M Rosenbaum, V Prieto, J Hellmer et al. An exploratory investigation of the morphology and biochemistry of cellulite. Plast Reconst Surg 07(101):1934–39, 1998.

32. DM Hexsel, R Mazzuco. Subcision: a treatment for cellulite. Int J Dermatol 39:539–44, 2000.

33. DM Gruber, JC Huber. Gender-specific medicine: the new profile of gynecology. Gynecol Endocrinol 13(1):1–16, 1999.

34. LHC Paschoal. Tratamento da "celulite"- lipodistrofia ginóide (LDG). In: EK Horibe (eds). Estética Clínica e Cirúrgica. Revinter Rio de Janeiro; 2000: 257–60.

35. D Hexsel, T Dal Forno, CL Hexsel. Severity Scale of Cellulite. JEADV 23:523–28, 2009.

36. C Bertin, H Zunino et al. A double-blind evaluation of the activity of an anti-cellulite product containing retinol, caffeine, and ruscogenine by a combination of several non-invasive methods. J Cosmetic Sci 52:199–210, 2001.

37. WP Coleman. Liposuction. In: RG Wheeland (ed.) Cutaneous Surgery. Philadelphia: WB Sauders Company; 1994: 549–67.

38. A Matarasso, SL Matarasso. When does your liposuction patient require an abdominoplasty? Dermatol Surg 23:1151–60, 1997.

39. A Benaiges, P Marcet, R Armengol et al. Study of the refirming effect of a plant complex. Int J Cosm Sci 20(4):223–33, 1998.

40. JF Fernandes. Avaliação Antropométrica. In: JF Fernandes A prática da Avaliação Física. Shape. São Paulo; 2003: 99–100.

41. RI Wellens, AF Roche, HJ Khamis et al. Relationships between the body mass index and body composition. Obes Res 4 (1): 35–44, 1996.

42. R Radie, V Nikolic, I Karner et al. Ultrasound measurement in defining the regional distribution of subcutaneous fat tissue. Coll Antropol 26:59–68, 2002.

43. F Perin, JC Pittet, S Schnebert et al. Ultrasonic assessment of variations in thickness of subcutaneous fat during the normal menstrual cycle. Eur J Ultrasound 11(1):7–14, 2000.

44. M Ferland, JP Depres. Assesment of adipose tissue by computed axial tomography in obese women: association with body density and anthropometric measurements. Br J Nutr 61(2):139–48, 1989.

45. R Ross, KD Shaw, J Rissanen et al. Sex differences in lean and adipose tissue distribution by magnetic resonance imaging: anthropometric relationships. Am J Clin Nutr 59:1277–85, 1994.

46. EL Thomas, N Saeed, JV Hajnal et al. Magnetic resonance imaging of total body fat. J Appl Physiol 85:1778–85, 1998.

47. M Querleux, C Cornillon et al. Anatomy and physiology of subcutaneous adipose tissue by in vivo magnetic resonance imaging and spectroscopy: relationships with sex and presence of cellulite. Skin Res Technol 8(2):118–24, 2002.

48. F Mirrashed. Pilot study of dermal and subcutaneous fat structures by MRI in individuals who differ in gender, BMI, and cellulite grading. Skin Research and Technology 10: 161–68, 2004.

49. DM Hexsel, M Abreu, TC Rodrigues et al. Side-by-side comparison of areas with and without cellulite depressions using magnetic resonance imaging. Dermatol Surg 35(10):1471–7, 2009.

50. PC Gruber, LC Fuller. Lipoatrophy semicircularis induced by trauma. Clin Exp Dermatol 26(3):269–71, 2001.

51. H Perrot. Localized lipo-atrophies. Ann Dermatol Venerol 115(4):523–7, 1988.

APPENDIX A

CELLULITE ASSESSMENT PROTOCOL

Name:
Age:
Color:
Phototype:
Descent:
Height:
Weight:
BMI:
Cellulite family history: ( ) Yes ( ) No
Age of onset:
Compromised areas:
Previous treatments:
Concomitant Diseases:
Drugs Utilization:
Assessed Region:
Hexsel & Hexsel e Dal´Forno Cellulite Severity Scale

A) Number of evident depressions

This item refers to the total number of evident depressions by visual inspection in the area to be examined. The scores are expressed as:

ZERO = None/no depressions

1 = A small amount: 1 to 4 depressions are visible
2 = A moderate amount: 5 to 9 depressions are visible
3 = A large amount: 10 or more depressions are visible

B) Depth of depressions

This item evaluates the depth of depressions by visual inspection of the affected areas; comparison to the pictures of CSS is recommended.

ZERO = No depressions

1 = Superficial depressions
2 = Medium depth depressions
3 = Deep depressions

C) Morphological appearance of skin surface alterations

Item C assesses the different morphological patterns of skin surface alterations; comparison with the pictures of CSS is recommended.

ZERO = No raised areas

1 = "Orange peel" appearance
2 = "Cottage cheese" appearance
3 = "Mattress" appearance

D) Grade of laxity, flaccidity, or sagging skin

Laxity, flaccidity, or sagging skin confers the affected skin a draped appearance. This effect aggravates the appearance of cellulite. Item D assesses the grade of flaccidity, and comparison to the pictures of CSS is recommended.

ZERO = Absence of laxity, flaccidity, or sagging skin

1 = Slight draped appearance
2 = Moderate draped appearance
3 = Severe draped appearance

E) Classification by Nürnberger and Müller [10]

This item is based on the current classification of cellulite, shown in Box 1. Patients should be evaluated in the standing position with relaxed gluteus muscles. However, if the patient has no evident depressions, they should be asked to contract their gluteus muscles or the *pinch test* should be applied (by pinching the skin between the thumb and index finger) in order to differentiate between scores zero and 1.

ZERO = Zero grade

1 = First grade
2 = Second grade
3 = Third grade

Scoring system of Cellulite Severity Scale and cellulite new classification

Points	Cellulite New Classification
1 to 5	MILD
6 to 10	MODERATE
11 to 15	SEVERE

Photonumerical Scale

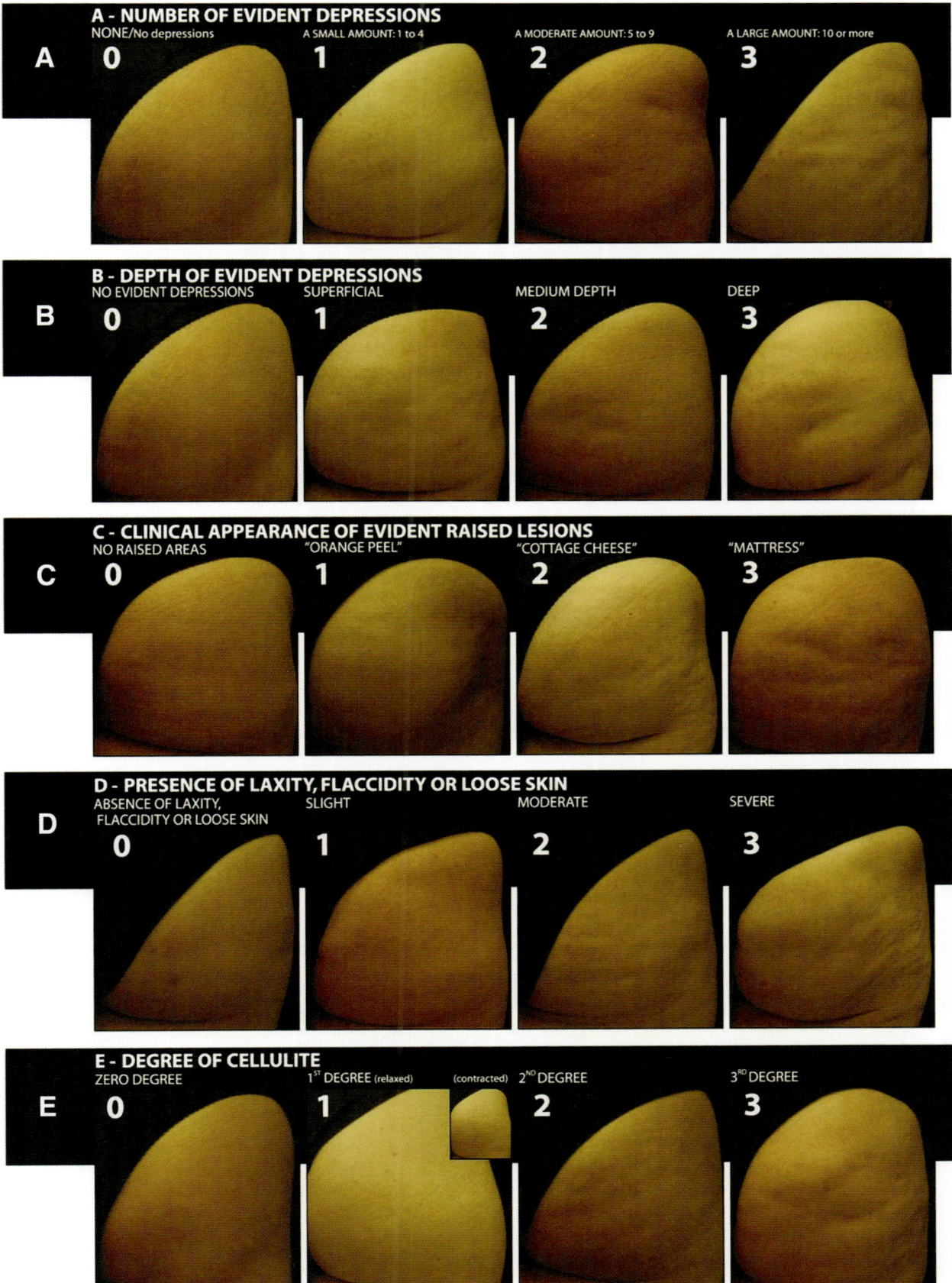

Figure 4.16 CSS – Cellulite Severity Scale.

5 Cellulite Pathophysiology
Zoe Diana Draelos

Introduction
Cellulite is the most common poorly understood aesthetic condition affecting females worldwide [1]. This can be verified by the many names ascribed to this uneven bumpy skin texture on the buttocks and thighs including adisposis edematosa, dermopanniculosis deformans, status protrusus cutis, and gynoid lipodystrophy (Fig. 5.1) [1]. Under ultrasound visualization, cellulite appears as low-density fat herniations into the denser dermal tissue [2]. There are many theories purported to describe the pathophysiology of cellulite, none can be verified however. These theories include: dietary influences, genetically determined fat deposition, vascular insufficiency, excess adipose tissue, and chronic inflammation (Table 5.1) [3]. This chapter will present the currently espoused theories allowing the reader to determine which most closely approximates clinical experience.

Dietary Influences
The theory that diet contributes to the pathophysiology of cellulite has been popularized by the consumer press. Articles abound stating that a low carbohydrate, low fat, low salt, high fiber diet can minimize cellulite. A controlled medical study to verify the effect of diet on cellulite minimization has never been conducted; however, a low calorie diet, which might be low in high calorie carbohydrates and fats, may decrease adipose tissue and improve cellulite [4]. Low salt, high fiber diets may indeed decrease extracellular fluid volume thus minimizing vascular effects.

When considering how diet affects the pathophysiology of cellulite, it is interesting to look at how cultural eating habits may contribute. Cellulite is more commonly seen in Caucasian females than Oriental females. It is true that visualization of skin texture irregularities is easier in fair skin, yet Oriental females seem to demonstrate less cellulite. One theory regarding the pathophysiology of cellulite is the affect of diet on circulating estrogens. The consumption of cow's milk in the Orient is low; however, much of the milk consumed in the United States contains estrogens that enter the milk from the food fed to the cows. Anther possible explanation is reduced endogenous estrogen production in Oriental females who consume large amounts of fermented soy in the form of tofu or soy nuts. Fermented soy is high in phytoestrogens, which may suppress adrenal and ovarian estrogen production, which is not the case with the estrogens ingested in cow's milk.

Thus, one explanation for cellulite is a poor diet leading to the deposition of excess fat, fluid retention, and a high circulating estrogen level [5]. Another theory is that cellulite is present due to predetermined genetic influences.

Genetically Determined Fat Deposition
Many researchers believe that the pattern of adipose deposit that leads to cellulite is genetically determined [6]. Thus, women will age and deposit fat in the same areas as their mother regardless of diet or estrogen stimulation [7]. This may be due to a hormone

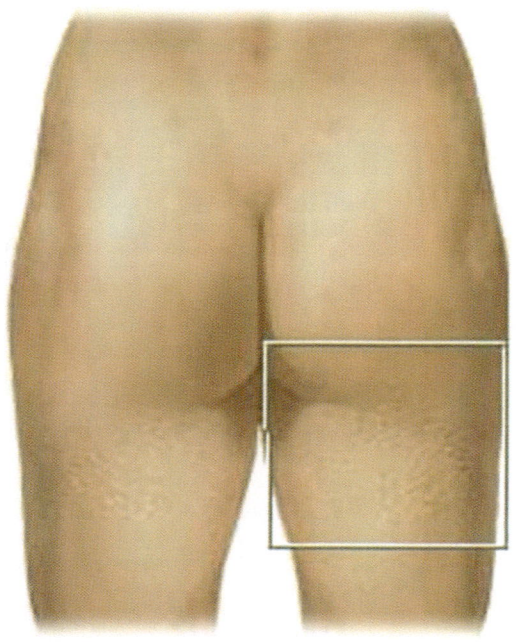
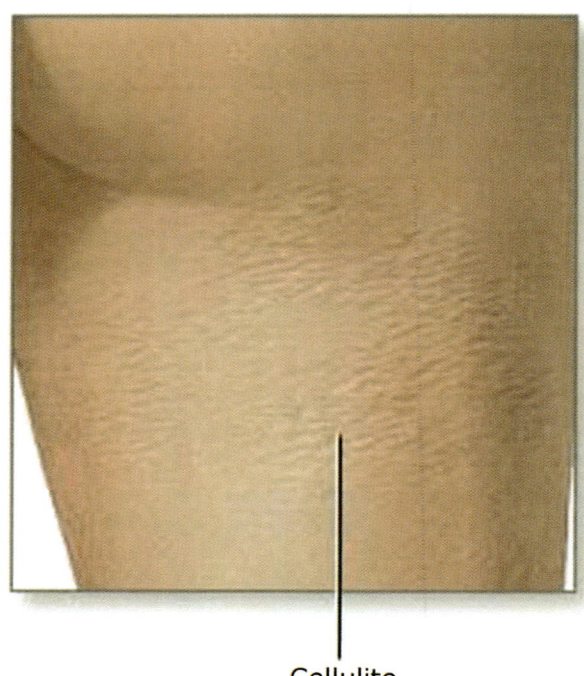

Cellulite

Figure 5.1 The most common location for cellulite is the upper posterior thighs. It may also occur on the upper posterior arms, buttock, and anterior thighs. Source: Wikipedia.

Table 5.1 Cellulite Pathophysiology Controversy

Cellulite theory	Pros	Cons
Dietary Influences	Oriental women who consume phytoestrogens in soy exhibit less cellulite	80% of women worldwide exhibit cellulite regardless of diet
Genetically Determined Fat Deposition	Daughters of mothers with cellulite are also likely to exhibit cellulite	Cellulite can be minimized by less body fat, which is self-determined
Vascular Insufficiency	Deterioration of dermal vasculature results in increased fluid retention and cellulite appearance	Ultrasound imaging of cellulite shows adipose tissue impinging on dermis, not only fluid
Excess Adipose Tissue	Women with more body fat tend to exhibit more cellulite	Weight loss does not eliminate cellulite
Chronic Inflammation	Inflammation from collagenase breaks down dermal collagen allowing for adipose herniations	Not all menstruating women exhibit cellulite to the same degree

receptor allele that determines the receptor number and sensitivity to estrogen. This may determine the distribution of subcutaneous fat. Pierard espoused this theory noting that cellulite is not a result of increased body mass, but rather can be influenced by the inherited waist-to-hip ratio [8].

Vascular Insufficiency

One of the most widely held theories regarding the pathophysiology of cellulite is the effect of vascular insufficiency. Smith postulates that cellulite is a degradation process initiated by deterioration of the dermal vasculature, particularly loss of the capillary networks [9]. As a result, excess fluid is retained with the dermal and subcutaneous tissues [10]. This loss of the capillary network is thought to be due to engorged fat cells clumping together and inhibiting venous return [11].

After the capillary networks have been damaged, vascular changes begin to occur within the dermis resulting in decreased protein synthesis and an inability to repair tissue damage. Clumps of protein are deposited around the fatty deposits beneath the skin causing an "orange peel" appearance to the skin as it is pinched between the thumb and forefinger. At this stage, however, there is no visual evidence of cellulite.

The characteristic appearance of cellulite is only seen after hard nodules composed of fat surrounded by hard reticular protein form within the dermis. Ultrasound imaging of skin affected by cellulite at this stage reveals thinning of the dermis with subcutaneous fat pushing upward, which translates into the rumpled skin known as cellulite.

Thus, this theory holds that hormonally mediated fat deposition, fat lobule compression of capillary vasculature, decreased venous return, formation of clumped fat lobules, and deposition of protein substances around clumped fat lobules leads to the appearance of cellulite.

Excess Adipose Tissue

Some investigators have observed that cellulite is more common in overweight and obese women. This felt to be due to the presence of copious fat lobules within the subcutaneous tissue encased in fibrous septae with dermal attachments (Fig. 5.2) [12]. These fibrous attachments surrounding abundant fat lead to the rumpled appearance of the skin characteristic of cellulite [13]. Thus, weight loss, which reduces the size of the fat lobules and removes the metabolic influences of excess adiposity, improves the appearance of cellulite [14]. Improvement can also be achieved with exercise, since improved muscle tone creates a better foundation to support the overlying fat.

Chronic Inflammation

The final theory espouses that cellulite is an inflammatory process resulting in breakdown of the collagen in the dermis providing for the subcutaneous fat herniations seen on ultrasound. The onset of cellulite with puberty and menstruation has caused some researchers to evaluate the hormonal changes necessary for sloughing of the endometrium [15]. It appears that menstruation requires the secretion of metalloproteases, (MMP) such as collagenase (collagenase-1, MMP-1) and gelatinase (gelatinase A, MMP-2) [16]. The endometrial glandular and stromal cells secrete these enzymes to allow menstrual bleeding to occur. Collagenases cleave the triple helical domain of fibrillar collagens at a neutral pH and are secreted just prior to menstruation. However, the collagenase may not only break down the fibrillar collagens present in the endometrium, but also in the dermis.

Furthermore, gelatinase B is produced by stromal cells or mast cells during the late proliferative endometrial phase and just after ovulation. Gelatinase B is associated with an influx of polymorphonuclear leukocytes, macrophages, and eosinophils, which also contribute to inflammation [17]. A marker for this inflammation is the synthesis of dermal glycosaminoglycans, which enhance

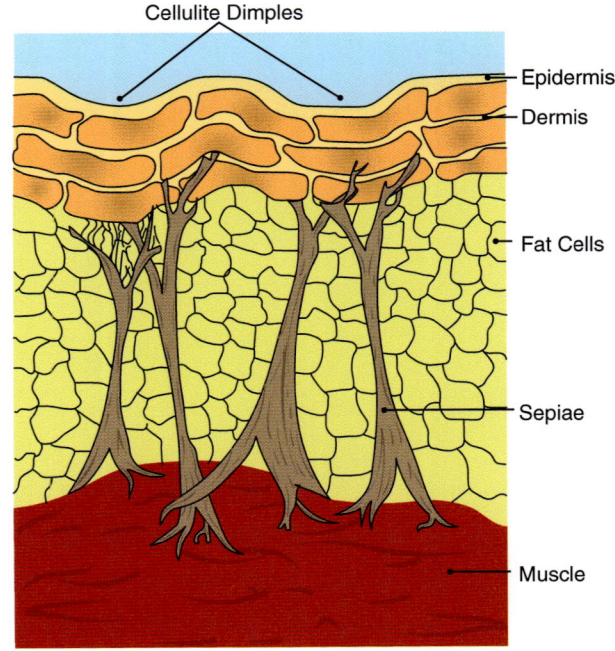

Figure 5.2 The organization of the adipocytes between fibrous septae results in the dimpling of the skin characteristic of cellulite.

water binding further worsening the appearance of the cellulite through swelling. The presence of these glycosaminoglycans has been observed on ultrasound as low-density echoes at the lower dermal/subcutaneous junction [18].

The secretion of endometrial collagenase to initiate menstruation also provides for collagen breakdown in the dermis [19]. With repeated cyclical collagenase production, more and more dermal collagen is destroyed accounting for the worsening of cellulite seen with age [20]. Eventually enough collagen is destroyed to weaken the reticular and papillary dermis and allow subcutaneous fat to herniate between the structural fibrous septa found in female fat. Obviously, if more subcutaneous fat is present, more pronounced herniation can occur.

Summary

The pathophysiology of cellulite is indeed controversial. Perhaps if the pathophysiology were understood, more effective treatments could be developed. It is most likely that cellulite is due to a combination of all the factors discussed including hormones, genetics, adipose tissue, microcirculation, and chronic inflammation. It cannot be denied that cellulite is a widespread human condition more commonly observed in females that worsens with advancing age. Further research will be needed to elucidate the rest.

REFERENCES

1. F Nurnberger, G Muller. So-called cellulite: an invented disease. J Dermatol Surg Oncol 4:221–9, 1978.
2. PR Dahl, MJ Salla, RK Winkelmann. Localized involutional lipoatrophy: a clinicopathologic study of 16 patients. J Am Acad Dermatol 35:523–8, 1996.
3. F Mirrashed, JC Sharp, V Krause et al. Pilot study of dermal and subcutaneous fat structures by MRI in individuals who differ in gender, BMI, and cellulite grading. Skin Res Technol 10(3):161–8, 2004.
4. MM Avram. Cellulite: a review of its physiology and treatment. J Cosmet Laser Ther 6(4):181–5, Dec 2004.
5. AV Rawlings. Cellulite and its treatment. Int J Cosmet Sci 28(3):175–90, Jun 2006.
6. ZD Draelos, KD Marenus. Cellulite-etiology and purported treatment. Dermatol Surg 23:1177–81, 1997.
7. C Scherwitz, O Braun-Falco. So-called cellulite. J Dermatol Surg Oncol 4:230–4, 1978.
8. JP Ortonne, M Zartarian, M Verschoore et al. Cellulite and skin ageing: is there any interaction? J Eur Acad Dermatol Venereol 22(7):827–34, Jul 2008; Epub 2008 Feb 27.
9. GE Pierard. Commentary on cellulite: skin mechanobiology and the waist-to-hip ration. J Cosmet Derm 4(3):151–2, 2005.
10. WF Smith. Cellulite treatments: snake oil or skin science. Cosmet Toilet 110:61–70, 1995.
11. SB Curri. Cellulite and fatty tissue microcirculation. Cosmet Toilet 108:51–8, 1993.
12. SB Curri, E Bombardelli. Local lipodystrophy and districtual microcirculation. Cosmet Toilet 109:51–65, 1994.
13. P Quatresooz, E Xhauflaire-Uhoda, C Pierard-Franchimont, GE Pierard. Cellulite histopathology and related mechanobiology. Int. J Cosmet Sci 28(3):207–10, Jun 2006.
14. GE Pierard, JL Nizet, C Pierard-Franchimont. Cellulite: from standing fat herniation to hypodermal stretch marks. Am J Dermatolpathol 22(1):34–7, Feb 2000.
15. F Terranova, E Berardesca, H Maibach. Cellulite: nature and aetiopathogenesis. Int J Cosmet Sci 28(3):157–67, Jun 2006.
16. E Marbaix, I Kokorine, P Henriet et al. The expresssion of interstitial collagenase in human endometrium is controlled by progesterone and by oestadiol and is related to menstruation. Biochem J 305:1027–30, 1995.
17. CF Singer, E Marbaix P Lemoine et al. Local cytokines induce differrential expression of matrix metalloproteinases but not their tissue inhibitors in human endometrial fibroblasts. Eur J Biochem 259(1-2):40–5, 1999.
18. M Jeziorska, H Nagasae, LA Salamonsen, DE Woolley. Immunolocalization of the matrix metalloproteinases gelatinase B and stromelysin 1 in juman endometrium throughout the menstrual cycle. J Reprod Fertil 107(1):43–51, 1996.
19. T Lotti, MD Ghersetich, C Grappone, G Dini. Proteoglycans in so-called cellulite. Int J Dermatol 29:272–4, 1990.
20. E Marbaix, I Kokorine, J Donnez et al. Regulation and restricted expression of interstitial collagenase suggest a pivotal role in the initiation of menstruation. Hum Reprod 11 (Suppl 2):134–43, 1996.

6 Diagnostic Techniques

Molly Wanner and Mathew Avram

Any layperson can recognize cellulite as the dimpled appearance of the thighs, abdomen, and buttocks of most women. Yet assessment of cellulite has not been well characterized in the medical literature, and studies of cellulite treatments do not utilize one consistent modality to evaluate it. The evaluation of cellulite is confused by the fact that a clear pathogenetic mechanism has not been proven and by practical difficulties, such as capturing the dimpling of cellulite on camera.

Even diagnostic techniques are controversial. The percentage of body fat in an area and the surface area of the dermal-subcutaneous border (an indicator of the extent of fat protrusions into the dermis) using ultrasound were shown to predict cellulite severity in one study [1]. On the other hand, the degree of protrusion of fat lobules into the dermis on biopsy was not correlated with severity of cellulite in another study [2,3].

Yet clinical evaluation, while paramount, can often be subjective. There is no agreed upon clinical criteria for establishing cellulite, further complicating matters. Diagnostic techniques, therefore, provide important additional tools. We will review existing and potential diagnostic modalities, as well as the clinical studies that have utilized these techniques.

Clinical Evaluation

The classification systems for cellulite have been reviewed elsewhere in this book [4–7]. In practice, many investigators have not used classification systems, and instead, use other variety of grading scales to evaluate improvement from baseline [8–14]. Grading scales that utilizes objective measures such as number and depth of dimples [13] may be more reliable than those that rely on subjective assessment. Regardless of classification or grading, evaluation of cellulite before and after treatment should occur in constant lighting.

In an effort to have a more objective measure of cellulite, investigators reference change in circumference to prove efficacy [8,10–12,15–21]. In fact, cellulite severity has been correlated with thigh circumference as well as BMI and percentage of fat [1]. Although circumference may be a proxy for the amount of subcutaneous fat, the severity of cellulite is dependent on both the amount of fat and the number of dimpled areas in a given area [1]. A change in circumference alone will not necessarily indicate an improvement in cellulite. In one study of LPG endermologie, 33 subjects had a loss in circumference, while only five had a reduction in cellulite grade [22]. Thus, other objective measures are preferred.

Biopsy

Nurnberger and Muller first described the anatomic appearance of cellulite on biopsy in 150 cadavers and 30 healthy subjects [4]. They found that women have radial fibrous connective tissue surrounding fat such that fat can herniate into the dermis and cause cellulite. Men have criss-crossed septa that divide the subcutaneous tissue in smaller and better reinforced units. Rosenbaum evaluated biopsies of five cadavers and seven healthy subjects including women (affected and unaffected) and men [23]. Skin with cellulite had thin connective tissue septa in a more radial orientation as compared with unaffected skin. As in the Nurnberger and Muller study, men had smaller fat lobules.

Pierard reviewed biopsies of 39 autopsy specimens and found that the connective tissue network, which he defines as fibrous strands as opposed to septa, was much more complex than Nurnberger suggested [2]. Like Nurnberger, he confirmed that men had a smooth dermal fat border compared with the lumpy appearance of the border in the female patient. On the other hand, his study also found a lack of correlation between herniation of fat into the dermis and the severity of cellulite. He suggested that it is the variation of thickness of these strands, which tethers the dermis and creates cellulite, rather than the orientation. He found a few α-actin+ myofibroblasts and reduced factor XIIIa+ dendrocytes in the most abnormal, enlarged fibrous stands.

In studies of cellulite treatment, findings on biopsy have been variously described. Adipocyte changes including lysis or thickening of the adipocyte membrane have been seen [24,25]. Dermal thickening or a more organized dermis has been reported after therapy [25,26]. A decrease in fat herniations in the hypodermis has been described [17]. Alteration of the connective tissue septa or change in dendrocytes or myofibroblasts within the hypodermal fibrous strands has been seen after therapy [27,28]. Dermal fibrosis has been described [15]. In some cases, no change has been seen before or after treatment, perhaps due to the small biopsy size [10,11].

In practice, the use of biopsy as a diagnostic technique has a role, but often is a cosmetically unacceptable alternative, particularly given the other options available. The *ex vivo* state may be different from the *in vivo* appearance, especially for small biopsies. Features such as dermal organization or epidermal thickening can vary greatly depending on sampling choice and processing after biopsy. Lastly, just as with clinical evaluation, biopsies are often evaluated subjectively, with qualitative rather than quantitative descriptions.

Photography

Photography can be useful for evaluating the degree of cellulite. In one study, black and white photographs of areas of cellulite were analyzed by grey level processing to create a shadow index that related the number of shadows to the total surface area. The shadow index was used as a quantitative measure of cellulite and found to relate to Nurnberger and Muller grade [29].

Cellulite is particularly difficult to photograph. Uniform lenses, filters, camera distance, consistent relationship of the camera with lighting, absence of jewelry, use of identical underclothing such as dark bikini underwear, and background are all important to photographing cellulite [30]. Cellulite changes with position, so photographing subjects in the same position for before and after photographs is necessary.

Lighting is paramount, and a variety of lighting strategies have been employed. Even if subjects are evaluated in person, lighting can change the appearance of cellulite. Bielfeldt used a neon ring light placed below the knee and attached a camera to and above the ring light to accentuate the depressions of cellulite [18]. In this article, there are photographs that illustrate when illumination or background is changed, the appearance of cellulite changes. Overhead lighting without flash and lateral light at both low angles and at 75°–90° angles have been suggested [29,30]. Photography at multiple angles has also been reported [31,32].

Some authors use a compression system to accentuate the mattress phenomenon and the appearance of cellulite for photography [1,33]. Perin used a compression system and took photographs with a 30° incident lighting system, a camera mounted perpendicular to the skin surface at a constant height, and a 60 mm focal length lens [33]. Inter-observer agreement was found using these methods. Some authors have used Canfield digital photography systems (Canfield Scientific, Fairfield, NJ) [15,32,33].

Optical Imaging

Three dimensional modeling of an area of cellulite to quantify the severity of cellulite may prove to be an important diagnostic tool. Smalls used a Cyberware Rapid 3D Digitizer laser scanner with data acquisition software on a linear platform to obtain 3D imaging of cellulite [1]. This laser scanning technology generated images that were scored and compared with scores generated after live patient viewing sessions. Scores on a 0–9 scale

of cellulite severity were in agreement. Depth of depressions and the ratio between the roughness of the skin surface (a measure of the difference between the cellulite surface and the reference plane) and the area of a flat plane were the parameters most correlated to visual appearance of cellulite severity.

Other optical systems including PRIMOS (GFMesstechnik, Teltow, Germany) that have been devised to measure wrinkles may prove useful [1,34,35]. (Akazaki, Smalls, Callaghan) 3D imaging with a CLINIPRO Antiaging SD camara (Barcelona, Spain) has been used in studies of cellulite devices [20,25]. This imaging system computes a measure of skin roughness which is based on the difference between the peaks and valleys of the skin affected with cellulite. This type of imaging may offer a more objective analysis of the appearance of cellulite than clinical evaluation. However, it will reflect surface improvement, not establish definitive evidence of structural change.

Imaging systems that may prove useful in the future include Optical Coherence Technology (OCT) and confocal microscopy. OCT reflects infrared light waves off of tissue structures to create an image of the underlying skin, magnifying skin structures [35]. OCT has been used to dynamically visualize the effects of the 1210 nm laser on *ex vivo* adipose tissue [36]. An even more magnified view is provided by *in vivo* confocal microscopy. Confocal microscopy has been used to characterize cellulite at the microscopic level [35]. Like OCT, this technology is not widely available. Both technologies are currently limited by depth of penetration.

Ultrasound

Ultrasound utilizes acoustic waves to generate echos of skin structures that can be transduced into an image [37]. Ultrasound machines such as the Dermascan C (Cortex Technology, Hadsund, Denmark) or the Collagenoson® (Minhorst, Germany)

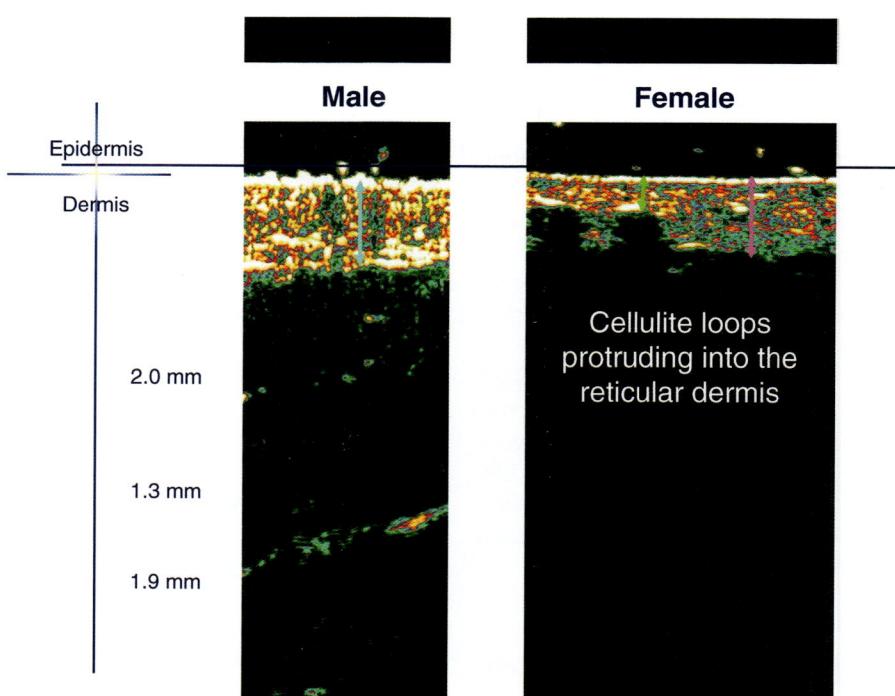

Figure 6.1 A high resolution ultrasound image of (A) male and (B) female subcutaneous fat. Note the fat herniation into the dermis for the female (asterisks), which is not present in the male (courtesy of Dr Agustina Vila Echague and Dr Avram).

produce cross-sectional images of cellulite (Rona, Kuhn) [26,37]. Ultrasound has been used to measure epidermal, dermal, and fat thickness and to assess the morphology of the dermis, dermal-fat border, and the subcutaneous layer.

With ultrasound, dermal thickness has been found to be thinner and fat thickness has been found to be thicker in subjects with cellulite [5,29]. As a result, investigators have used change in epidermal, dermal, or fat thickness as markers for treatment effect [17,28,38–40]. Fat thickness, alone, is not a good measure of cellulite; a thick fat layer may be seen in subjects with both mild and severe cellulite and the impact of fat thickness may depend on body mass index (BMI) [41,42].

Based on the theory that treatments for cellulite may alter or shorten the connective tissue septa, depth of skin structures has been measured. The distance between the dermis to the fascia or muscle has been measured to assess for the degree of improvement of cellulite after radiofrequency [43].

The density of the dermis has been evaluated in studies of cellulite. Decreased dermal density, thought to be due to dermal degradation, has been reported to affect cellulite severity in subjects over age 30 [29]. Density can be evaluated both qualitatively with visual scoring systems or quantitatively with computer derived measures of echogenecity of the ultrasound image [44–46].

Although some do not consider border irregularity to be a good measure of cellulite severity [2,3,28], an irregularity of the dermal-fat border has been correlated with the appearance cellulite [18,23] (Fig. 6.1). Border irregularity can be quantified on ultrasound and can be represented by the dermal-subcutaneous surface area, the length of the dermal-subcutaneous border, or by a parameter of unevenness that is calculated from ultrasound images [1,18,29]. A study by Smalls found that cellulite severity could be predicted by the percentage of fat in an area and by the ultrasound-measured dermal-subcutaneous surface area in a region [1]. Increased length of the dermis-hypodermis border was found to be associated with cellulite in another study [29]. The area of the dermal-hypodermal border has been used gauge response to treatment [47].

While the ability to quantify skin and subcuticular characteristics such as thickness, dermal density, and border irregularity makes ultrasound a valuable diagnostic option, the drawback of ultrasound is that it is heavily operator dependent. Even a 1 mm change in the position of the ultrasound can yield a drastically different appearance of the dermal fat border on ultrasound [18]. A variation of pressure on the ultrasound handpiece will change thickness, depth, and density.

MRI

High resolution MRI is a useful tool for cellulite imaging [48]. Querlex described the use of high resolution MRI to evaluate cellulite [49]. MRI images were taken using a 1.5 T whole-body MRI system in combination with a home built high intensity surface gradient coil and a small surface radiofrequency coil. Images of 67 subjects comprised of men, women without cellulite, and women with cellulite were taken. Women with cellulite seemed to have a thicker dermis and thicker adipose layer. Cellulite on MRI was characterized by indentations of adipose tissue into the dermis, a higher percentage of fibrous septa that are perpendicular rather than parallel to the surface, and a thick deep adipose layer. Water content of the subcutaneous layer was not related to cellulite.

Mirrashed also described the use of high resolution MRI to evaluate cellulite [42]. MRI images were compared to a clinical grading system based on the presence of dimples. Images were obtained with a 3T MRI plus a radiofrequency coil which had a single ring surface coil inductively coupled with a matching ring strapped to the subject's thigh. Clinical appearance of cellulite was described in low and high BMI groups. In high BMI subjects with cellulite, a thinner dermis with weakly reinforced and sparse fibrous septa of the fat yielded extrusion of fat into the dermis. In low BMI subjects, the thickness of the layer of fat beneath the dermis played the largest role.

MRI was used in a study of cellulite treatment with a unipolar radiofrequency device [15]. In this study, MRI was used to evaluate gross changes in the subcutaneous fat layer and no changes were seen. In a study of a dual wavelength low level laser, MRI revealed a decrease in fat thickness [21].

High resolution MRI has the benefit of providing clear images of the subcutaneous layer. Multiple cross-sectional areas can be evaluated at once, preventing the sampling error associated with ultrasound and biopsy. MRI is also less operator dependent than ultrasound. The quantitative measurements to assess MRI, rather than qualitative descriptors would enhance the usefulness of this tool. Nevertheless, the cost of MRI may be prohibitive.

Vascular Imaging

Based on the theory that cellulite is characterized by abnormal circulation, vascular imaging has been used to study cellulite. Vascular imaging techniques include laser doppler flowmetry, thermography, and video capillaroscopy. Doppler applies laser light to the skin which is then scattered and reflected to generate an image of arterial and venous activity [37]. Thermography measures circulation indirectly, through temperature [37]. Videocapillaroscopy uses a magnifying lens in oil immersion and a halogen light source to obtain capillary images [50,51]. Light reflection rheography has been used to evaluate venous activity, and lymphatic flow has been measured by lymphoscintigraphy [50]. Blood flow in cellulite subjects has been evaluated using microdialysis probes [23].

Curri studied 14 female patients who were undergoing liposuction with an optic probe video capillaroscope, laser-Doppler flowmetry, and histology [52]. She measured 1500 capillaries, venules, and fat cells and found a statistically significant correlation between dilation of capillaries and venules and hypertrophy of fat cells. She also reported a statistically significant correlation between severity of cellulite of the lower limbs and breast and symptoms of chronic venous insufficiency, although she emphasized that the role of circulatory damage in the development of cellulite is difficult to confirm. Similarly, Smith described decreased blood flow using laser-Doppler in 10 subjects with cellulite who were compared with control subjects [5]. Changes in circulation due to cellulite have not been uniformly substantiated [23].

Circulatory parameters have been evaluated in studies of cellulite treatments. A change in circulation with increased capillary density and increased flow after treatment with an oral formulation of plant substances has been reported using video-capillaroscopy, laser-Doppler, and thermography [50]. Doppler analysis has confirmed increased blood flow after application of topical cellulite products [18,38]. Change in circulation after treatment with extracorporeal shock wave therapy has been

Table 6.1 Diagnostic Techniques

Technique	Pro	Con
Circumference measurements	Easy to do	May not be representative
Photography	Readily available	Small changes in environment change image
		Complex to standardize
Biopsy	Reveals cellulite and treatment response at a microscopic level	Cosmetically unacceptable
		Architecture may change *ex vivo*
		Sampling error
		Evaluation often qualitative
Optical imaging-3D	Standardizes visual images	Evaluated in few studies
	Provides quantitative measure	Reflects surface change, not deep architecture change
Optical imaging-OCT & confocal	High magnification view *in vivo*	Limited availability
	May provide real time imaging during treatment	Limited depth of penetration
Biomechanical measurements	Easy to do with standardized instruments	May not be representative
		Difficult to compare measurements between studies
Ultrasound	Provides *in vivo* view of dermal and hypodermal structures	Sampling error
	Provides quantitative measure	Operator dependence
MRI	Less sampling error	Cost
	Not operator dependent	
Vascular imaging	Some imaging techniques (Doppler) are widely available	May not be representative

described using liquid crystal contact thermography [26]. On the other hand, circulatory changes have not always been noted [53]. Some studies using thermography have found results that are either difficult to interpret or that show no change in circulation after cellulite treatment [14,54].

Biomechanical Measurements

Biomechanical Tissue Characterization (BTC-2000) technology (SRLI Technologies; Nashville, TN) has been used to evaluate the biomechanical properties of skin with cellulite [1,55]. A Cutometer (Courage and Khazaka; Germany) and ballistometer have been used as well [5,18,28]. The use of these diagnostic devices is based on the theory that lax skin will enhance the severity of cellulite, and biomechanical measurements will quantitatively capture skin laxity [1,7,29,55,56].

Subjects with cellulite do appear to have greater skin laxity with more compliant skin and less stiffness or firmness of the skin [1,5,55]. However, laxity may not play as large a role as other factors in cellulite. In one study, compliance and stiffness were not found to influence the severity of cellulite as much as other features (the percentage of fat in an area and the total surface area of the dermal-subcutaneous border) [1].

A number of studies have evaluated biomechanical measures after treatment of cellulite [5,18,29,54]. One study evaluated elasticity with an elasticity meter and found an increase in elasticity following treatment with low-fluence laser and suction massage device for cellulite [54]. Others have used a Cutometer (Courage and Khazaka; Germany) and found a change in elasticity after application of topical cellulite products [18,28].

Since laxity seems to play a role in cellulite severity, this diagnostic technique may be helpful in the evaluation of cellulite. Since biomechanical measures do not provide the best overall measure of cellulite severity, these measures are most appropriately used in conjunction with other diagnostic techniques. This diagnostic technique is also limited by the fact that measurements of biomechanical properties may not be compared between studies unless the same measurement system is used [57].

Other Techniques

Given the potential role of percent body fat in the appearance of cellulite, measures of body fat may have an adjunctive role in the evaluation of cellulite. Measurements of body fat using a caliper or plicometry or the use of a Dual-Energy X-ray Absorptiometry (DEXA) scan may be helpful [1,37,58]. Lipolysis in cellulite and after treatment with a cellulite device has been more directly evaluated using microdialysis probes to measure glycerol output [23,59].

Another technique is an ultrasonic pain test, a test that measures the amount of compression it takes to elicit pain. This test uses pain as a proxy for the edema and inflammation purported to be related to cellulite. A study of cellulite treatments compared with placebo revealed a reduction in pain after treatment but not after placebo [50].

Conclusion

There are multiple modalities, each with pros and cons, used to evaluate cellulite (Table 6.1). The ideal diagnostic technique captures the entire picture of cellulite, as opposed to one characteristic such as fat thickness; provides objective measures that can be compared between studies; is reliable; has limited sampling error; and is not operator dependent. As of yet, there is no gold standard, although there are good options available.

3D imaging seems to be an excellent alternative as it can provide quantitative measures that are correlated with cellulite severity. This diagnostic technique reflects surface change. Although the surface appearance is ultimately what matters to the patient, and this technique may imply deeper change, it does not prove it. 3D imaging, therefore, may be less reliable as a proof of concept for new device or therapy.

Ultrasound and MRI do provide deep images of the underlying skin and subcutaneous structure. Ultrasound can be used quantitatively, although it is limited by operator dependence and the potential for sampling error. MRI may prove useful in the future, but to date has been used either in a more qualitative manner or to measure fat thickness only. It is also costly.

Other options such as photography can be unreliable; small changes in lightening can have a dramatic effect. Biopsy, while providing perhaps the clearest image of anatomy, is typically described qualitatively, is subject to sampling error, and may be cosmetically unacceptable for the evaluation of a cosmetic issue. Biomechanical measurements, circumference measurements and measures of circulation don't capture certain elements of cellulite that contribute to the severity. OCT and confocal microscopy are limited by depth of penetration.

In the future, the ideal technique would enable the physician or investigator to diagnose cellulite *in vivo* at the bedside and visualize the effects of cellulite treatment in real time. Yet despite the flaws in the currently available diagnostic techniques, these modalities provide important and useful alternatives to clinical evaluation and offer objective data that improve our understanding of cellulite and its treatment.

REFERENCES

1. LK Smalls, CY Lee, J Whitestone et al. Quantitative model of cellulite: three dimensional skin surface topography, biophysical characterization, and relationship to human perception. J Cosmet Sci 56:105–20, 2005.
2. G Pierard, JL Nizet, C Pierard-Franchimont. Cellulite: From standing fat herniation to hypodermal stretch marks. Am J dermatopathol 22:34–37, 2000.
3. G Pierard. Commentary on cellulite: skin mechanobiology and the waist-to-hip ratio. J Cosmet Dermatol 4:151–52, 2005.
4. F Nurnberger, G Muller. So called cellulite: An invented disease. J Dermatol Surg Oncol 4:221–29, 1978.
5. WP Smith. Cellulite Treatments: Snake oils or skin science. Cosmetics and Toiletries 110:61–70, 1995.
6. ABR Rossi, AL Vergnanini. Cellulite: a review. J Eur Acad Dermatol Venereol 14:251–62, 2000.
7. DM Hexsel, T Dal'Forno, CL Hexsel. A validated photonumeric cellulite severity scale. J Eur Acad Dermatol Venereol 23:523–28, 2009.
8. TS Alster and EL Tanzi. Cellulite treatment using a novel combination readiofrequency, infrared light, and mechanical tissue manipulation device. J Cosmetic Laser Ther 7:81–85, 2005.
9. M Kulick. Evaluation of the combination of radio frequency, infrared energy and mechanical rollers with suction to improve skin surface irregularities (cellulite) in a limited treatment area. J Cosmet Laser Ther 8:185–90, 2006.
10. NS Sadick, RS Mulholland. A prospective clinical study to evaluate the efficacy and safety of cellulite treatment using the combination of optical and RF energies for subcutaneous tissue heating. J Cosmet Laser Ther 6(4):187–90, 2004.
11. NS Sadick, C Magro. A study evaluating the safety and efficacy of the Velasmooth™ system in the treatment of cellulite. J Cosmet Laser Ther 9:5–20, 2007.
12. R Wanitphakdeedecha, W Manuskiatti. Treatment of cellulite with a bipolar radiofrequency, infrered heat, and pulsatile suction device: a pilot study. J Cosmet Dermatol 5:284–88, 2006.
13. M Alexiades-Armenakas, JS Dover, KA Arndt. Unipolar radiofrequency treatment to improve the appearance of cellulite. J Cos Laser Ther 10:158–53, 2008.
14. Birnbaum L. Addition of conjugated linoleic acid to a herbal anticellulite pill. Advances in Therapy 5:225–29, 2001.
15. DJ Goldberg, A Fazeli, AL Berlin. Clinical, laboratory, and MRI analysis of cellulite treatment with a unipolar radiofrequency device. Dermatol Surg 34:204–09, 2008.
16. PK Nootheti, A Magpantay, G Yosowitz et al. A single center, randomized, comparative, prospective clinical study to determine efficacy of the velasmooth system versus the triactive system for the treatment of cellulite. Lasers Surg Med 38:908–12, 2006.
17. GH Sasaki, K Oberg, B Tucker, M Gaston. The effectiveness and safety of topical PhotoActif phosphatidylcholine-based anti-cellulite gel and LED (red and near-infrared) light on Grade II-III cellulite: A randomized, double-blinded study. J Cosmet Laser Ther 9:87–96, 2007.
18. S Bielfeldt, P Buttgereit, M Brandt et al. Non-invasive evaluation techniques to quantify the efficacy of cosmetic anti-cellulite products. Skin Res Technol 14:336–46, 2008.
19. MP Goldman. Cellulite: A review of current treatments. Cos Dermatol 15:17–20, 2002.
20. C Romero, N Caballero, M Herrero et al. Effects of cellulite treatment with RF, IR light, mechanical massage and suction treating one buttock with the contralateral as control 10:193–201, 2008.
21. E Lach. Reduction of subcutaneous fat and improvement in cellulite appearance by a dual-wavelength, low-level laser energy combined with vacuum and massage. J Cos Laser Ther 10:202–09, 2008.
22. AT Gulec. Treatment of cellulite with LPG endermologie. Int J Dermatol 48:265–70, 2009.
23. M Rosenbaum, V Prieto, Hellmer Johan et al. An exploratory investigation of the morphology and biochemistry of cellulite. Plast Reconstr Surg 101:1934–9, 1998.
24. MA Trelles, SR Mordon. Adipocyte membrane lysis observed after cellulite treatment is performed with radiofrequency. Aesth Plast Surg 33:125–28, 2009.
25. C Van der Lugt, C Romero, D Ancona et al. A multicenter study of cellulite treatment with a variable emission radio frequency system. Dermatol Ther 22:74–84, 2009.
26. C Kuhn, F Angehern, O Sonnabend, A Voss. Impact of extracorporeal shock waves on the human skin with cellulite: A case study of an unique instance. Clinical Interventions in Aging 3:201–10, 2008.
27. A Goldman, RH Gotkin, DS Sarnoff et al. Cellulite: A new treatment approach combining subdermal Nd:YAG laser lipolysis and autologous fat transplantation. Aesth Surg J 28:656–62, 2008.
28. C Pierard-Franchimont, GE Pierard, F Henry et al. A randomized, placebo-controlled trial of topical retinol in the treatment of cellulite. Am J Clin Dermatol 1:369–74, 2000.
29. JP Ortonne, Z Zartarian, M Verschoore et al. Cellulite and skin ageing: is there any interaction? J Eur Acad Dermatol Venereol 22:827–34, 2008.
30. G Gherardini, A Matarasso, A Serure et al. Standardization in photography for body contour surgery and suction-assisted lipectomy. Plas Reconstr Surg 100:227–37, 1997.

31. J Rao, KE Pabbo, MP Goldman. A double-blinded randomized trial testing the tolerability and efficacy of a novel topical agent with and without occlusion for the treatment of cellulite: a study and review of the literature. J Drugs Dermatol 3:417–25, 2004.

32. J Rao, MH Gold, MP Goldman. A two-center, double-blinded, randomized trial testing the tolerability and efficacy of a novel therapeutic agent for cellulite reduction. J Cosm Dermatol 4:93–102, 2005.

33. F Perin, C Perrier, JC Pittet et al. Assessment of skin improvement treatment efficacy using the photograding of mechanically-accentuated macrorelief of thigh skin. Int J Cos Sci 22:147–56, 2001.

34. S Azazaki, H Nakagawa, H Kazama et al. Age-related changes in skin wrinkles assessed by a novel three-dimensional morphometric analysis. Br J Dermatol 147:689–95, 2002.

35. T Callaghan, KP Wilhelm. An examination of non-invasive imaging techniques in the analysis and review of cellulite. J Cosmet Sci 56:379–93, 2005.

36. CG Rylander, TE Milner, JS Nelson, NJ Kemp. OCT imaging of ex vivo porcine skin and adipose tissue during 1210 nm laser irradiation. Presented at ALMS, Washington DC; 2009.

37. C Rona, M Carrera, E Berardesca. Testing anticellulite products. Int J Cos Sci 28:169–73, 2006.

38. AM Kligman, A Pagnoni, T Stoudemayer. Topical retinol improves cellulite. J Dermatol Treat 10:119–25, 1999.

39. JS Fink, H Mermelstein, A Thomas, R Tro. Use of intense pulsed light and a retinyl-based cream as a potential treatment for cellulite: a pilot study. J Cosmet Deratol 5:254–62, 2006.

40. DA Buscaglia, ET Conte, W McCain, S Friedman. The treatment of cellulite with methylxanthine and herbal extract based cream: An ultrasonographic analysis. Cosmet Dermatol 11:30–40, 1996.

41. N Collis, LA Elliot, C Sharpe, D Sharpe. Cellulite Treatment: A myth or reality: A prospective randomized, controlled trial of two therapies, endermologies, and aminophylline cream. Plast Reconstruct Surg 104:1110–14, 1999.

42. F Mirrashed, JC Sharp, V Krause et al. Pilot study of dermal and subcutaneous fat structures by MRI in inidividuals who differ in gender, BMI, and cellulite grading. Skin Res Tech 10:161–68, 2004.

43. ME Pino, RH Rosado, A Azuela et al. Effect of controlled volumetric tissue heating with radiofrequency on cellulite and the subcutaneous tissue of the buttocks and thighs. J Drugs Dermatol 5:714–22, 2006.

44. C Christ, R Brenke, G Sattler et al. Improvement in skin elasticity in the treatment of cellulite and connective tissue weakness by means of extracorporeal pulse activation therapy. Aesth Surg J 28:538–44, 2008.

45. F Angehrn, C Kuhn, A Voss. Can cellulite be treated with low energy extracorporeal shock wave therapy? Clinical Interventions in Aging 2:623–30, 2007.

46. R Bousquet-Rouaud, M Bazan, J Chaintreuil, AV Echague. High-frequency ultrasound evaluation of cellulite treated with the 1064 nm Nd:YAG laser. J Cosmet Laser Ther 11:34–44, 2009.

47. GW Lucassen, WLN van der Sluys, JJ van Herk et al. The effectiveness of massage treatment on cellulite as monitored by ultrasound imaging. Skin Res Technol 3:154–60, 1997.

48. D Gensanne, G Josse, J Theunis et al. Quantitative magnetic resonance imaging of subcutaneous adipose tissue. Skin Res Technol 13:45–50, 2009.

49. B Querleux, C Cornillon, O Jolivet, J Bittoun. Anatomy and physiology of subcutaneous adipose tissue by in vivo magnetic resonance imaging and spectroscopy; Relationships with sex and presence of cellulite. Skin Res Tech 8:118–24, 2002.

50. F Distante, PA Bacci, M Carrera. Efficacy of a multifunctional plant complex in the treatment of the so-called 'cellulite': clinical and instrumental evaluation. Int J Cos Sci 28:191–206, 2006.

51. SB Curri. Cellulite and Fatty Tissue microcirculation. Cosmetics and Toiletries 108:51–58, 1993.

52. SB Curri, E Bombardelli. Proposed etiology and therapeutic management of local lipodystrophy and districtual microcirculation. Cosmetics and Toiletries 109:51–65, 1994.

53. O Lupi, IJ Semenovitch, C Treu et al. Evaluation of the effects of caffeine in the microcirculation and edema on thighs and buttocks using the orthogonal polarization spectral imaging and clinical parameters. J Cosmet Dermatol 6:102–07, 2007.

54. S Boyce, A Pabby, P Chucchaltkaren et al. Clinical evaluation of a device for the treatment of cellulite: Triactive. Am J Cos Surg 22:233–37, 2005.

55. MK Dobke, B DiBernardo, C Thompson, H usal. Assessment of biomechanical properties: is cellulitic skin different? Aes Surg J 22:260–66, 2002.

56. LK Smalls, M Hicks, D Passeretti et al. Effect of weight loss on cellulite: gynoid lypodystrophy. Plast Reconstr Surg 118:510–16, 2006.

57. C Christ, R Brenke, G Sattler et al. Improvement in skin elasticity in the treatment of cellulite and connective tissue weakness by means of extracorporeal pulse activation therapy. Aesth Surg J 28:538–44, 2008.

58. T Lesser, E Ritvo, LS Moy. Modification of subcutaneous adipose tissue by a methylxanthine formulation: a double blind controlled study. Dermatol Surg 25:455–62, 1999.

59. C Monteux, M Lafontan. Use of microdialysis technique to assess lipolytic responsiveness of femoral adipose tissue after 12 sesssion of mechanical massage technique. J Eur Acad Dermatol Venereol 22:1465–70, 2008.

7 Cellulite-Associated Clinical Conditions of Aesthetic Interest

Rosemarie Mazzuco and Taciana de Oliveira Dal'Forno

Introduction

A few clinical conditions that are of aesthetic interest are commonly observed in association with cellulite. Since they share the same physiopathogenic bases, it is rare for one of these conditions to occur alone. Very often two, three or all of these conditions may be associated in the same patient.

Depending on their influence on cellulite, they may be classified as triggering or worsening conditions and co-existing conditions. This chapter will discuss flaccidity, localized fat, stretch marks and cosmetic sequelae post-liposuction.

SKIN FLACCIDITY
General Aspects

One of the functions of skin concerns mechanical factors—elasticity and tone—that protect the organism against damage caused by hard knocks [1]. While skin elasticity is the responsibility of collagen fibers, its tone is maintained mainly by the elastic fibers. Over the years, both elasticity and skin tone are considerably diminished, an effect of the so-called intrinsic aging which occurs in all organs [2], and whose molecular mechanisms have become better known in the last decade [3]. The fragmentation of the dermal matrix fibers as a result of the action of the metalloproteinase matrix, and the consequent collapse of fibroblasts, is the process that triggers a "self-perpetuating, never-ending deleterious cycle" [4], which can be clinically perceived as progressive skin aging, in which flaccidity is one of the most important alterations.

Cutaneous flaccidity or loose skin are the names given to the appearance of skin excesses in relation to the underlying tissues. It may have several clinical manifestations ranging from a slight softening of the skin to the touch, to the apron-like appearance of the affected areas. It occurs in all people during their lifetime, and no differences are identified regarding sex. In addition, with the evolution of bariatric surgery techniques and as this procedure has been more frequently performed, severe flaccidity is, nowadays, a condition which is relatively often seen in doctors' offices, and the most common unaesthetic condition in patients with great weight loss.

Factors predisposing or worsening cutaneous flaccidity include genetic factors, photoexposure [5], frequent weight variances during lifetime, rapid and excessive loss of weight in obese patients, excessive liposuction, presence of multiple atrophic striae, and use of some medications (e.g. penicillamine [6]). Some genetic diseases in collagen and/or elastin, such as cutis laxa [7] may result in early appearence of loose skin, and must be considered in investigation of flaccidity in young people.

A few specific body areas are more predisposed to develop flaccidity. It has already been known for a long time that the thickness and degree of skin elasticity vary according to the body area. Recently published studies show that flexure areas, such as the inner part of the forearm and legs, have thinner skin and a higher elasticity index [8], which could explain the greater tendency to flaccidity in these areas.

Diagnosis and Differential Diagnosis

The diagnosis is clinically performed. The patient should be examined in the orthostatic position. Characteristically, flaccidity is diagnosed by the appearance of excess of skin, which ranges from light changes in the relief, of "draping" kind, especially on the extension aspects of the proximal portion of the limbs, to the exuberant apron look.

In differential diagnosis, the collagen and elastic fiber diseases, such as the various types of cutis laxa and elastic pseudoxanthoma, may be considered. Among these unaesthetic changes, the presence of old striae may be observed. When they occur in great number, the affected area may look flaccid. This results from breaking and destructuring the elastic and collagen fibers during the stria formation process, and from the resulting dermal atrophy. In this case, treating the stria improves the aspect of the flaccid skin.

Flaccidity may worsen cellulite, due to the effects of gravity and weight of subcutaneous fat over the connective septa. Often the patient's complaint is cellulite, and actually the diagnostic is skin flaccidity (Fig. 7.1). A commonly used maneuver to confirm the diagnosis of flaccidity is to traction the skin of the affected area against gravity or cephalically. In order to do it, the patient must still be in the orthostatic position. Cases in which the changes in relief are the result of flaccidity, present improvements of these changes with traction.

Treatment

The treatment of skin flaccidity may be a great challenge for a physician who treats aesthetic conditions. So far there has not been a simple, adequately effective treatment. The best results are obtained in the mild and initial flaccidity conditions, with procedures performed periodically over long periods of time.

The most widespread treatment options are surgical procedures to remove excess skin—face lift or body dermolipectomy—and skin tightening procedures. The latter procedures are more useful nowadays, as they are non-invasive techniques that stimulate collagen and elastic neoformation by epidermal ablation or, more recently, by direct dermal stimulation.

Dermolipectomy is the most widely used procedure to correct intense body flaccidity. In this case, especially in patients who were submitted to bariatric surgery and have lost much of their body weight, dermolipectomy is the most suitable procedure [9]. However, even nowadays, there is a high risk of complications, the most frequent being long healing time due to suture dehiscence or seroma [10]. Especially in surgeries performed in several areas of the body at the same time (total body lift) [9,11], the rate of complications is up to 50% [12]. Other factors limiting this procedure are general, prolonged anesthesia, the risk of bleeding

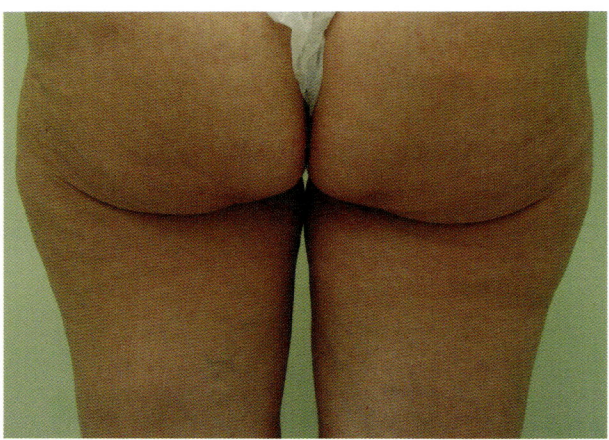

Figure 7.1 Woman with skin flaccidity, who was looking for treatment for cellulite. Observe the relief alterations, which can cause confusion in the diagnosis.

and postoperative infection, besides the long downtime and the unaesthetic large scars which are always formed. The latter, when on the lower abdomen or on the breasts, can be hidden by clothes, which unfortunately does not happen in the scars on the upper and lower limbs.

The skin-tightening procedures arose precisely with the intention of completely or partly replacing the need for conventional surgery. All the existing techniques and devices were developed aiming to promote collagen and elastic neoformation in the dermis. This effect can be achieved in two ways: by epidermal ablation with consequent scar formation and dermal contraction, the case of laser and pulsed intense light equipment; or by direct dermal stimulation with protection of the epidermis, which is achieved using devices with infrared radiation (IR) and/or radiofrequency (RF).

In the first case, limitations are pain during the procedure, the need for some type of anesthesia, downtime, and the risk of infection, dischromias or unaesthetic scars, besides the cost of the equipment and/or consumables. As a result, this is a procedure that can only be performed on small areas with good healing, such as the face.

Because devices that use RF or IR do not cause any damage to the epidermis, they can be more easily used on large areas such as the abdomen, thighs, arms and flanks, as often as necessary to achieve an optimal result. However, precisely as the epidermis acts as a barrier that does not allow the RF and IR waves to reach the dermis, it strongly diminishes the efficacy of the device, making it necessary to perform several sessions at fortnightly or monthly intervals. When devices are used with consumables, the need for repetitions adds a high financial cost to treatment. In order to increase the potency of these devices and consequently diminish the number of sessions required, equipment was developed that associates modalities such as RF and IR [13]. More recently, some authors demonstrated intense neocollagenesis and neoelastogenesis after using a new device that releases radiofrequency waves directly on the dermis through microelectrodes inserted into the skin [14]. Possibly, in future, this will be a good modality of non-surgical correction of body flaccidity over large areas.

Since poly-L-lactic acid stimulates neocollagenesis, it can also be considered for the treatment of flaccidity in localized, small

areas, such as the neck and chest [15], as well as for some selected lesions of cellulite.

Other procedures that cause some kind of dermal trauma were also proposed to correct flaccidity and other alterations associated with skin aging, such as micropunctures obtained by passing a roller with microneedles on the skin [16], carboxytherapy [17] and mesotherapy [18].

Although systemic medications have been proposed by some authors, their use is still controversial, both in cutaneous flaccidity prevention and the treatment.

LOCALIZED FAT
General Aspects
In women some places present a greater predisposition to fat deposition, like the buttocks, hips and thighs, a condition that is responsible for the female body contour, differentiating it from the male android shape. This characteristic deposition is regulated by the female sexual hormones [19] and suffers genetic influence. Some women, especially those with a greater BMI (Body Mass Index), may deposit excess fat in one or more of these areas, a condition known as localized fat. Men, because of the cortisol's effect (stress-associated hormone), tend to have more fat deposition in the abdomen and flanks.

Localized fat is responsible for a large part of the demand for aesthetic procedures for dermatologists and plastic surgeons. These fat deposits have little tendency toward mobilization, compared with the rest of the body fat, and as a consequence, patients can frequently become thinner, lose subcutaneous thickness all over the body, including the face, and the localized fat is practically unaffected.

Diagnosis and Differential Diagnosis
The patient must be weighed initially, to calculate the Body Mass Index (BMI). If the BMI is below 25, the excess fat deposits at specific sites may be diagnosed as localized fat. The circumference of the sites affected should be measured with a tape measure and with an adipometer for purposes of therapeutic control.

Localized fat is one of the conditions that worsen the aspect of the cellulite, due to the bulging effect of the fat lobes that are tractioned by the connective septa, resulting in the mattress aspect of the skin (Fig. 7.2).

Treatment
Liposuction is the first line treatment for localized fat and it will be described in another chapter. Even using the tumescent technique, a few adverse effects and/or complications are inevitable, and inherent to the very nature of the procedure: hematomas and ecchymosis, long recovery periods with increased postoperative discomfort, changes in relief and skin laxity [20].

In 1996, the first article was published in which a laser source was used as an adjuvant to perform liposuction [21]. In 2006, a 1064 nm Nd:YAG laser was approved by the United States Food and Drug Administration for the surgical incision, excision, vaporization, ablation, and coagulation of all soft tissues [20]. This device, as well as the 980 nm diode laser [22] has been used for a new modality of liposuction: the so-called laser-assisted lipolysis [23,24].

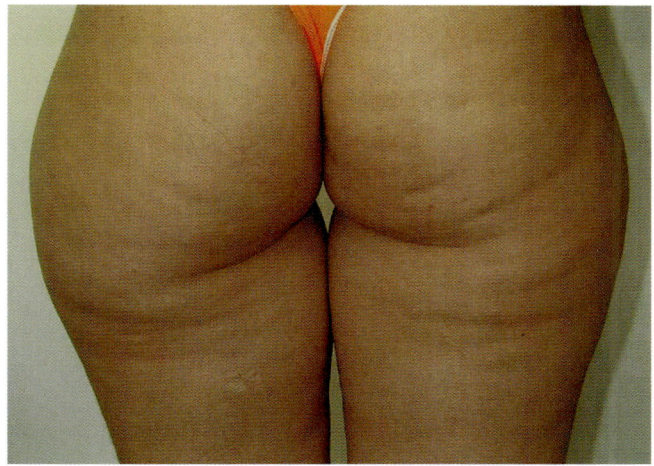

Figure 7.2 Woman presenting localized fat in the lateral aspects of the thighs, with secondary relief alterations, minimizing cellulite.

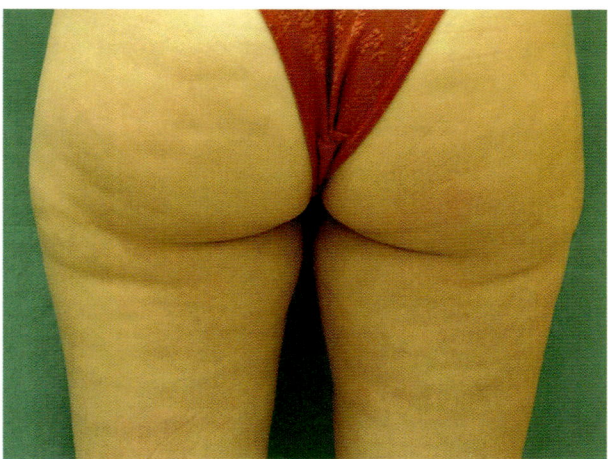

Figure 7.4 Same patient as Fig. 3, after four sessions of sodium desoxycholate' injections in the localized fat areas.

Other devices use ultrasound as an adjuvant to conventional liposuction technique, with a view to making the surgeon's work easier, and also to prevent adverse effects, by diminishing tissue trauma [25].

Phosphatidylcholine (PPDC) [26], a phospholipid extracted from soy lecithin, and sodium deoxycholate (SDC) [27] are used in several countries as lipolytic agents [28]. Although there is a clear clinical effect [29] (Figs. 7.3 and 7.4), the real lipolytic action mechanism of PPDC and SDC has not been completely elucidated yet. Histological studies performed on rats [30] and on biopsy materials show a moderate inflammatory reaction in the subcutaneous tissue, with consequent fibrosis [31] after injecting PPDC.

Finally, in recent years, devices were introduced for non-invasive lipolysis, which utilize focused ultrasound [32,33] with encouraging results and a good safety profile. Radio-frequency, besides the already known effect on flaccidity, also acts on lipolysis [34]. The latter is a good treatment option for patients with flaccidity, associated with small deposits of localized fat.

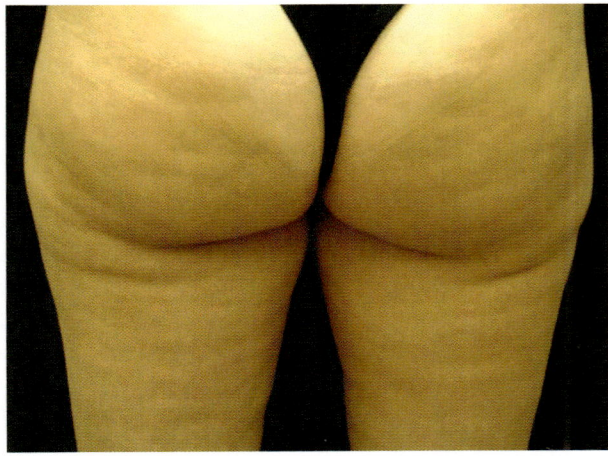

Figure 7.3 Patient with localized fat worsening the aspect of cellulite, before treatment.

STRETCH MARKS
General Aspects
Stretch marks are also known as striae distensae and striae atrophicans. They are visible as linear scars that are formed in areas of dermal damage produced by stretching of the skin [35]. They are associated with various physiologic states including puberty, pregnancy, growth spurts, rapid weight gain or loss, obesity, and states leading to excess of cortisol [36,37].

The factors that rule the development of striae are poorly understood. Many authors have suggested that striae develop as a result of stress rupture of the connective tissue framework, but others disagree. It has been suggested that they develop more easily in skin that has a critical proportion of rigid cross-linked collagen, as they occur in early adult life [35]. Many factors including hormones (particularly corticosteroids), mechanical stress, and genetic predisposition also seem to play a role [36].

In adolescence, some factors are directly related to the increase in local volume in risk areas, causing distention of the skin, with the consequent appearance of stretch marks. Factors of particular note in this age range are: the greater accumulation of fat in certain areas of the body, making the body lines more curved, mainly in women; weight gain and the increase in the 17-cetosteroids [38].

In pregnant women a combination of hormonal factors (e.g., adrenocortical hormones, estrogen, relaxin) associated with increased lateral stress on the connective tissue due to increased size of the various portions of the body is thought to be important [39]. An observational analysis of 324 primiparae observed striae in 52% at delivery and concluded that the most significant risk factor was low maternal age [40]. Another study evaluated the risk factors for the development of striae in 112 primiparae women, showing that women who developed striae were significantly younger and had gained significantly more weight during pregnancy. Moderate and severe striae were associated with lower maternal age, higher birth weight, more advanced gestational age at delivery and family history of striae [41].

They are a feature of Cushing's disease, and they may be induced by local or systemic steroid therapy [35]. Topical corticosteroids, especially when used in larger areas and under occlusion, favor the appearance of stretch marks in the area or even at some distance [42]. Striae have been reported in human immunodeficiency virus (HIV)-positive patients receiving the protease inhibitor indinavir [35].

Diagnosis and Differential Diagnosis

Stretch marks occur in areas of reduced skin resistance and greatest accumulation of adipose tissue. They are linear atrophic depressions of the skin that are formed in areas of dermal damage. Striae are usually multiple, well-defined linear atrophic lesions that follow the lines of clivage. Initially, striae appear as red-to-violaceous elevated lines that can be mildly pruritic and are called striae rubra (Fig. 7.5). Over time, the color gradually fades, and the lesions become atrophic, with the skin surface exhibiting a fine wrinkled appearance, the striae alba (Fig. 7.6) [36]. These characteristics of atrophy are permanent in stretch marks [43].

They are common during adolescence and they seem to be associated with rapid increase in size of a particular region [35]. Women are most commonly affected, with marks occurring predominantly on breasts and other areas also affected by cellulite, like hips and abdomen, while in males, they more frequently occur on the back, lower back and outer edge of the thighs [43,44]. They may develop on the shoulders in young male weight lifters when their muscle mass rapidly increases [35].

Striae occur in up to 90 percent of pregnant women. They are very common over the abdomen and breasts in pregnancy, but they can occur on hips, buttocks, thighs and flanks. The striae associated with systemic corticosteroid therapy and Cushing's syndrome can be larger and more widely distributed [36].

From a clinical and histological point of view, there are no significant differences between stretch marks of different etiology or localization, or between stretch marks of patients of different sexes or age groups. Basically they differ with time of evolution and are classified as recent or old. They are similar to early scars. Therefore, for clinical, histological and therapeutic purposes, a very simple classification was suggested [43]:

Recent stretch marks: narrow (up to 5 mm) and wide (>5 mm), onset up to six to 12 months, usually pink, eritematous, sometimes hyperpigmented.

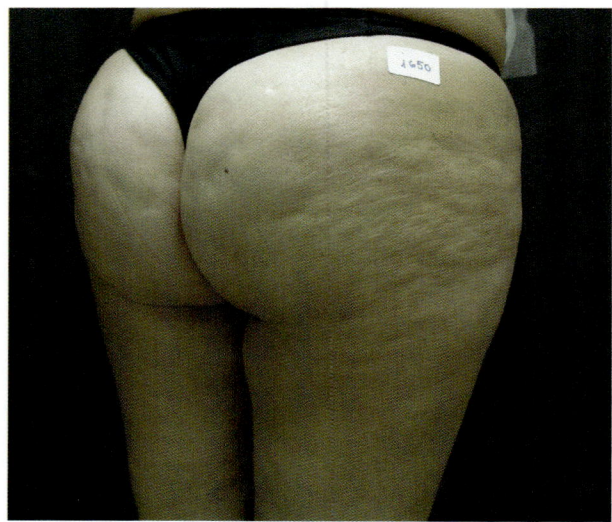

Figure 7.6 Clinical aspect of multiple striae alba associated with cellulite on the buttocks in a female patient age 47.

Old stretch marks: narrow (up to 5 mm) and wide (>5 mm), onset more than six to 12 months, usually hypocromic or same color as non-affected skin.

Histopathological findings suggest that stretch marks are like scars. The epidermis may be normal in recent, and atrophic in old stretch marks. In the dermis the inflammatory process causes destruction of the collagen and elastic fibers characterized by the fragmentation of these fibers, with perivascular lymphohistiocyte infiltration and telangiectatic vessels [43].

Striae must be differenced from linear focal elastosis that is characterized by rows of yellow palpable striae-like bands on the lower back. Unlike striae, these lesions are raised and yellow rather than depressed and white. Elderly men are most commonly affected, although cases in teenagers have been described. Histologically, there is a focal increase in the number of elongated or fragmented elastic fibers and a thickened dermis [36].

Treatment

Different treatments may be indicated for recent (rubra) or old (alba) stretch marks. As stretch marks tend to regress spontaneously over time, the usefulness of treatments that have been tried without case controls was not well established [36]. Early therapeutic interventions may guarantee better results by preventing or at least minimizing the structural alterations in the epidermis [43].

The treatment of recent striae with 0.1% tretinoin cream can improve their appearance, and it has been shown to decrease their length and width [45,46]. However, a study shows that a lower tretinoin concentration (0.025%) seems not to improve early stretch marks [38]. Other topical treatments including 0.05% tretinoin/20% glycolic acid and 10% ascorbic acid/20% glycolic acid may also improve the appearance of stretch marks [47].

In pregnant women, preventive application of a water/oil massage cream seems to be effective [48]. A study evaluating treatment with a cream containing Centella asiatica extract, alpha

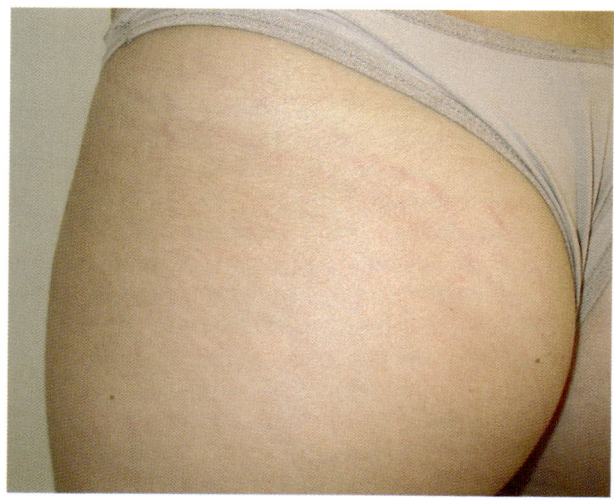

Figure 7.5 Clinical aspect of striae rubra on the buttocks in a female patient age 13 without cellulite.

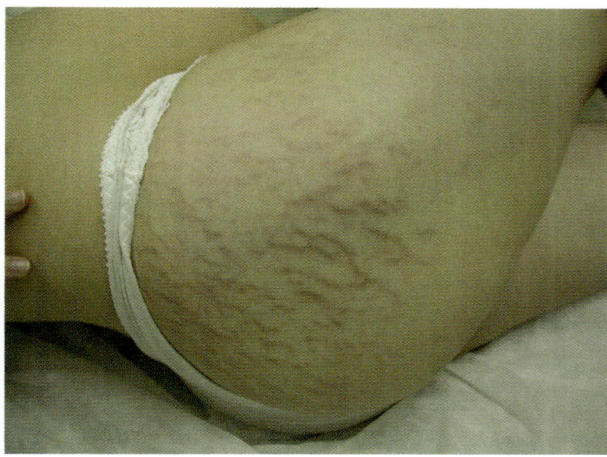 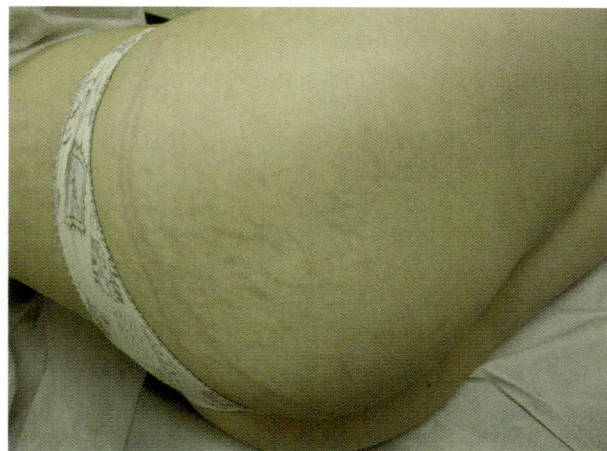

Figures 7.7 and 8 Recent stretch marks aspect before and after serial superficial dermabrasion in a pregnant woman.

tocopherol and collagen-elastin hydrolysates, showed less development of stretch marks in pregnancy [49].

Treatment with the 585 nm pulsed dye laser at low energy densities seems to improve the appearance of old striae. The use of the 10 mm spot size with 3.0 J/cm^2 fluence improved the appearance of striae better than the other parameters. Apparent increased dermal elastin was also observed eight weeks post therapy [50]. Nonetheless, another study showed only moderate beneficial effect in reducing the degree of erythema in striae rubra and no apparent clinical change on striae alba, recommending this laser only for striae rubra in patients skin types II to IV [51].

A study that evaluated the effects of 585 nm pulse dye laser and the short pulsed CO_2 laser in old striae in patients with types IV, V, and VI skin, showed no improvement, hyperpigmentation and persistent erythema. This study concluded that, in patients with higher skin phototypes, laser treatment of striae should be avoided or used with great caution [52].

Only one study evaluated the effect of intense pulsed light in the treatment of striae. Fifteen women with old striae were treated showing clinical and microscopical improvement in all patients [53].

Treatment with the 308 nm excimer laser seems to be safe and effective in pigment correction of hypopigmented scars and striae alba. Final averages of pigment correction rates relative to control sites were approximately 60% to 70% by visual assessment and 100% by colorimetric analysis after nine treatments administered biweekly. Maintenance treatment every one to four months seems to be required to sustain the cosmetic benefit [54]. Light sources emitting ultraviolet B (UVB) and narrow band UVB/UVA1 therapy irradiation also have been shown to repigment old striae [55,56]. The repigmentation after UVB occurs due to increase in melanin pigment, hypertrophy of melanocytes, and an increase in melanocytes [55].

In a study, a radiofrequency (RF) device in combination with a pulsed dye laser was used to treat abdominal striae in 37 patients. Almost 90% percent of the patients showed overall improvement. All the biopsies of nine patients showed an increase in the amount of collagen fibers, and increased elastic fibers were found in six specimens [57]. Bipolar RF device seems also to be effective, with

clinical, histological, and immunohistochemical improvement of treated striae [58].

The 1,064 nm long-pulsed Nd:YAG laser was evaluated in a study with recent stretch marks. The improvements were considered excellent by 55% of the patients, showing that this laser should be effective on recent stretch marks [59].

The non-ablative 1,450 nm diode laser has been shown to improve atrophic scars, but in a study was ineffective in improving the clinical aspect of recent or old stretch marks in Asian patients with skin types IV to VI. A high percentage of patients (64%) had postinflammatory hyperpigmentation [60].

Recent preliminary studies have showed that fractional photothermolysis with 1550 nm erbium-doped fiber laser seems to be safe and effective in the treatment of recent and old stretch marks [61,62,63].

Subcision® may be useful when the striae surface is very depressed, because it favors the formation of neocollagen, when performed in the dermis. However, this procedure is not very effective as an isolated method, because it does not structurally alter the epidermis [43]. In a preliminary study, there was necrosis in a high percentage of striae treated with Subcision, with subjective results [64].

Microdermabrasion was also decribed to treat recent and old stretch marks, but no study was conducted [65]. A report of a series of cases treated by a combination treatment (sand abrasion and a patent mixture containing 15% trichloracetic acid) followed by 6–24 h of a patent cream under plastic occlusion in the striae of 69 patients showed clinical improvement by 70% [66]. Superficial dermabrasion gives good results on recent narrow stretch marks. In a study, 28 patients, with mean ages of 16 years and multiple recent stretch marks on the abdomen, hips, thighs or breasts, underwent a weekly serial superficial dermabrasion treatment with a dermabrasion device (10,000 rpm) with 3 mm round diamond fraises. On the dermatologic evaluation, all patients had some clinical improvement of the recent stretch marks, but those that had only or in the majority narrow stretch marks improved more (82,1% had moderate to accentuate improvement) (Figs. 7.7 and 7.8) [67]. As it is only a mechanical treatment, it may also be useful in pregnant women.

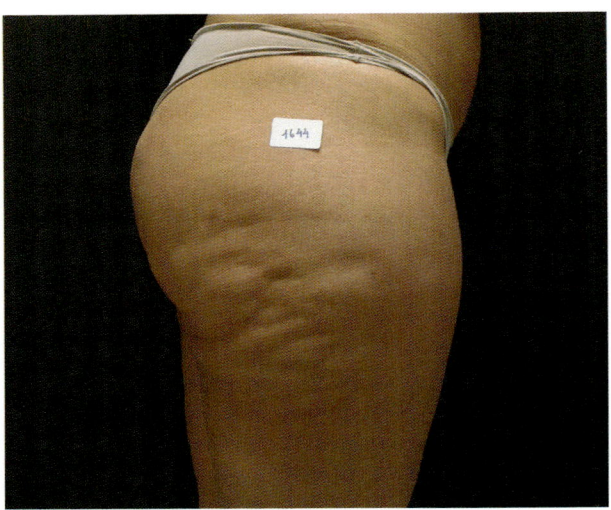

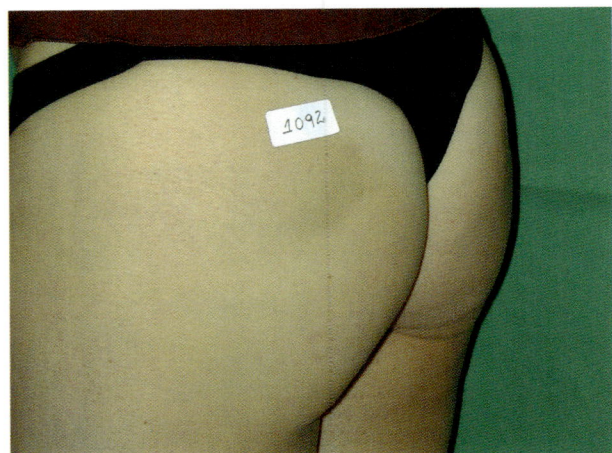

Figure 7.9 Depressed lesions of liposuction sequelae causing cutaneous surface alterations that are clinically similar to depressed lesions of cellulite in a female patient age 45.

Figure 7.10 Lipoatrophy secondary to previous injections causing a depressed lesion clinically similar to depressed lesions of liposuction sequelae in a female patient age 26.

COSMETIC LIPOSUCTION SEQUELAE
General Aspects

The most common and least serious cosmetic liposuction sequelae consist of harmonious undercorrection, asymmetry, residual bulge, large- or small-step contour deformity, and pigmentation. The more serious cosmetic sequelae are the following:

- dimple or dimples in a crenellated, checkerboard, or waffle pattern;
- groove or multiples grooves, either parallel to one another or in a fanlike arrangement;
- simple or high-volume overcorrection, which may produce a cavity or poor cosmetic results;
- wrinkles, which may be layered, parchment-like, padded, or serrated;
- a variable combination of the above-listed sequelae that produces a moonscape appearance;
- excess skin, of variable size;
- tissue collapse;
- postoperative "banana roll";
- double fold;
- ptosis, which is common after excessive removal of fat from the buttocks [68].

Superficial liposuction, in which the cannula comes into contact with the dermis, creates a surface dent or divot. Upon physical examination, the dent persists in the supine position. Similarly, subdermal liposuction that uses small cannulas causes wrinkling by destroying or damaging the subcutaneous septa, which may be responsible for skin contraction. Deep liposuction damages the muscle and fascia, and causes retractile fibrosis with adhesion of the skin to the underlying tissue [68].

The subcutaneous fibrosis caused by a previous surgery of the subcutaneous, mainly liposuction, is also one of the more common causes of cutaneous surface alterations that are clinically similar to depressed lesions of cellulite. Depressed lesions of liposuction sequelae cause secondary cellulite or aggravate cellulite [69].

Diagnosis and Differential Diagnosis

Alterations to the cutaneous surface resulting from liposuction usually appear late, from three months to one year after surgery. They may be slight, moderate or severe, and always emerge in previously treated areas, such as the lateral and posterior thighs, buttocks, abdomen, flanks, and the region above the knees [69].

Like cellulite, the cutaneous sequelae from liposuction are predominantly depressed lesions, but raised and depressed areas may intercalate and vary in number and shape as a reflection of the number and variety of liposculture cannula insertions, as well as the size and type of cannulas. Generally, they form larger depressions with bizarre shapes and, unlike cellulite, they do not necessarily follow the direction of the relaxed skin tension lines. Instead, they follow the direction of cannula insertion (Fig. 7.9) [69]. As occurs in cellulite, muscle contractions worsen the deformities. In patients who have redundant skin before liposuction, the procedure worsens the skin flaccidity [68].

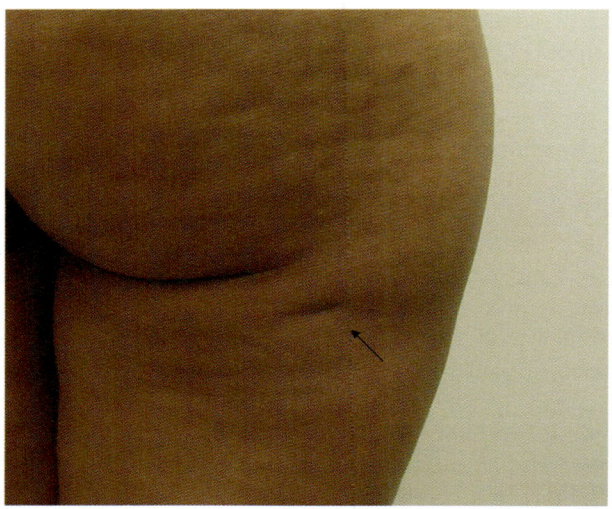

Figure 7.11 Liposuction scar causing a depressed lesion clinically similar to depressed lesions of cellulite in a female patient age 31.

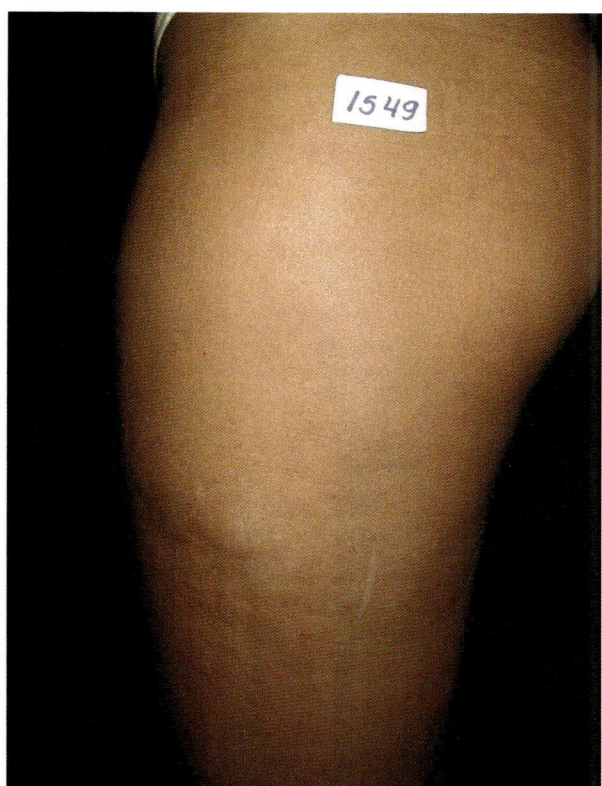

Figure 7.12 Localized scleroderma causing depressed lesions clinically similar to depressed lesions of liposuction sequelae in a female patient age 24.

exhibited hemosiderosis, most of them lasting up to three months. Four percent had hemosiderosis for six months and two percent for two years. Thirteen percent had painful palpable nodules until three months after the procedure, in some treated areas. Four percent had bulging in some treated areas after 30 days. No patient had infection or cutaneous necrosis. The patient self-assessment showed improvement of the depressed lesions in all patients (mild in 10.8%; moderate in 39.1%; and accentuate in 50%) [75]. Special pre- and post-surgical care is important in obtaining successful results.

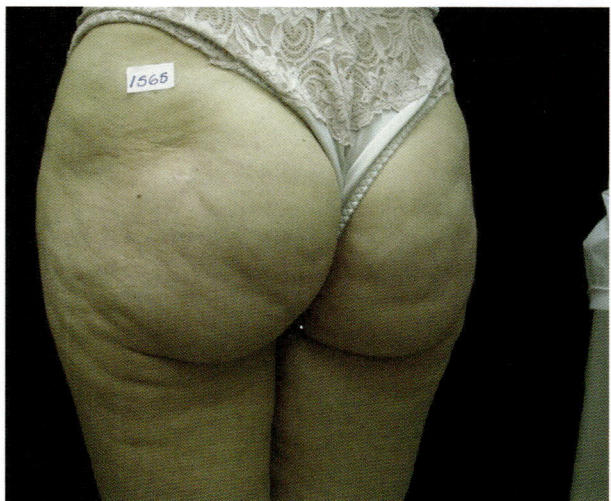

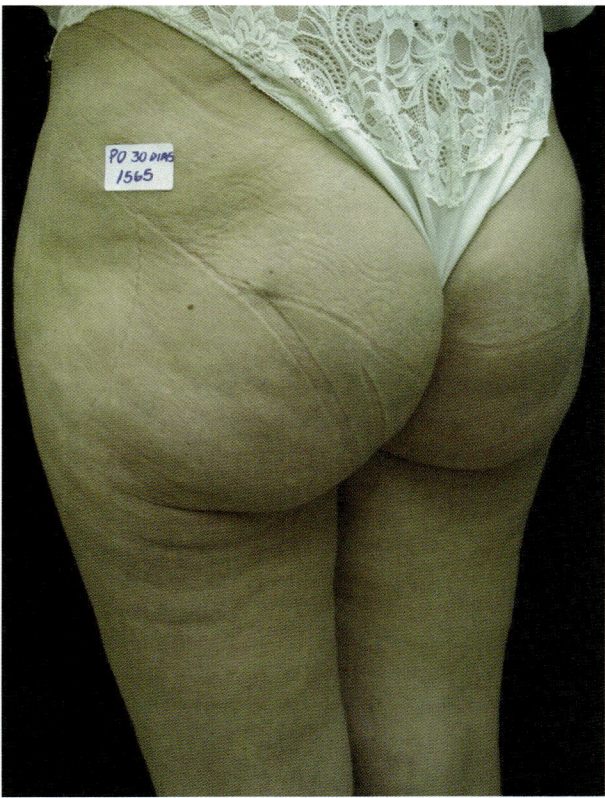

Figures 7.13 and 14 A 47-year-old female patient with cutaneous depressed lesions on thighs and buttocks secondary to liposuction, pre and 30 days post 1 session of Subcision®.

The liposuction sequelae should be differentiated from subcutaneous fibrosis originating from trauma or from previous injections in the affected area (such as corticosteroid or insulin-induced lipoatrophy) (Fig. 7.10) [70,71], atrophic scars (Fig. 7.11), worsened flaccidity caused by the aging process, lipodystrophies, cutaneous localized scleroderma (Arkachaisri) (Fig. 7.12) and lipomatosis [72].

Treatment

The risk of liposuction cosmetic sequelae must be minimized through careful patient selection, in which presence of cellulite, false bulges and flaccidity should be considered. The use of appropriate technique and cannulas, and rigorous postoperative care are also very important.

Touch-up liposuction allows correction of sequelae that are characterized by excess residual fat, such as bulges, undercorrection, step deformity or asymmetry. A six-month wait allows complete ceasing of the edema, as well as recovery of tissue flexibility at the treated site [68].

Similarly to cellulite, Subcision® may be used to treat depressed lesions that occur after liposuction [73,74]. Hexsel and Dal'Forno treated 46 female patients with depressed lesions secondary to liposuction with Subcision® technique. Liposuctions had been performed by plastic surgeons from eight months to 14 years previously. The patients were submitted to one to three sessions of Subcision® only on the cellulite-like depressions. On the dermatologic evaluation all patients had some improvement of the treated depressed lesions (Figs. 7.13, 7.14, 7.15 and 7.16). All patients

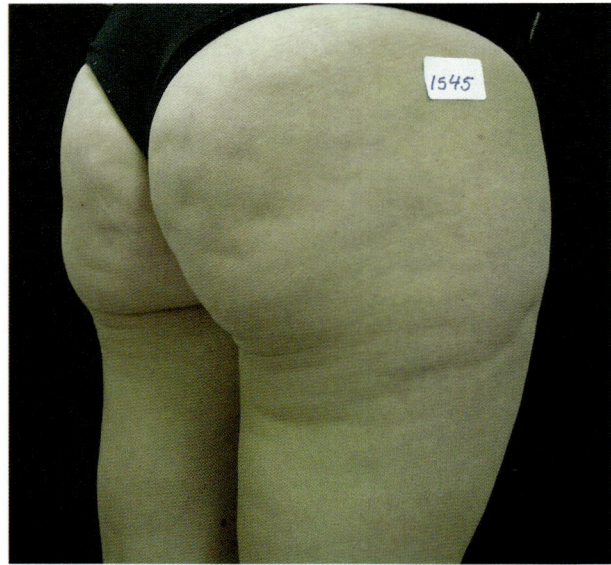

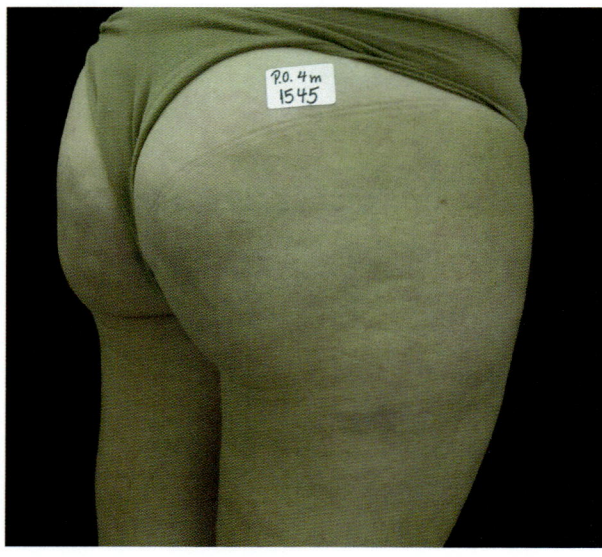

Figures 7.15 and 16 A 26-year-old female patient with cutaneous depressed lesions on thighs and buttocks secondary to liposuction, pre and 4 months post 1 session of Subcision®.

Conclusion

A number of clinical conditions or circumstances frequently accompany or aggravate cellulite, especially skin flaccidity, localized fat, stretch marks and cosmetic liposuction sequelae. These conditions should be evaluated in cellulite patients, because they may require different treatments. Improvement of these associated conditions generally is very important in the treatment of patients with cellulite.

REFERENCES

1. CB Archer. Functions of the skin. In: T Burns, S Breathnach, N Cox, C Griffiths (eds). Rook's Textbook of Dermatology, Blackwell Publishing 7th ed; 2004: 4.1–4.12.
2. J Uitto. Connective tissue biochemistry of the aging dermis. Age related alterations in collagen and elastin. Dermatol Clin 4:433–46, 1986.
3. GJ Fisher, S Kang, J Varani, Z Bata-Csorgo, Y Wan, S Datta, JJ Voorhees. Mechanisms of photoaging and chronological skin aging. Arch Dermatol 138(11):1462–70, 2002.
4. GJ Fisher, J Varani, JJ Voorhees. Looking older: fibroblast collapse and therapeutic implications. Arch Dermatol 144(5): 666–72, 2008.
5. N Sadick. Tissue tightening technologies: fact or fiction. Aesthet Surg J 28(2):180–8, 2008.
6. E Poon, GH Mason, C Oh. Clinical and histological spectrum of elastotic changes induced by penicillamine. Austr J of Dermatol 43:147–51, 2002.
7. L Rodriguez-Revenga, P Iranzo, C Badenas et al. A Novel Elastin Gene Mutation Resulting in an Autosomal Dominant Form of Cutis Laxa. Arch Dermatol 140:1135–9, 2004.
8. S Diridollou, D Black, JM Lagarde et al. Sex- and site-dependent variations in the thickness and mechanical properties of human skin in vivo. Int J Cosmet Sci 22(6):421–35, 2000.
9. JF Capella. Body lift. Clin Plast Surg 35:27–51, 2008.
10. SO Sozer, FJ Agullo, AA Santillan, C Wolf. Decision Making in Abdominoplasty. Aesth Plast Surg 31:117–27, 2007.
11. DJ Hurwitz, S Agha-Mohammadi, K Ota, J Unadkat. A clinical review of total body lift surgery. Aesthet Surg J 28:294–303, 2008.
12. RB Nemerofsky, DA Oliak, JF Capella. Body lift: an account of 200 consecutive cases in the massive weight loss patient. Plast Reconstr Surg 117:414–30, 2006.
13. C Romero, N Caballero, M Herrero et al. Effects of cellulite treatment with IR light, mechanical massage and suction treating one buttock with the contralateral as a control. J Cosmet Laser Ther 10:193–201, 2008.
14. BM Hantash, AA Ubeid, H Chang et al. Bipolar fractional radiofrequency treatment induces neoelastogenesis and neo-collagenesis. Lasers Surg Med 41:1–9, 2009.
15. R Mazzuco, DM Hexsel. Poli-L-lactic acid for neck and chest rejuvenation. Dermatol Surg 2009 (in press).
16. MC Aust, D Fernandes, P Kolokythas et al. Percutaneous collagen induction therapy: an alternative treatment for scars, wrinkles, and skin laxity. Plast Reconstr Surg 121:1421–9, 2008.
17. JC Ferreira, A Haddad, SA Tavares. Increase in collagen turnover induced by intradermal injection of carbon dioxide in rats. J Drugs Dermatol 7:201–6, 2008.
18. BS Atiyeh, AE Ibrahim, SA Dibo. Cosmetic mesotherapy: between scientific evidence, science fiction, and lucrative business. Aesthetic Plast Surg 32:842–9, 2008.
19. P Björntorp. Adipose tissue distribution and function. Int J Obes 15:67–81, 1991.
20. B Katz, J McBean, JS Cheung. The new laser liposuction for men. Dermatol Ther 20:448–51, 2007.
21. DB Apfelberg. Results of multicenter study of laser-assisted liposuction. Clin Plast Surg 23:713–9, 1996.
22. JP Reynaud, M Skibinski, B Wassmer et al. Lipolysis using a 980-nm diode laser: a retrospective analysis of 534 procedures. Aesthetic Plast Surg 33:28–36, 2009.
23. KH Kim, RG Geronemus. Laser Lipolysis Using a Novel 1,064 nm Nd:YAG Laser. Dermatol Surg 32:241–48, 2006.

24. A Goldman, DE Schavelzon, GS Blugerman. Laserlipolysis: liposuction using Nd:YAG laser. Rev Soc Bras Cir Plast 17:17–26, 2002.

25. MW Mann, MD Palm, RD Sengelmann. New advances in liposuction technology. Semin Cutan Med Surg 27:72–82, 2008.

26. D Hexsel, M Serra, R Mazzuco et al. Phosphatidylcholine in the treatment of localized fat. J Drugs Dermatol 2:511–8, 2003.

27. AM Rotunda, H Suzuki, RL Moy et al. Detergent effects of sodium deoxycholate are a major feature of an injectable phosphatidylcholine formulation used for localized fat dissolution. Dermatol Surg 30:1001–8, 2004.

28. M Palmer, J Curran, P Bowler. Clinical experience and safety using phosphatidylcholine injections for the localized reduction of subcutaneous fat: a multicentre, retrospective UK study. J Cosmet Dermatol 5:218–26, 2006.

29. G Salti, I Ghersetich, F Tantussi et al. Phosphatidylcholine and sodium deoxycholate in the treatment of localized fat: a double-blind, randomized study. Dermatol Surg 34:60–6, 2008.

30. PG Rittes, JC Rittes, MF Carriel Amary. Injection of phosphatidylcholine in fat tissue: experimental study of local action in rabbits. Aesthetic Plast Surg 30:474–8, 2006.

31. A Salles, C Valler, MC Ferreira. Histologic Response to Injected Phosphatidylcholine in Fat Tissue: Experimental Study in a New Rabbit Model. Aesth Plastic Surg 30:479–84, 2006.

32. J Moreno-Moraga, T Valero-Altés, AM Riquelme et al. Body contouring by non-invasive transdermal focused ultrasound. Lasers Surg Med 39:315–23, 2007.

33. KW Foster, DJ Kouba, J Hayes et al. Reduction in thigh and infraumbilical circumference following treatment with a novel device combining ultrasound, suction, and massage. J Drugs Dermatol 7:113–5, 2008.

34. MA Trelles, SR Mordon. Adipocyte membrane lysis observed after cellulite treatment is performed with radiofrequency. Aesth Plast Surg 33:125–8, 2009.

35. NP Burrows, CR Lovell. Disorders of connective tissue. In: RH Champion, JL Burton, FJG Ebling, (eds). Rook's Textbook of Dermatology. 7th edition. Oxford: Blackwell; 2004: 46.1–71.

36. C Maari, J Powell. Atrophies of connective tissue. In: JL Bologna, JL Jorizzo, RP Rapini (eds). Dermatology. London: Mosby; 2003: 1539–48.

37. G Yosipovitch, A DeVore, A Dawn. Obesity and the skin: skin physiology and skin manifestations of obesity. J Am Acad Dermatol 56(6):901–16; quiz 917–20, Jun 2007.

38. S Pribanich, FG Simpson, B Held et al. Low-dose tretinoin does not improve striae distensae: a double-blind, placebo-controlled study. Cutis 54:121–124, 1994.

39. TJ Lawley, KB Yancey. Skin changes and diseases in pregnancy. In: IM Freedberg, AZ Eisen, K Wolff et al (eds). Fitzpatrick's Dermatology in General Medicine. 6th edition. New York: Mc Graw Hill; 2003: 1361–6.

40. GS Atwal, LK Manku, CE Griffiths, DW Polson. Striae gravidarum in primiparae. Br J Dermatol 155(5):965–9, Nov 2006.

41. H Osman, N Rubeiz, H Tamim, AH Nassar. Risk factors for the development of striae gravidarum. Am J Obstet Gynecol 196(1):62.e1–5, 2007.

42. K Beer, J Downie. Sequelae from inadvertent long-term use of potent topical steroids. J Drugs Dermatol 6(5):550–1, 2007.

43. D Hexsel. Body repair. In: LC Parish, S Brenner, M Ramos-e-Silva. Women's Dermatology. From Infancy to Maturity. Parthenon, London; 2001: 586–95.

44. H Frédérique. FC Piérard et al. Striae distansae of pregnancy: in vivo biomechanical evaluation. Int Journal Dermatol (36): 506–08, 1997.

45. S Kang. Topical tretinoin therapy for management of early striae. J Am Acad Dermatol 39(2 Pt 3):S90–2, Aug 1998.

46. O Rangel, I Arias, E García, S Lopez-Padilla. Topical tretinoin 0.1% for pregnancy-related abdominal striae: an open-label, multicenter, prospective study. Adv Ther 18(4):181–6, 2001.

47. K Ash, J Lord, M Zukowski, DH McDaniel. Comparison of topical therapy for striae alba (20% glycolic acid/0.05% tretinoin versus 20% glycolic acid/10% L-ascorbic acid). Dermatol Surg 24(8):849–56, 1998.

48. F Wierrani, W Kozak, W Schramm, W Grünberger. Attempt of preventive treatment of striae gravidarum using preventive massage ointment administration. Wien Klin Wochenschr 104(2):42–4, 1992.

49. GL Young, D Jewell. Creams for preventing stretch marks in pregnancy. Cochrane Database Syst Rev (2):CD000066, 2000.

50. DH McDaniel, K Ash, M Zukowski. Treatment of stretch marks with the 585-nm flashlamp-pumped pulsed dye laser. Dermatol Surg 22(4):332–7, 1996.

51. GP Jiménez, F Flores, B Berman, Z Gunja-Smith. Treatment of striae rubra and striae alba with the 585-nm pulsed-dye laser. Dermatol Surg. 29(4):362-5, 2003.

52. K Nouri, R Romagosa, T Chartier et al. Comparison of the 585 nm pulse dye laser and the short pulsed CO2 laser in the treatment of striae distensae in skin types IV and VI. Dermatol Surg 25(5):368–70, 1999.

53. E Hernández-Pérez, E Colombo-Charrier, E Valencia-Ibiett. Intense pulsed light in the treatment of striae distensae. Dermatol Surg 28(12):1124–30, 2002.

54. MR Alexiades-Armenakas, LJ Bernstein, PM Friedman, RG Geronemus. The safety and efficacy of the 308-nm excimer laser for pigment correction of hypopigmented scars and striae alba. Arch Dermatol. 140(8):955–60, 2004.

55. DJ Goldberg, ES Marmur, C Schmults et al. Histologic and ultrastructural analysis of ultraviolet B laser and light source treatment of leukoderma in striae distensae. Dermatol Surg 31(4):385–7, 2005.

56. NS Sadick, C Magro, A Hoenig. Prospective clinical and histological study to evaluate the efficacy and safety of a targeted high-intensity narrow band UVB/UVA1 therapy for striae alba. J Cosmet Laser Ther 9(2):79–83, 2007.

57. DH Suh, KY Chang, HC Son et al. Radiofrequency and 585-nm pulsed dye laser treatment of striae distensae: a report of 37 Asian patients. Dermatol Surg 33(1):29–34, 2007.

58. G Montesi, S Calvieri, A Balzani, MH Gold. Bipolar radiofrequency in the treatment of dermatologic imperfections: clinicopathological and immunohistochemical aspects. J Drugs Dermatol 6(9):890–6, 2007.

59. A Goldman, F Rossato, C Prati. Stretch marks: treatment using the 1,064-nm Nd:YAG laser. Dermatol Surg 34(5): 686–91, 2008.

60. YK Tay, C Kwok, E Tan. Non-ablative 1,450-nm diode laser treatment of striae distensae. Lasers Surg Med 38(3):196–9, 2006.

61. AF Taub. Fractionated delivery systems for difficult to treat clinical applications: acne scarring, melasma, atrophic scarring, striae distensae, and deep rhytides. J Drugs Dermatol 6(11):1120–8, 2007.

62. BJ Kim, DH Lee, MN Kim et al. Fractional photothermolysis for the treatment of striae distensae in Asian skin. Am J Clin Dermatol 9(1):33–7, 2008.

63. M Stotland, AM Chapas, L Brightman et al. The safety and efficacy of fractional photothermolysis for the correction of striae distensae. J Drugs Dermatol 7(9):857–61, 2008.

64. P Luis-Montoya, P Pichardo-Velázquez, MT Hojyo-Tomoka, J Domínguez-Cherit. Evaluation of subcision as a treatment for cutaneous striae. J Drugs Dermatol 4(3):346–50, 2005.

65. JM Spencer. Microdermabrasion. Am J Clin Dermatol, 6(2):89–92, 2005.

66. MA Adatto, P Deprez. Striae treated by a novel combination treatment–sand abrasion and a patent mixture containing 15% trichloracetic acid followed by 6–24 hrs of a patent cream under plastic occlusion J Cosmet Dermatol 2(2): 61–7, 2003.

67. DM Hexsel, T Dal'Forno, R Mazzuco. Superficial dermabrasion in the treatment of recent stretch marks (striae rubra). J Am Acad Dermatol poster P350, 2009.

68. YG Illouz. Complications of liposuction. Clin Plast Surg 33(1):129–63, 2006.

69. D Hexsel, T Dal'Forno, S Cignachi. "Definition, clinical aspects, associated conditions, and differential diagnosis", In: M Goldman, PA Bacci, Leibaschoff, et al. Cellulite – Pathophysiology and Treatment. New York, NY: Taylor & Francis; 2006: 7–28.

70. JA Avilés-Izquierdo, MI Longo-Imedio, JM Hernánz-Hermosa, P Lázaro-Ochaita. Bilateral localized lipoatrophy secondary to a single intramuscular corticosteroid injection. Dermatol Online J 30:12(3):17, 2006.

71. AJ Ramos, MA Farias. Human insulin-induced lipoatrophy: a successful treatment with glucocorticoid. Diabetes Care 29(4):926–7, 2006.

72. V Pandzic Jaksic, M Sucic. Multiple symmetric lipomatosis - a reflection of new concepts about obesity. Med Hypotheses. 71(1):99–101, 2008.

73. DS Orentreich, N Orentreich. Subcutaneous incisionless (subcision) surgery for the correction of depressed scars and wrinkles. Dermatol Surg 21(6):543–9, 1995.

74. DM Hexsel, R Mazzuco. Subcision: a treatment for cellulite. Int J Dermatol 39:539–44, 2000.

75. DM Hexsel, T Dal'Forno. Subcision in the treatment of liposuction sequelae. J Am Acad Dermatol Poster P3526, 2009.

8   Medical Therapy

Fabrizio Angelini, Carmine Orlandi, Pietro Di Fiore, Luca Gatteschi,
Mirko Guerra, Fulvio Marzatico, Massimo Rapetti, and Attilio Speciani

Introduction

The term cellulite is often used improperly to define clinical and morphological ailments. In fact it would be correct when talking about this syndrome to distinguish between localised adiposity (AL) and edemato-fibro-sclerotic pannicolopatia (PEFS). Localised adiposity should be considered a female secondary sexual characteristic, which in general does not require therapeutic treatment except in the case of excessive growth (hypertrophy or hyperplasia). Whereas PEFS is a degenerative process of the subcutaneous fatty tissue as a consequence of a localised microangiopathy of the lower limbs with the formation of edema and subsequent fibro-sclerotic evolution. It often runs in families mainly due to chronic venous-lymphatic insufficiency. It may be worsened or sparked off by many conditions such as being Caucasian, postural alterations resulting from alterations of the rachis and lower limbs, overweight and obesity, incorrect diet, some endocrinopathies (hypothyroidism, hyperthyroidism, micropolycystic ovary syndrome) [1,2] alterations of the alimentary tract, alterations of the intestinal bacterial flora, mood swings with alterations of food intake, reduced physical exercise, taking hormones (estro-progestinic), smoking, constipation and wearing tight clothing. It is in any case a chronic disease that may evolve into a phlebolymphopathy and therefore requires adequate and prompt remedies. Cellulite, despite its frequent misuse as a term, may be classified into various clinical forms: the adipose, edematous, mixed (adipo-edematous), edematous-adipose, fibrous, sclerotic and fibro-sclerotic types [3]. It is also important to distinguish cellulite from various diseases and/or syndromes which have clinical characteristics that are very similar to those of cellulite. Among these are lipo-edema, lymph edema, phlebedema, phlebolymphedema, lipolymphedema, cyclical edema, localised adiposity, various syndromes (Barraquer-Simmons, Vilain, Dercum, Whipple, Weber-Christian), lipomatosis, lipodistrophy, lipolymphedema of the ankle and dermatological diseases such as pigmentation. A special mention should be given to lipoedema as a syndrome with an as yet unknown etiology, characterised by the deposit of fat in the subcutaneous tissue often associated with the appearance of edema in the erect position localised on the legs and buttocks. Lipoedema unlike lipolymphedema, always starts from the legs and does not affect the feet or ankles. It is not affected by weight and may run in families. This is a very common ailment in which the appearance of the edema is the consequence of the deposit of fat in tissues revealing an endocrine-metabolic disorder of the interstitial matrix and is not accompanied by obesity or overweight. In this case the edema is the result of an altered distance ratio between the adipose cell and the connective structure with consequent loss of support. This type of edema tends to worsen with deambulation and in the erect position. Moreover, an important differential feature compared to the lymph edema is that the lipoedema is soft when touched with possible folding of the skin, which does not appear doughy.

Bearing in mind that the disorders illustrated above and cellulite in particular are sometimes characterised by an accumulation of adipose tissue and by inflamed tissue with reduced vascularisation the nutritional therapy of these ailments must aim primarily at the objectives which may be summarised as follows:

1. The preventive aspect to attempt to limit the nutritional factor as one of the causes of the degenerative disease;
2. The correction of overweight as one of the causes or as the trigger;
3. Moreover, given that in these disorders and in cellulite in particular there is an increase of phlogistic factors and hypo-vascularisation of the tissues, the nutritional approach should, as far as possible, try to improve tissue trophism and blood flow.

To reach the three above objectives it is our conviction that a nutritional approach should be used with a low insulinemic stimulus, moving from a quantitative concept (diet = fewer calories) to a qualitative concept (diet = stimulus or decrement of some hormones essential for health).

The idea of pharmacy-nutrition, in other words food seen as a medicine, is thus strengthened as is nutritional endocrinology, that is to say the stimulation using macro nutrients (carbohydrates, fats and proteins) of specific hormonal systems (insulin-glycogeneicosanoids), which may favour or damage the state of health in general and, in the case of cellulite, the worsening of the state of the tissues involved (adipose, connective, interstitial) in the glutei-femoral areas or on the inside of the knee.

Nutritional treatment of cellulite therefore is not just a hypo-caloric approach but is aimed at improving the state of tissue trophism and, in particular at preventing and in some cases reducing the tissue phlogosis characteristic of the disease

To conclude, we can set three targets for the efficacious nutritional therapy of cellulite:

1. Correcting overweight and obesity if present;
2. Increasing the blood flow;
3. Reducing inflammation.

The first objective, in other words the correction of overweight and/or obesity, may be reached by means of a reduction of the calorie intake, especially of that deriving from carbohydrates with a high glycemic index, in other words those carbohydrates which raise blood sugar levels with a consequent increase in levels of insulin.

The other two objectives may be reached by means of a balanced diet of carbohydrates, proteins and fats through a diet that is rich in fruit and vegetables, lean meat, fish and monounsaturated fats such as olive oil. It has become not only important to choose healthy foods now, but also to avoid substances contained in foods, such as hydrogenated fats, inter-esterified oils, monosodium glutamate and aspartame. It is also fundamental to propose nutritional models that are valid for a lifetime and not just for brief periods, so that the yo-yo is avoided, which would cause a worsening of the initial state of the cellulite. In conclusion, the use of integrators, such as omega-3, vitamins and minerals, must be evaluated to reduce the inflammation further.

Subcutaneus Adipose Tissue as Endocrine Organ

The subcutaneous adipose tissue, along with the visceral tissue, is regarded as an endocrine organ, or rather the adipose tissue isn't just a connective tissue specialised in storing triglycerides, but also a tissue that is able to communicate externally.

The adipose tissue can communicate on various levels. It can communicate through hormones such as leptin, adiponectin and resistin or through citokines like IL-6 and TNF-α.

We should also not forget the adipose tissue's ability to free up free fatty acids and its enzymic action as set out by aromatases.

As regards the relationship of the subcutaneous tissue with hormones, it has a negative correlation with SHBG and a positive correlation with the availability of estradiol accommodated for the total amount of testosterone. The subcutaneous tissue, like the visceral, also has an inverse correlation with the total testosterone and DHT [4].

The hormonal component is therefore strongly linked to the pathogenesis of cellulite and the different levels of estradiol and testosterone, which explains why cellulite is mainly a female problem.

The ability of the adipose tissue to generate cytokines is associated to the need to communicate its state and the excessive cellular expansion caused by a poor diet causes stress, which is why the adipose cell sends 'signals' of cellular sufferance.

The signals are given, for example, by IL-6, a cytokine known to many for its stimulation of acute stage inflammatory proteins.

IL-6 pulls macrophages towards the adipose tissue, which in turn pull other macrophages and other inflammatory cytokines [5].

On a systemic level, one-third of the circulating level of IL-6 comes from the production of adipose tissue. These levels are associated with the plasmatic levels of fatty acids and metabolic factors, such as the increase in the oxidation of fatty acids and lipolysis by the adipocytes [6].

In the pancreas IL-6 also acts on the α cells deputised to the production of glucagon, where IL-6R is present. The presupposition for what happens is a state of overnutrition causes resistance to insulin and therefore creates a supplementary job for the pancreatic islets that produce insulin. That is why IL-6 stimulates the α cells thereby causing the cells to expand, balancing the function of the β cells in this way [7].

IL-6 is also a precursor for stress by the muscles. In fact in the muscles doing the physical exercise, IL-6 promotes the use and release of fatty acids. In treating cellulite undoubtedly the first thing to do is to prescribe a diet and physical exercise to ensure that fatty acids are released and consumed by the muscles [8].

Another molecule that is extremely important for the etiopathogenesis of cellulite is TNF-α, a cytokine involved in the inflammation, apoptosis and production of other cytokines, like IL-6 and IL-1, and causes insulin resistance. The adipose cell responds to the production of TNF-α, under the stress of a volumetric

expansion. TNF-α also causes the expression of adhesion molecules in the vascular endothelium and the secretion of chemokines by the macrophages and endothelial cells [9]. The expression of TNF-α by the adipose tissue is directly related with the insulin-dependent processes, including glucidic homeostasis and lipidic metabolism [4]. TNF-α has a multiple effect on the lipidic metabolism on a paracrine level on the adipocytes and on an endocrine level, such as the effects on the liver. In the adipose tissue TNF-α promotes the lipolysis and inhibits the lipogenesis, causing an increase in the level of fatty acids in the blood [10]. TNF-α also causes an increase in the genetic expression in the liver for the production of de novo fatty acids and a reduction in the oxidation of fats. The production of the VLDL by the liver increases as a result of this, leading to hypertriglyceridemia [11]. TNF-α also acts on other molecules, such as insulin, actually on the insulin receptors, making them less visible on the surface of the cell and leading to insulin resistance [12]. TNF-α acts on a local level, altering the secretion of adipokines, considerably reducing their expression [13].

Among the hormones produced by the adipose tissue, adiponectin is actually the most abundant molecule. It has many effects, such as the increase in the sensitivity to insulin and the inhibition of TNF-α. There is also an inverse correlation between adiponectin, the risk of obesity, insulin resistance and cardiovascular illnesses. Adiponectin levels are higher in women, and this constitutes a sexual dimorphism. The circulating adiponectin does not fluctuate much and this suggests that the liberation isn't acute, but is regulated in the long term by metabolic changes. The clinical result is regained with the adiponectin that is inversely correlated to the BMI, and the insulin resistance also inhibits its production [7].

Adiponectin has many vascular effects that cause an improvement in the subcutaneous adipose tissue [7].

For the clinical picture of cellulite, the microvascular component assumes an important factor and the adiponectin is intimately related to the working of the endothelium. It is worth remembering that the adipose tissue isn't richly vascularised as others may be, therefore the endothelial function, albeit reduced yet efficient, must be an objective that can be achieved in treating cellulite.

Techniques for Measurement of Adipose Tissue

We use the term "overweight" to indicate an excess of 20–30% over the ideal weight; beyond 30% we speak of obesity. It is easy to determine the body weight, but often this is not correctly interpreted with the concept of obesity. There are particular physical conditions (bodybuilding) or pathological conditions (ascetes, heart failure) in which the body weight is above normal without configuring a state of obesity. For this reason it is necessary to adopt specific methods to calculate the exact percentage of the fatty mass in order to make a correct diagnosis of overweight or obesity.

Direct measurement techniques are: body impedance analysis (see Fig. 8.1), density measurement, ecography, computerized tomography, magnetic nuclear resonance, measurement of total body water, measurement of total body potassium, neutronic activation, method of absorption with single or double photon, uptake of a liposoluble inert gas. Indirect measurement techniques: index of body mass, plicometry, waist-hip ratio, standard tables,

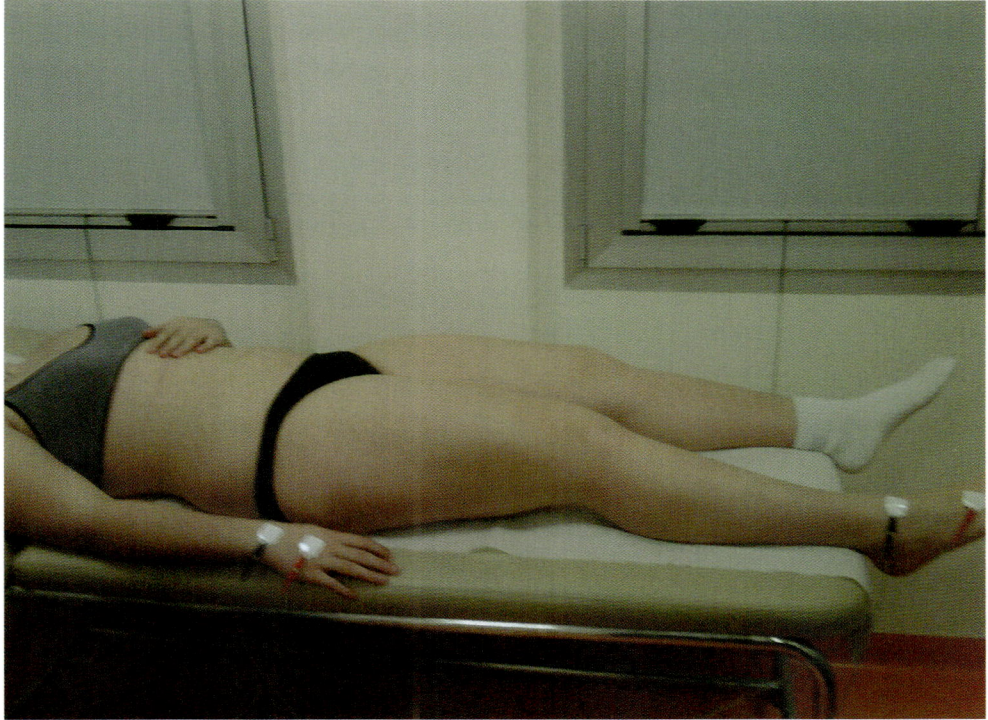

Figure 8.1 Body impedance analysis.

anthropometric methods, creatinine clearance [14,15]. The direct techniques are certainly characterized by greater accuracy of measurement, but are often difficult to perform and in any case they often require highly specialized personnel and can be very expensive. Indirect techniques can often be correlated to the direct methods with the important advantage of being easy to perform at no cost, which makes them usable in common clinical practice.

Indirect Techniques

These measurements are designed to provide values similar to those found in the tables of desirable weight.

Table 8.1 Vascular effect of adiponectin in the subcutaneous adipose tissue

Vascular effect of adiponectin in the subcutaneous adipose tissue
Increased endothelium-dependent vasodilation
Increased endothelium-independent vasodilation
Antiatherosclerotic effect
Suppression of the expression of receptors known as scavengers of vascular adhesion molecules
Reduced expression of TNF-α and reduction of the effects of this adipokine on the endothelial inflammatory response
Amelioration of the effect of growth factors on vascular smooth musculature
Inhibition of the effects of oxidized low density lipoproteins (oxLDL) on the endothelium, with suppression of cell proliferation, of generation of superoxides and of activation of mytogen activated protein kinase (MAP)
Increased production of NO
Stimulation of angiogenesis
Reduction of the thickness of the tunica intima and smooth musculature that is secondary to artery wall injury
Inhibition of migration and proliferation of endothelial cells

Formulas for the ideal weight:

Broca Formula: Ideal weight (kg) = height (cm) − 100 (men) or 104 (women)

Lorenz Formula: Ideal weight (kg) = height (cm) − 100 −[(height-150)/4].

These formulas were used for a long time, without taking account of the fact that weight is a three-dimensional parameter. They were eventually replaced by other measurements such as the Buffon, Roher and Bardeen formula and then by that of Quetelet and Martin. However, since these formulas are based solely on theoretical factors, from the clinical point of view the formula for the index of body mass is the one most widely used:

Body Mass Index (BMI) = weight (kg)/height (mt)

This parameter correlates very well with body fat especially when we consider the age of the patient. It tends to remain constant in patients with a certain degree of thinness or obesity in a rather broad range of height, so that variations of the BMI can provide a valid measurement of body fat regardless of height. Evaluation of the body mass index is now the most widely used method in outpatient practice to measure the degree of obesity.

Plicometry

The percentage of adipose mass can be estimated through the measurement of skin folds using a special instrument called a Harpenden plicometer. For a correct assessment it would be advisable to measure the thickness of the subcutaneous tissue in folds at the bicipital, tricipital, subscapular and suprailiac levels. Though this method is still used, it is fraught with difficulties due to the poor standardization of the test (diversity of pressure and difficulty in locating the exact points to measure in some patients, especially severely obese ones). The difficulty can be increased by different distribution of the adipose tissue from one patient to another (generalized, abdominal). With this method the threshold values obtained, with the sum of the thickness of the subscapular and tricipital fold are 52 mm for men and 70 mm for women.

Waist-Hip Ratio (WHR)

On the basis of the distribution of the adipose tissue, it is possible to distinguish three types of obesity: android, intermediate and gynoid. The use of this method is a simple and valid index of the central or peripheral distribution of the adipose tissue and is related to the appearance of different and multiple metabolic complications. Android obesity (centripetal, of the trunk, apple-like, abdominal, visceral) is characteristic of the male sex with a distribution of the adipose tissue in the upper part of the body (face, neck, shoulders, upper abdomen) and is aggravated by various complications such as diabetes mellitus, hyperlipidemies, hyperuremia and high blood pressure. Gynoid obesity (subcutaneous, pear-like) is characteristic of the female sex, with distribution of the adipose tissue in the lower part of the body (hips, buttocks, thighs, lower abdomen) and is related to complications such as venous insufficiency and cellulitis. On the basis of the waist-hip ratio we can establish parameters that indicate the various types of obesity [16,17]:

Gynoid obesity WHR < 0.78
Intermediate obesity WHR between 0.79 and 0.84
Android obesity WHR > 0.85

Direct Techniques

Computerized analysis of body composition by body impedance analysis

When we speak of B.I.A. we refer to a method that is easy to perform and is considered the most reliable to provide an exact estimate of the body composition. It succeeds in overcoming the error of assessment that can be made using other methods still in use today (BMI, plicometry) that, while undoubtedly valid, do not provide an exact measurement of the components of our body. First discovered in 1962 by Thomasett, who discovered the relationship between total body water and a particular physical parameter called impedance, it was not until 1983 that Nyboer, through complex calculations (predictive equations) was able to apply the principles of impedance to the study of the body composition. A few years later other scholars defined the utility and reliability of measurement of body impedance to determine the amount of water in the organism and thus to calculate the exact composition of the body.

Body impedance analysis is based on physical principles through the quantification of the amount of water in the body. Water is a good conductor of electricity and, as the lean mass consists mainly of water, by measuring the water content of the body it is possible to determine the amount of lean and fatty mass, the intracellular and extracellular content of water, the quantity of cellular mass (a fundamental parameter to define the patient "in good health" and the basal calorie consumption. Body impedance analysis does not require any special preparation of the patient (it is sufficient not to drink and not to perform any physical

activity for 4 hours prior to the examination) [18]. The fields of application of this method have developed in recent years to the point that this examination has become fundamental even in pathologies heretofore considered at risk (kidney failure). It has become particularly important for the correct assessment of the body composition of the obese patient both at the beginning of the dietetic and/or pharmacological treatment, but also and above all for a dynamic determination of the variation of the bodily parameters in time, with particular attention to conservation of the lean mass. However, in view of the capacity of this method to assess, mainly, the body water content, it has found application also in pathologies in which water exchange may be altered. Among these are water retention, kidney failure (the first studies on impedance measurement were made on patients undergoing dialysis, when the first database was created), high blood pressure (especially in patients being treated with diuretics with particular attention to the more drastic ones like furosemide), dehydration, denutrition, glandular diseases (particularly those affecting the surrenal glands or hypothyroidism), pregnancy and menstrual disorders [19].

DXA

The DXA (dual energy X-ray absorptiometry) scan is mainly used to evaluate bone mineral density, and furthermore, can also be used to measure total body composition and fat content. The DXA is the latest and most accurate way of testing and determining body composition; it is generally considered the current gold standard for this purpose.

This method applies the concept that lean tissue and fat tissue have different density and therefore, using special formulas, it is possible to convert the density value to that of the percentage of body fat.

The DXA is useful for getting information about bone density, body fat percentage, lean body mass, fat mass, and distribution of fat and lean mass in trunk, legs and arms.

In women with cellulite, DXA can help to evaluate the amount of adipose tissue of the legs. This information is very important for medical therapy and also patients, who with a great understanding of how the body is responding to the changes made, are more inspired to persist with this therapy and maintain their newly adopted lifestyle.

The investment level needed to buy the medical device is still high but DXA is a safe, painless and quick test that provides detailed information about patient's lifestyle; as a consequence, DXA analysis is still costly for patients.

Macro-Nutrients

Macro-nutrients are proteins, lipids (fats) and carbohydrates. They are the main ingredients of the diet and the basic material that our body is composed of (proteins and fats normally account for 44% and 30% respectively of the body's dry weight), or the fuel required to make it work (carbohydrates and fats in theory supply about 55% and 30% respectively of the energy we need).

Proteins

Proteins are the macromolecules derived from the union of much simpler units, the amino acids. They constitute the category of macromolecules most common in nature, given that they represent about 50% of the dry weight of cells. The basic ingredients of proteins are, as we have said, the amino acids or rather the alpha-L amino acids. From a biological point of view these compounds divide into two main categories: essential amino acids (EAA) and nonessential amino acids (NEAA). Proteins perform numerous and very varied functions in the body that constitute most of the essential life processes. For the sake of convenience proteins are classified into various groups depending on their characteristics: simple proteins composed only of amino acids (fibrous, globular) and combined proteins composed in part of amino acid and in part of a non-proteic group called prosthetic (chromoprotein, metalloprotein, nucleoprotein, glycoprotein, lipoprotein). The daily dietary need has not yet been defined with absolute certainty since there are many parameters to consider. Protein intake is not only correlated with growth and maintenance of body weight but with many vital processes. Enzymes and some proteic hormones need to be synthesised continuously [20]. The osmotic pressure of the organism must be maintained and there may be further variations in requirements linked to changes in temperature or the activities performed or even to varied physiological states, such as in pregnancy or when breast-feeding. There are however some widely accepted notions of daily protein requirements that recommend at least 1.2 g/day of protein per kg of body weight for women and 1.5 g/day per kg of body weight for men. However a quantitative indication alone is not sufficient. The quality of the protein is important too. The distinction between EAA and NEAA is fundamental since the body is unable to synthesise EAA which therefore need to be eaten as they are, while it can synthesise NEAA albeit at the expense of other amino acids. The role attributed to these substances nowadays is obviously a structural one but amino acids may also be used for other purposes such as producing energy as happens whenever a dietary deficit (a diet low in glucides) or prolonged fasting (amino acids deriving from the breakdown of cellular and tissue structures) occurs. They may also be transformed into stores (glycogen or lipid) when the diet is too rich and the intake of amino acids exceeds the actual requirement. Proteins are digested and absorbed in the small intestine even though the digestive process involves the mouth, stomach and large intestine. The absorption of intact proteins occurs only in the breast-fed baby by means of pinocytosis while in the adult this process is so limited as not to be of particular significance. The absorption of digested proteins takes place at the beginning of the small intestine and is practically complete by the time it gets to the empty intestine.

Carbohydrates

Carbohydrates are a class of compounds very plentiful in nature and include sugars, starch and cellulose. Various divisions have been proposed for the purpose of classifying carbohydrates although they are commonly divided into four groups: mono-saccharides, disaccharides, oligosaccharides and glycans. Among the most important simple sugars are glucose (commonly known as dextrose), fructose (also called levulose) and galactose. A diet free of carbohydrates provokes serious metabolic alterations and absolutely harmful biochemical imbalances in laboratory animals. In fact, while glucides can also be produced using alternative metabolic procedures from proteins and lipids, a dietary deficiency will inevitably affect the ability to maintain a stable level of blood sugar (glycemia), an essential element for the correct per-formance of all vital processes. The caloric requirement for the survival of an individual depends on many factors, of which age and the type of work performed are important, but is generally around 2000–4000 calories per day. Carbohydrates provide about 4 kcal/g (roughly the same as proteins) against the 9 kcal/g of fats and may make up over 50% of the calorie requirement depending on the diet [21,22]. Once carbohydrates have been introduced through the diet they undergo a process of separation into mono-saccharide components so as to be absorbed and metabolised. The main glycans consumed in the diet are starch and glycogen which begin to be broken down by enzymes as soon as they are masticated. The monosaccharides are thus liberated and can be absorbed by the intestinal villi. Absorption may be passive (by mere diffusion) or active (through the consumption of energy). The monosaccharides are then sent to the portal vein and hepatic artery through which they arrive at the liver. It is through these mechanisms, controlled by the endocrine and nervous systems, that the concentration of glucose in the blood is kept constant. In man, in conditions of fasting, the glycemia level oscillates between 70 and 90 mg/100 ml and must not go under 40 mg/100 ml, a limit below which the body enters an extremely serious clinical and metabolic situation called "hypoglycaemic coma" deriving from the particular sensitivity of nervous tissue to the level of blood sugar in the body.

Lipids

Fats and oils represent the commonest and sole category of compounds known as lipids. The term lipid may be used to define any compound of a group of substances that are generally soluble in ether, chloroform or other solvents for fats but soluble only to a limited degree in water. Foods may contain all or some of these substances but the ones we are most affected by are the fats or glycerides and the phosphates. Fats and oils are the most highly concentrated source of energy. They provide about 40 kJ of energy per gram which is about double that of proteins or carbohydrates. They are carriers of liposoluble vitamins and contribute to the sense of taste and the palatability of foods as well as to the sense of fullness. Lipids in the form of triglycerides, phospholipids, cholesterol and cholesterol esters are essential for the structure, composition and permeability of the cellular membrane and walls. Lipids are the main component of adipose tissue which also acts as a thermal insulator for the body [23]. On average an adult eats from 60 to 150g of lipids a day composed of 90% of triacil-glycerols and for the remainder by phospholipids, unbound and estered cholesterol and unbound fatty acids. As well as these, 1–2 g of cholesterol and 7–20 g of lecithin are excreted in the lumen of the duodenum as constituents of bile. The metabolic importance of fatty acids is mainly energetic. In fact their oxidative breakdown results in the production of large quantities of energy in the form of ATP and triglycerides constitute the main energy reserve of the body. Most of the fats used by man are supplied through the diet by means of digestive and absorption processes. Fatty acids are absorbed by the various tissues in variable quantities and may be used to produce energy. This process comes about mainly in the mitochondrions. The extent to which fatty acids are used to produce energy varies considerably from one tissue to another and depends on the metabolic state, state of nourishment, of fasting and of physical exercise. For example while nervous tissue hardly uses fatty acids at all to produce energy, muscle tissue, whether skeletal or cardiac, uses them to a considerable degree. In conditions of prolonged fasting moreover many tissues become capable of using ketone bodies too, including the nervous system. Polyunsaturated fatty acids deserve a special mention. Lately much attention has been focused on these acids with regard to their purported ability to prevent or delay the atherosclerotic process. The human body is able to produce most of those present in the organism except for those belonging to the linoleic and linolenic series. The function of the fatty acids of the linoleic series became clear when arachidonic acid was identified as the precursor of prostaglandin, while a derivative, C22, of the linolenic series has been found in high concentrations in the membrane of nervous cells and those of the retina. An important function of all unsaturated fatty acids is to maintain a certain fluidity of cellular membranes.

NUTRITIONAL TREATMENT
Food Hormones
Glucagon is secreted by the alpha cells of the pancreas when the level of glucose in the blood falls below the normal level (i.e. 4.5 mM). It triggers a series of reactions at the level of the liver that lead to the release of glucose from the glycogen reserves and block the production of triglycerides. The ingestion of proteins, as a result an increase of amino acids in the blood, leads to a postprandial physiological increase of glucagon. Blood levels of glucagon are higher in glucagonoma, endocrine polyadenomatosis, liver and kidney failure, untreated diabetes and Cushing's disease. Traumas, prolonged fasting, infections, excessive physical exercise, pancreatitis, pheochromocytoma, untreated diabetes mellitus, uremia and chronic kidney failure also cause an increase in the levels of glucagon. A reduction in the blood levels of glucagon occurs in patients with cystic fibrosis, chronic pancreatitis, pancreatitis caused by tumour or surgical removal of the pancreas.

Insulin is also secreted by the pancreas, by the beta cells, under the opposite conditions from those which cause glucagon secretion, that is, an abundance of glucose in the blood, a condition known as "hyperglycemia". It is a protein-synthesized hormone in the form of inactive proinsulin, consisting of two polypeptide chains, A and B, connected by a polypeptide (peptide C), from the detachment of which active insulin originates. The concentration of insulin may be elevated in patients with insulinoma and acromegalia, in obesity, in Cushing's disease and in women taking oral contraceptives [24]. The task of insulin is to eliminate the excess sugars in the blood by facilitating their absorption at the muscular level and by the liver. Insulin also stimulates the synthesis of triglycerides and their "storage" in the form of fatty droplets that join together to form fatty tissue, and if the accumulation is excessive, what is known as a "paunch" will form, and in extreme cases it can result in obesity. Insulin is secreted mainly because of an excess of glucose (carbohydrates) in the blood (and a negligible increase of amino acids), while glucagon is secreted only in response to an increase in the concentrations of amino acids (proteins). Fats do not seem, however, to affect the synthesis of these two hormones. After a meal, the pancreas secretes as much insulin as necessary to maintain the proper concentration of sugars in the blood. A meal rich in carbohydrates causes a higher rate of production of insulin to be secreted into the blood.

If this occurs, it upsets the balance between insulin and glucagon. The diet should therefore be well-balanced and should provide us with the proper amount of carbohydrates, proteins and fats to meet the needs of the organism. Many studies of obese patients have shown that these patients have a low response to insulin and it has been shown that insulin-resistance is a major factor of risk for diabetes [25].

Resistance to insulin is the inability to regulate the action of insulin at the level of the muscles and fatty tissue. The excess of insulin is associated with an increased synthesis of fats (triglycerides) and their reduced fission, and an increase in PAI-1, a factor that regulates fibrinolysis and coagulation [26–30]. Studies made on groups at high risk for the development of diabetes, such as the Pima Indians of North America or the relatives of patients affected by type 2 diabetes, have shown how insulin-resistance precedes and predicts the subsequent development of diabetes. On the other hand, insulin-resistance is one of the components of the so-called "X-Syndrome" or endocrine-metabolic syndrome, clinically characterized by high arterial blood pressure, insulin-resistance, hyperinsulinemia, hyperlipoproteinmia and alterations of blood coagulation [31,32].

Clinical and epidemiological studies suggest a close correlation between the X syndrome and risk for ischemic heart disease. There is also substantial evidence indicating that insulin-resistance and the resulting compensatory hyperinsulinemia are major risk factors for vascular atherosclerotic disease, which is one of the most frequent medical pathologies connected with aging [33–39]. The pathogenesis of insulin-resistance appears to be quite complex and is caused by a combination of genetic defects and environmental factors. Some of the genetically predetermined molecular defects can be considered the pathogenetic "prime mover" which is followed by a sequence of secondary metabolic alterations that conspire to cause the many clinical expressions of insulin-resistance. Like oncogens, these primitive genetic factors could be called diabetogens. Up to the present time, almost 100 proteins involved in the biological response to the action of insulin have been identified and characterized at the muscular level. The first reaction to the secretion of insulin consists of its interaction with its receptor on the plasma membrane of the target cells (Fig. 8.2).

The insulin receptor is an integral glycoprotein of the membrane formed by two alpha or two beta chains joint by three sulphide bridges and an enzyme belonging to the family of the tyrosine-kinases. The sites of the bond for insulin are on the extracellular side and the domains of tyrosine-kinase are on the cytosolic side [40]. The insulin receptor (HIR) has two isoforms that differ as regards the presence (HIRB) or absence (HIR-A) of a chain of 12 amino acids located on the COOH-terminal end of the extracellular subunit (Fig. 8.3).

The expression of the two isoforms is tissue-specific and is regulated by a mechanism of alternative "splicing" of exon 11 of the gene of the insulin receptor. Recent studies have reported that the two receptor isoforms possess a different affinity for the bond with insulin and different kinetics of internalization, thus suggesting the possibility that the two receptor isoforms may have a different biological activity, going so far as to cause specific modulation of different tissues in the cellular response to the stimulus of insulin. The action of insulin on the transport of glucose involves the translocation of carrier proteins, called transporters, from the

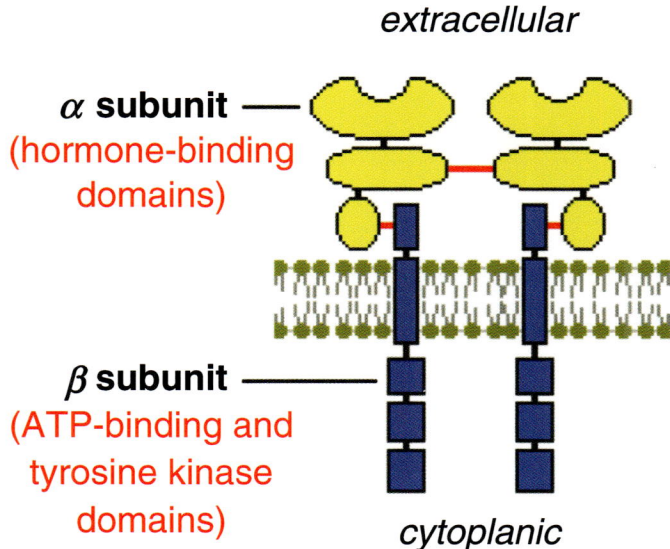

Figure 8.2 Insulin receptor.

intracellular compartment to the plasma membrane, and the subsequent activation of the translocated transporters on the cell surface. The transporters of glucose are a family of proteins with five different tissue-specific isoforms called GLUT (Fig. 8.4).

The insulin-sensitive isoform, present in the two main target organs, the muscle and fatty tissue, is GLUT 4. The transporters of GLUT 4 are positioned on the plasma membrane where they facilitate the entrance of a larger quantity of glucose in the muscle and fat cells. Furthermore, no significant alterations of the gene expression of GLUT 4 have been shown under conditions of preclinical insulin-resistance such as obesity and a reduced tolerance to carbohydrates.

Overweight/Obese Patients and the Metabolism of Sugars and Fats

Hyperinsulinemia causes a reduction in the surface density of insulin receptors and a reduction of their bonding affinity for insulin, giving rise to a condition known as insulin resistance. This

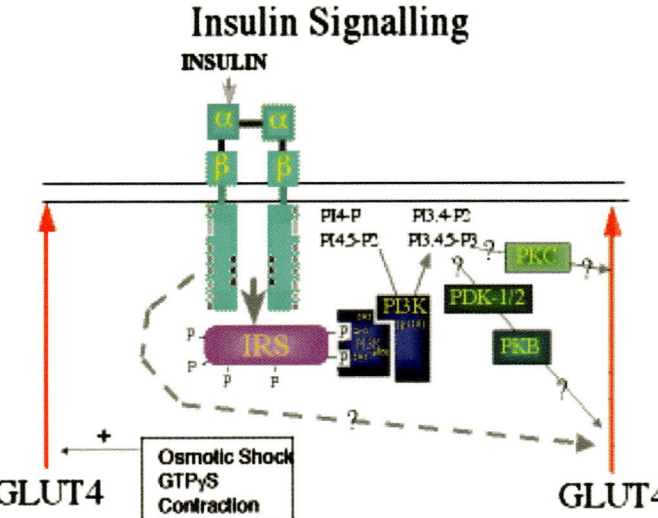

Figure 8.3 Insulin-induced Glut4 expression.

in turn further stimulates the secretion of insulin with gradual exhaustion of the pancreatic reserves and a possible development of type 2 diabetes mellitus. It is well known, in fact, that obesity is one of the main factors of risk for the development of type 2 diabetes mellitus and that the risk of this pathology increases with the increase of the BMI (Fig. 8.5).

Insulin resistance causes a reduction of glycogen synthesis in the liver and an increase of neo-glucogenesis. This condition is aggravated by the increased release in the portal bloodstream of FFA (free fatty acids) by the visceral adiposites, which are particularly sensitive to lipolithic stimuli [41,42]. The increase in the concentration of FFA in the portal circulation facilitates production by the liver of VLDL (very low density lipoproteins). Consequently, we can observe the alterations characteristic of the

- increase of triglycerides appearance of small, dense LDL (low density lipoproteins)
- increase of apolipoprotein B, decrease of HDL (high density lipoproteins).

This is associated with an approximately 20-fold increase in the risk of cardiovascular disease [43–45].

The presence of an altered balance between the synthesis of triglycerides and their mobilization by the hepatocyte, in the form of VLDL is a cause of hepatic steatosis, characterized by a fat accumulation that exceeds 5% of the weight of the organ. This accumulation translates, on the cytological plane, into the appearance of fatty droplets in the hepatocyte.

From the ecographic point of view it can be seen that there is an increase in the ecogenicity of the organ that acquires the typical appearance described as bright liver, with an increase in the volume and rounded margins. The possible appearance of inflammation and fibrosis characterizes a condition that has a potential for rapid degeneration and that is defined as non-alcoholic steatohepatitis (NASH) [46–48,28].

This condition has been observed mainly in obese patients, particularly middle-aged women and/or type 2 diabetics. Factors that foster the process are hyperlipoproteinmia, the use of drugs and some of the surgical procedures that are used to treat severe obesity. A diet rich in sugars causes an increase in the production of insulin by the beta cells of the pancreas. By consuming too many proteins we force it to secrete glucagon. Both situations of imbalance cause their own specific problems.

Many studies of obese patients have shown that these patients have a low response to insulin and it has been shown that insulin resistance is a major factor of risk for diabetes [25].

Resistance to insulin is the inability to regulate the action of insulin at the level of the muscles and fatty tissue. The excess of insulin is associated with an increased synthesis of fats (triglycerides) and their reduced fission, and an increase in PAI-1, a factor that regulates fibrinolysis and coagulation [26–30]. Studies made on groups at high risk for the development of diabetes, such as the Pima Indians of North America or the relatives of patients affected by type 2 diabetes, have shown how insulin resistance precedes and predicts the subsequent development of diabetes. On the other hand, insulin resistance is one of the components of the so-called "X-syndrome" or endocrine-metabolic syndrome, clinically characterized by high arterial

Insulin and the regulation of glucose transporters

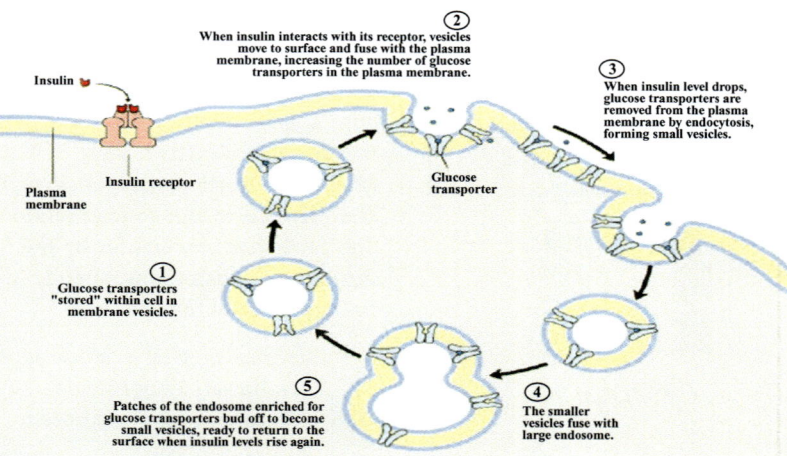

Figure 8.4 Glucose Transporters on membrane surface.

blood pressure, insulin resistance, hyperinsulinemia, hyperlipoproteinmia and alterations of blood coagulation [31,32]. Clinical and epidemiological studies suggest a close correlation between the X-syndrome and risk for ischemic heart disease. There is also substantial evidence indicating that insulin resistance and the resulting compensatory hyperinsulinemia are major risk factors for vascular atherosclerotic disease, which is one of the most frequent medical pathologies connected with aging [33–39].

The pathogenesis of insulin resistance appears to be quite complex and is caused by a combination of genetic defects and environmental factors. Some of the genetically predetermined molecular defects can be considered the pathogenetic "prime mover" which is followed by a sequence of secondary metabolic alterations that conspire to cause the many clinical expressions of insulin resistance. Like oncogens, these primitive genetic factors could be called diabetogens. Up to the present time, almost 100 proteins involved in the biological response to the action of insulin

have been identified and characterized at the muscular level. The first reaction to the secretion of insulin consists of its interaction with its receptor on the plasma membrane of the target cells (See Fig. 8.2).

Insulin and Inflammation

In cellulite treatment, as well as wanting to achieve a drop in subcutaneous fat, the objective must also be a reduction in inflammation.

There is a strong link between insulin and inflammation since the insulin resistance is associated with an excessive production of inflammatory cytokines [49].

The relationship between insulin resistance and cytokines is complicated since they influence each other. In fact, as stated above, TNF-α inhibits insulin receptors that lead to greater insulin secretion to provide the inhibition; on the other hand, the excessive insulin response in turn inhibits the number of the receptors expressed on the surface.

TNF-α also has a clear influence on the endothelium and therefore the insulin resistance is also associated with the cardiovascular risk.

It has been demonstrated that, in the subcutaneous adipose tissue of moderately obese women, women with insulin resistance had a greater amount of inflammation compared to the obese group, but not insulin resistant [50].

In some research, the inflammatory process seems to be mainly linked to the subcutaneous adipose tissue (although not all publications are in agreement on this point). In treating cellulite this reflects the importance of modulating the inflammation through nutritional treatment aimed at reducing the insulin response [51].

An appropriate diet that controls the insulin and reduces the body fat does not only cause a reduction in the inflammatory cytokines, but also an increase in the anti-inflammatory cytokines such as interleukin 10, interleukin 1 receptor antagonist [52].

It has now become clear that the first step in treating cellulite, excess adipose tissue and inflammation is to control insulin through diet and physical exercise.

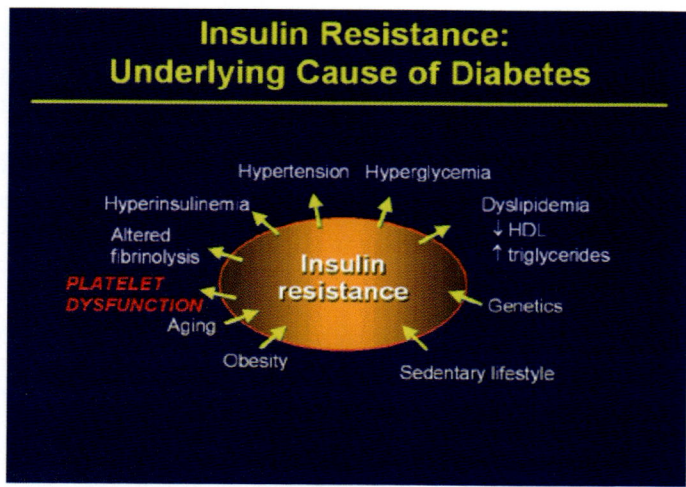

Figure 8.5 Insulin and Disease.

The Food Pyramids

There is increasing talk of "healthy eating". There is no longer any doubt about the link between nutrition and the diseases of the rich countries: obesity, arterial sclerosis, diabetes, hypertension, etc. [53]. 40% of oncological disease and 60% of cardiovascular disease depends in fact on bad nutrition. There is widespread evidence to show in particular that the incidence of breast cancer is directly linked to a high consumption of fats and with obesity. Just as much evidence has been found from research to show that a constant intake of fruit and vegetables, which provide the body with antioxidant substances, vitamins and fibre, discourage a whole series of neoplasia [54,55].

In 1992 the United States Department of Agriculture (USDA) published the now famous food pyramid which aimed at helping the American public choose a diet that would keep them healthy and reduce the risk of chronic illness.

The USDA pyramid has complex carbohydrates at the bottom: bread, pasta, rice, refined cereals and so on to be eaten without moderation and in quantities decidedly superior to the other foods [56].

This is followed by vegetables and fruit, potatoes (another source of carbohydrates), then dairy products, animal and vegetable proteins such as red meat, poultry, fish, beans and eggs.

At the top of the list are foods to be eaten in moderation: sweet foods, fats and oils. Since 1992, further research has shown how this pyramid had many defects. By promoting the consumption of complex carbohydrates and excluding fats and oils, the pyramid was a deceptive guide. Not all fats are in fact harmful nor are all complex carbohydrates good for one's health.

Two authoritative American epidemiologists with specific and recognised expertise in the field of nutrition, Walter Willett and Meir Stampfer, published their proposed revision of the pyramid in the journal *Scientific American* containing, compared to the previous version, several significant changes [57]. Willett and Stampfer's pyramid got a lively debate going among the experts. The authors, in fact, "broke away" from the established thinking of the past in some spheres and, as often happens, this decision was subject to differing evaluations in the scientific community [58,59]. See Fig. 8.6.

The new pyramid includes, first of all, two concepts that have clearly emerged in recent years and that is that not all fats have the same nutritional value and that the classic differentiation between simple and complex carbohydrates, in fashion for many decades, is probably no longer sufficient to enable consumers to choose the healthiest foods.

As regards fats in particular, the new pyramid has adopted drastic choices. While all the fats were placed near the top in the old version (meaning, as everyone knows, that they were to be eaten in moderation), currently only saturated fats, and specifically butter, are still in this "uncomfortable" position.

Fats of vegetable origin such as olive, corn and rape oil, known in the USA as "canola," are situated towards the bottom of the pyramid, with a specific suggestion that they be eaten every day and probably during meals. Margarines, relatively rich in "trans" type fats are excluded from the pyramid altogether, not even being present in the upper part.

This approach regarding the consumption of fats presumably derives from the information gathered by the authors, who have been conducting three extensive epidemiological studies for many years now (the study of nurses, the study of health professionals, the study of doctors) which has provided an enormous quantity of information also relating to the correlation between specific aspects of nutrition and the risk of cardiovascular events [60].

In the study of the nurses in particular, which is the one with the longest follow-up, one can observe how with the increase in the consumption of monounsaturated fatty acids, and especially of polyunsaturated fats, the risk of cardiovascular events continually decreases. The fifth of the population with the highest intake of polyunsaturated fats (specifically of linoleic acid) show in the above study a risk of cardiovascular events which is 30–35% lower than the fifth of the population in the same study with a lower intake of these fatty acids.

At the extreme opposite of the scale, high consumers of trans fatty acids show a relevant and significant increase of cardiovascular events compared to women who consume a smaller quantity of these fats.

The authors therefore stigmatise the consumption of fats of animal origin or of hydrogenated vegetable fats, while they explicitly promote the consumption of vegetable oil, in all its forms (and therefore of olive oil and corn oil). Also as regards carbohydrates the choices adopted in the new pyramid are quite drastic and have in actual fact aroused some perplexity among those operating in the sector. The complex carbohydrates such as bread, pasta and rice, previously at the bottom of the state pyramid, have been repositioned, in this proposed revision, right at the top of the pyramid. In practice a total turnaround: a group of foods that in the previous guide were to represent the basis of daily nutrition is today classified as "to be eaten in moderation". In their place at the bottom of the pyramid are wholemeal cereals, rich in fibre, for which a daily intake is recommended.

Presumably the basis for differentiating between these two categories of foods should be looked for in their differing propensity to release sugar into the blood once consumed: in other words their glycemic index. Foods with a low glycemic index tend in fact to be associated with higher cholesterol/HDL values, reduced plasmatic values for certain indicators of inflammation (such as reactive protein C, or PCR, the levels of which are correlated to cardiovascular risk), to more favourable plasmatic levels of the triglycerides. The new pyramid has an added lowest step that underlines the need to perform an adequate amount of physical exercise every day and that presents, as an external suggestion, the consumption of a moderate amount of alcohol (where there are no counter indications) and of a vitamin supplement which the authors deem sufficient for most of the population [61]. The first of these factors is actually generally supported by the scientific community (physical exercise is well known for helping to maintain the right body weight, of improving the values for HDL and of exerting a pro-fibrinolytic effect); the consumption of moderate amounts of alcohol in turn has recognised positive effects on cardiovascular risk, mediated in this case too by the improvement of the plasmatic lipoprotein profile and by the induction of a favourable relationship between the metabolic processes of thrombosis and fibrinolysis; as far as the use by large parts of the population of vitamin and mineral supplements is concerned, opinions are more divided: specifically, it may well be that vitamin intake in

51

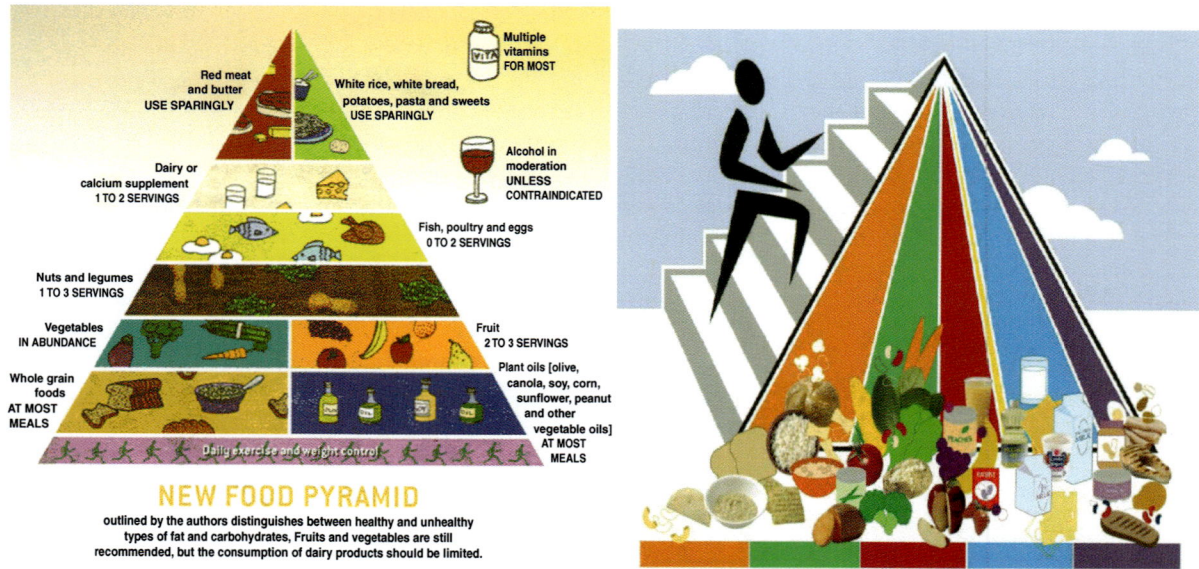

Figure 8.6 The USDA Food Pyramid.

Mediterranean areas like our own is superior and that therefore such intervention is less important than in areas where less fruit, vegetables and fresh plants are eaten, as one can observe in many Anglo-Saxon countries.

Anti-Inflammation Diet

The world of diets now seems to have become limitless. There are various types of diets: the Mediterranean, Atkins, the Zone, the Paleo Diet, the Blood Group Diet, and so on. The truth is that the human body has its own physiology and mechanisms that should be satisfied. The topics that have generated the most interest over the last few years have regarded the consumption of carbohydrates and protein. The questions have always been the same, how much carbohydrate? How much protein? Which carbohydrates? The answers are often different, but we can perhaps say that a milestone has been reached. At last we now talk about glycemic index and load and the distinction between simple and complex carbohydrates has almost been set aside.

The glycemic index was discovered in 1981 by Dr. David Jenkins, a professor of food science at the University of Toronto in Canada, who started to consider foodstuffs not only based on their quantitative content of carbohydrates, but also based on the different effect that these could have on glucose levels in the blood. In fact the glycemic index is a classification of the various foodstuffs containing carbohydrates on a scale from 0 to 100, based on the speed with which they cause an increase in glycemia (or rather the glucose levels in the blood). It is calculated by comparing the foodstuffs that contain equal quantities of carbohydrates with a control food, such as pure glucose. In practical terms, an amount of foodstuff being tested, containing 50 g of carbohydrates, is given to various volunteers, then their glycemia is measured at 15–30-minute intervals over the next two hours and a glycemic curve is created. This is then compared with the glycemic curve created based on taking 50 g of pure glucose (control foodstuff). A glycemic index equal or higher than 70 is regarded as HIGH, MEDIUM if between 56 and 69, and LOW if equal or less than 55. These values are stated in the reference tables. The foodstuffs

containing carbohydrates that are broken down rapidly during the digestive processes have a high GI, therefore following their absorption there will be a rapid and high glycemic response, producing high quantities of insulin (a hormone secreted by the pancreas in response to the glycemic increase), which facilitates its entrance into the adipose tissue, as well as into muscle, where it is converted into fat, to accelerate the disposal of the glucose. On the contrary, there are carbohydrates in low GI foodstuffs that are broken down slowly and cause a gradual release of glucose in the blood with a positive influence on the secretion of insulin. Slow digestion helps to keep one feeling full for longer and helps with weight loss. Keeping the glycemic index at lower levels during the day improves the health of the coronary arteries, reducing the oxidative stress associated with glycemic peaks, reduces the formation of lipidic deposits, atheromatous plaques and thrombi. However we should add that we cannot choose the foodstuffs purely based on the GI value stated in the reference tables as this can vary based on different factors, such as the variety, collection time, area and means of production, fat content, protein and fibre, preservation and drying, the method and cooking time and other ingredients in the recipe. High fat quantity slows down the gastric emptying and influences the digestion and absorption processes; therefore the foodstuffs with a high percentage of lipids have a reduced GI value compared to those in which there are minimal quantities of fat. For example, chips have a lower GI compared to potatoes cooked without fat, just as many biscuits have a lower GI than white bread. However, this does not mean that they are a better choice as the fat content has a negative effect on the general state of health in a greater measure compared to the benefits of a low glycemic index [1].

Therefore the GI is never considered in isolation and is above all connected also to quantity, that is to say, to the glycemic load (GL). The glycemic response of a foodstuff, that is to say the scale with which the glycemia increases and remains high after being taken, depends also on the amount of carbohydrates contained in it as well as its glycemic index. The glycemic load is an index that takes into consideration the amount and type of carbohydrates in the foodstuffs and is calculated by multiplying the glycemic index of the foodstuff by the amount of carbohydrates in a single portion and dividing it by 100.

CG = (IG * Carbohydrates in the portion): 100

The carbohydrate content of a foodstuff can easily be identified by observing the nutritional label and then comparing it with the portion consumed. As regards the GI, we must stick to the reference tables instead as it is still not common practice to show it on the labels of specific products. By calculating the glycemic load one has a more correct view of how much a certain portion of a given foodstuff goes on to influence one's glycemia. For example, melon has a high glycemic index, but in 100 g it contains a few grams of carbohydrates, so the glycemic load of one portion is modest. Therefore it is always important to consider the GI of every foodstuff in accordance with its GL [2].

Food Intolerance

Cellulite: Immunological Inflammation Function and Other Alimentary Aspects

Daily we have to examine patients who have complex manifestations that involve all body systems. Most doctors are often unprepared to handle these type of phenomenons.

If a patient presents unique symptoms as articular pain, abdominal pain, reflux disease (GERD), colitis, cough, asthma, and skin allergies that appeared after eating some food, the most common answer is: "It's impossible that everything is connected."

Today not only we are sure that it is so but we also know that overweight, obesity and cellulite (even in underweight patients or patients with alimentary behaviour disorders) are an integral part of this situation, one that finds its cause in inflammation determined by food intake.

This inflammation is at the same time the concause and also the main cause of all reactions, that lead lypodystrophy (cellulite). It may depend on a retarded allergic reaction to food as well as on altered relations among the meals and from the altered hormone balance established by the same adipokine production.

It is really important to consider the immunological scientific discoveries of recent years in order to understand the direct effect of food allergies and discuss all possible actions.

In considering a complex inflammatory disorder, a well-informed doctor asks his patient to undergo specific tests for IgE (Prick and RAST test), without realizing that in the last 5 years scientific research has taken a huge step forward on food allergies and their related causes. Thanks to this today we know that food allergies are divided in immediate food allergies (bound to immunoglobulin E) and delayed allergies (caused by a cellular reaction promoted by several types of antibodies) which up to now were considered food intolerancies. The latest scientific research, strong and unattackable, proves that:

a. Everyone is allergic to something and the only way to healing is monitoring the immune system (which is why almost everyone said to have an intolerance or an allergy when the real truth is that we have these diseases from birth and these symptoms are only the demonstration that we lost control of their regulation [62]).

b. Many allergies and all food intolerances are connected to delayed phenomena, modulated by cell reactions and not just by IgE antibodies (as it has been believed for decades) [63].

c. Recently some alternative reasons for the manifestation of classic allergies have been identified, that cause the same phenomena but are not revealed by classic tests. The diagnoses that have been carried out until now are very incomplete [64].

The scientific work that recently has upset the academic world is worth pointing out: the American Fred Finkelman discovered that at least two different ways of allergy activation exist showing the same identical symptoms. This means that every diagnosis carried out until 2007 has been rather incomplete, since the "alternative" one could not be excluded. The reaction to a food-delayed allergy is therefore a reaction caused primarily by the action of the cells rather than only the antibodies.

The description of this allergy showing two ways, the classic one (with presence of IgE), and the alternative one (without IgE, of cellular type), is close to the classic model of delayed food hypersensitivity (intolerance), as it supports the conviction that the second type of allergy is (as anticipated by Sampson) a model always present in the body system, more or less partnered with the type IgE reaction [63].

Let's observe in detail these two manifestations:

- Classic way modulated by IgE, by histamine, stimulated by few quantities of antigen, even in the presence of low quantities of antibodies
- Alternative way mediated by macrophages, with the participation of PAF (platelet activating factor), modulated by IgG (immunoglobulin G), and probably stimulated by high quantities of antigens repeated in more time, in the presence of elevated quantities of antibodies.

Therefore we are dealing with an extraordinary discovery that allows us to completely reconsider the way in which allergies develop and are controlled. We need to remember also that IgG are the antibodies that grow when the tolerance towards the classic allergy begins to develop, so IgG never need to be considered totally dangerous.

The Allergy and Intolerance Reactions: Global Involvement

In this context one cannot underestimate the continuous interaction, in the organism, among the different systems and apparatuses. It is not rare, for example, that in a person suffering from a thyroidal pathology, sooner or later, an antibody response that is related to the same gland is also activated. It has been shown that a person who has had Hashimoto thyroiditis, and is allergic to graminaceous plants, during springtime, when pollen stimulates the nasal response, points out a clear increase of thyroidal antibodies, that, in accordance with the official science, are not related to the pollen reaction. On the contrary the highlighted response depends on the fact that the entire body reacts, and not just a single part of it. The fact that the body's response appears in several areas offers also the possibility to work therapeutically starting from different areas; it happens, for example, that contact dermatitis heals thanks to an acarus allergy vaccine. Why? The immunologic therapy is educating the entire system (and

Table 8.2 Glicemic index and Glycemic load in different foods

Foodstuff	Glycemic index	Portion (G)	Carbohydrate per portion	Glycemic load per portion
Croissant	67	57	26	17
Water crackers	78	25	18	14
Soft drink with orange juice and sugar	68	250	34	23
White bread	70	30	14	10
White bread, gluten free	71	30	15	11
Corn flakes	77	30	25	20
Fresh apple	44	120	13	6
Fructose	19	10	10	2
Saccharose	68	10	10	7

not only the respiratory apparatus) to respond better to the provocation. The reason is that the system "thinks" in global terms, and it is in those terms that, as eminent researchers like Polly Matzinger and David Napier claim, one need to reconsider completely the allergic response. Let's think, for example, about the fact that the liver (usually not considered an allergy affected organ, unlike the nose, eyes, lungs) is the organ with the highest number of mast cells and with the maximum number of connections to the nervous system and is one of the greater producers of IL6 that, as we will see, represents one of the fattening signals induced by food. Until now nobody spoke about a real allergy of the liver, but some researchers began to point out the importance of the allergic reaction to explain the chronic inflammation of the liver.

Perhaps in the near future one can consider chronic hepatitis or cirrhosis as possible manifestations of allergic reaction. Today the interaction between chronic inflammatory statuses and allergy phenomena is getting more noted and studied. The disorder of the system represented by the presence of a persisting inflammation, even limited, can create the conditions for the development of some pathologies and mostly can contribute to their maintenance, or severely interfere with their healing. Regarding cellulite and fattening we are realizing that the type of nutritional choices, often independent of the quantity of calories eaten, causes the inflammatory responses that maintain the lipodystrophy and induce the adipose deposit even in presence of a low-calorie diet.

Food-Delayed Allergies: Signal of Adipose Build-Up
After some years of debate, of improper use and criticism, the phenomenon of food-delayed allergies, as per Sampson's definition since 2003 (food intolerances), has begun a path of greater scientific recognition. Food intolerances represent one of the most important defence mechanisms of the body and are involved in the management of food inflammation, in regulating hypothalamic signals and in fattening as well as in the induction of several degenerative pathologies. Thus a properly followed food intolerance diet, respectful of some nutritional principles, can help many persons who suffer from food-delayed allergies to find their own form and to lose weight, checking also the stimuli action to lipodystrophy.

Food intolerances spark in the body an inflammatory process that causes fattening and activates a danger signal for the whole system.

Storing fat (usually in the wrong areas) is everyone's correct response to a possible "low-grade" inflammation like the typical one of food intolerances or of chronic infective phenomenon or other immune-flogistic phenomena, events that the body interprets as a continuing in the time signal of danger and that cause insulin resistance and fat build-up in the adipocytes. The aim of a diet controlling food intolerances is cancelling the inflammatory aspect, eliminating the danger signal produced by the system and sending metabolism activation signals instead.

A nutritional plan that controls the existing allergies represents a powerful signal diet [65,66], that allows weight loss precisely in the areas in which the fat has been built-up wrongly and helps metabolism reactivation, restoring the proper sensitivity to insulin. The lipodystrophy control according to an individualized criterion needs to pass along this way.

In 2007 an important work by Solt explained that the presence of Interleukine 1 (IL1) one of the typical cytokines produced by the body during an allergic or inflammatory reaction, induced the NF-kB activation, provoking therefore a fat build-up in response to this danger signal, clearly to store in hope of better times. Evidently signals in the body are more powerful than calories.

Since 2007 Zeyda as well has highlighted that a low-intensity inflammatory stimulus, as the one of food intolerances, causes the activation of special white blood cells (macrophages) in fat tissue that lead to insulin-resistance induction and thus fattening [67]. Fattening caused by food intolerances (insulin resistance produced by IL1, IL6, TNF alfa) refers to the importance of IL6 produced by the liver as response to the inflammatory stimulus coming from the portal circulation related to the use of non-tolerated food. Also the liver participates in the immune-flogistic feedback causing the "defensive" response of fattening in the presence of a diet that repeatedly uses non-tolerated food.

Obviously an acute and violent allergic stimulus can cause malabsorption, but when the stimulus is extended in time and by low intensity, it becomes an important danger signal and the body reacts in a useful way, as it has since Palaeolithic times. It lowers the metabolism and increases the transformation of energy in fat, to defend itself from possible future famines.

In women (and also in men) followed until now with a food intolerances control diet and with the respect to adipokines production, the component that most characterized loss of weight has been the power of losing especially the fat mass instead of muscle mass or water.

In order to follow a food intolerances control diet one needs to have some available results from a food intolerances study test, to explain them on the basis of the "five large food groups theory," thus avoiding highlighting insignificant reactions (for example) to the cola nut or the mandarin, but enhances ones really important for the recovery of the dietetic tolerance of the average European, so: milk and milk products; wheat and cereals; yeast and fermented substances: nickel and hydrogenated vegetal fats; natural salicylates.

The test we prefer to use for our evaluations is the ALCAT test, but even other cell tests with special characteristics can be useful, also combined, if necessary, with assessments of generic type to clarify the hypersensitivity diagnosis. In direct contact with the person who wants to lose weight one explains the diet instructions and the nutritional planning that are useful to every single case [68].

The diet needs always to be a rotation diet and never an exclusion diet (it can produce opposite effects) and always with the purpose of the immunologic tolerance recovery on the basis of a correction of the food intolerances, allowing three to five diet-free meals per week, to help the recovery of the tolerance and make the path for getting over their own form of intolerance a joy. The diet needs always to be integrated with some nutritional rules as the prolonged mastication, that activates the fat melting and helps allergy control, starting every meal with a piece of raw fruit or vegetable ("raw, alive and colored" substances), a technique that speeds up the food intolerance and allergies control, allowing the tolerance recovery towards all types of food.

SUPPLEMENTATION
Dietary Supplementation and Cellulite
An important "cosmeceutic" action led by dietary supplements helps the topic treatment of cellulite. You need however to remember that "cellulite" is a pathology, and thus the effects of the cosmeceutic treatments both topical and systemic ones can operate and moderately relieve the conditions of skin alteration typical of the cellulite: orange peel skin, lumps, pain in palpating, color of the complexion.

Of course it is necessary to operate in a coordinated in-out way to get significant results in the struggle against cellulite, together with nutritional supplementation, the subjects undergo a regulation of their lifestyle, eliminating sedentariness, smoking and incorrect food.

The dietary supplements intake needs to follow some "pharmacologic" rules to be effective, but these rules are often ignored or underestimated. Every substance's systemic intake (in the case of supplements by mouth) is assumed to be given in the proper manner and quantity, and moreover "timed" to get the right bioavailability to develop its function in the organismic area where you want it to operate, in this case in the sub-derma of the glutei-femoral zone. The cellulite, with regards to its "pathologic" degree is characterized by a modified micro-vascular system and an adipoicitary fibro-occlusion one that obstructs the ideal bioavailability at cellular level. This is the reason that III and IV degree cellulite can react less positively to the in-out cosmeceutic treatment. Regarding this new opportunity to treat cellulite by a systemic intervention, today cosmetic houses suggest new

associations of topicals and supplements, that generally contain botanic origin substances, that can drain liquids, eliminate stagnation toxins, modulate positively the capillary tonicity, stimulate the microcirculation, operate a special lipolysis, prevent and lower the inflammatory processes mediated by free radicals and firm up and tone up the skin [68,70,71].

Bioflavonoides
Among the important substances that can be used in "anti-cellulite" supplements there are bioflavonoides that can help the modified microcirculation in a substantial way. The vegetal extracts mostly used are ginkgo, black bilberry, grape, centella asiatica, pineapple and melilot derivate ones. Substances contained in these vegetal extracts protect capillaries, can improve collagen and elastin synthesis, modulate the platelet aggregation, and lower the venous stagnation and the local edematous situation with an improvement of the peripheral circulation and of the skin biomechanical proprieties [69].

The Hamamelis virginiana extract, used by topic or systemic way, has an anti-inflammation and protective action against the peri-vasal connective matrix degradation, which is the cause of the rising of capillary permeability and of chronic inflammation maintenance in phlebo-lymphatic stasis situations. Several studies have demonstrated that this extract can inhibit the action of some hormones like alpha-glucosidasis which are able to degrade the connective [72].

Papaya (carica papaya) and pineapple (Ananas stivus, Ananas comosus) extracts have anti-inflammation and anti-edemigen activity. Especially bromelain extracted from the pineapple contains a series of proteinase with anti-edemigen, anti-inflammatory, anti-thrombotic, fibrinolytic and immune-modulator activity. It is used in systemic and topic preparations [73].

Butcher's broom (ruscus aculeatus) contains steroidal saponins like ruscogenin and neoruscogenin with the ability to increase the venous tone (alpha agonist activity) and reduce the edema [74]. It is used as an extract for systemic uses or in topical 3% preparations.

Very common among the "anti-cellulite" supplements is the othosiphon stamineus that, thanks to the presence of synaesthesia potentiate, which aids the draining and anti-edema effect, helps a better water turnover.

Cellulite, as above explained, can be tackled in different ways, thus also in the dietary supplements intake you can search and apply varied nutritional strategies. One of these is assisting a dietetic caloric reduction using vegetal substances and extracts which can negatively modulate carbohydrates and fats. Soluble dietary fibers like oligosaccharides (FOS, GOS, chitosan, glucomannan etc.) taken before meals can reduce fat absorption, other ones sugars (Gymnema sylvestre, Garcinia cambogia, Phaseolus vulgaris), thus by reducing the assumption of a specific caloric amount per meal and modulating the insulin induction you can obtain better results in the diet approaches.

Metabolic Activators
A third category of vegetal substances and extracts helping the cellulite systemic treatment is composed by "metabolic activators" like guarana (caffeine), green tea and cacao (catechine).

Coenzyme-L and L-carnitine aminoacyd increase the lipolytic effect of methylxantynes helping the free fatty acids' transportation through the membranes, in particular the mitochondrial ones, thus avoiding the level of the fatty acids concentration that gives a negative feed-back of the lipolysis and increases ATP which stimulates the lipase [75].

The majority of the extracts having metabolic activator potentials contain substances that in some way inhibit the adipocyte phosphodiesterase. The inhibition of this enzyme in the adipose cell allows it to maintain high levels of cAMP that in this case maintain protein-kinase (PCK) activity, that in turn, activates the intra-adipocyte lypase. The intra-adipocyte lypase stimulates the lypolise and so the triglycerides hydrolysis in fats and glycerol.

Through metabolism activators we try to obtain a kind of squeezing of the adipocytes, with an increase of circulating fatty acids that need to be used in order to obtain a positive anti-cellulite result. Consequently moderate physical exercise is a necessary factor to obtain important results, thanks to its direct effect on the caloric and lipidic consumption, but also to optimize the effectiveness of the cosmeceutical treatments both systemic (supplements) and topic.

Finally the cellulite improvement is noted also through the improvement of cutaneous aspect of the areas with cellulite. The complexion colour, the cutaneous elasticity and a better hydration can be obtained by polyunsaturated fatty acids oils and mainly by omega-3 (fish oil, borage, flax and wheat germs).

Omega-3

The fatty acids of the series omega-3 are normally present in seafood, in certain plants and also in a number of animal products such as chicken, turkey and eggs. Alpha-linolenic acid is the omega 3 fatty acid most extensively found in the vegetable world. This fatty acid has to be transformed into EPA and DHA in order to exercise those biological effects that we now know are essential for the correct functioning of certain organs and elements like the brain, retina and gonads, and that are protective against atherosclerosis and cardio-vascular disease. Alpha-lineolenic acid can be obtained in plants in higher quantities than linoleic acid, through a synthesis in the membrane of the chloroplasts, which is not possible in the animal world. EPA and DHA are present in phytoplankton and are concentrated in particular in a number of species of fish, especially those that live in cold waters.

Omega-6

The most significant acids of the omega-6 series are linoleic acid, gamma-linolenic acid, dihomo gamma-linolenic acid and arachidonic acid. The most widespread is linoleic acid which is predominant in seed oils; arachidonic acid is typical of the animal world, as it is a product of the conversion of linoleic acid; gamma-linolenic acid is the first intermediate step in the conversion of linoleic acid into arachidonic acid [76]; dihomo gamma-linolenic acid is difficult to find because of its high metabolic turnover of transformation into prostaglandin 1. Though the metabolic conversion of gamma-linolenic acid is typical of the animal world, significant quantities can also be found in several plants: Oenothera biennis, Boragob officinalis, Ribes nigrum, Mucorjavanicus (a fungus).

The biological role of omega-3 fatty acids

The long-chain polyunsaturated fatty acids of the omega-3 series can have a structural and functional role, especially EPA and DHA. DHA (22:6 omega-3) have a prevalently structural activity in the organism. It is represented, in particular, in the phospholipids of cerebral synaptosomes, in the retina and in the phospholipids of the intramembranary channels of sodium. DHA seems to be particularly important in the development and maturation of:

- the brain
- the reproductive organs
- the retina

EPA performs its prevailing action as the direct precursor of the prostaglandins of the series 3, which inhibit platelet aggregation. There is some evidence that the consumption of omega-3 fatty acids has important preventive and therapeutic effects.

Synthesis of the Main Action of Omega-3 Fatty Acids

The main actions of the omega-3 fatty acids (anti-atherogenetic, anti-inflammatory, anti-thrombotic action) depend on the prevalence of the protective factors over those causing the risk (see Fig. 8.7).

The functional activity of the omega-3 fatty acids on the cardio-vascular system reduces:

platelet aggregation
arterial blood pressure and the vasospastic response to vaso-constrictors, the linkage of albumin in type 1 diabetes
cardiac arrhythmia
hyperplasia of the blood vessels and hematic viscosity

It increases:

platelet survival
bleeding time
arterial vascular compliance and the function of the cardiac beta-receptors
coronary post-ischemic flow

The Biological Role of Omega-6 Fatty Acids

The long-chain polyunsaturated fatty acids of the omega-6 series can have either structural or functional roles. Arachidonic acid is the one that performs, in the organism, a prevalently structural action. It is largely found in the membrane phospholipids and is important, when appropriately balanced with DHA, in embryo development and in the growth and development of children (see Fig. 8.8).

From the functional point of view, arachidonic acid produces prostaglandins of the series 2, which give rise to the formation of mediators with pro-inflammatory activity and, partially, platelet aggregation. DGLA produces prostaglandins of the series 1 with anti-inflammatory action and immune-modulators.

Table 8.3 The effects of omega-3 supplementation

Consumption of omega-3 fatty acids increases:
The formation of prostaglandin PGI3
The production of Leukotrienes B5 which are much less inflammatory than Leukotrienes B4
The production of interleukin 2 and production of EDRF (endothelial derived relaxing factor)
Fibrinolytic activity, deformation of erythrocytes and an increase of HDL.

Omega-6 fatty acids: Linoleic acid (C 18:2)

Arachidonic acid (C 20:4)

Alpha-linolenic acid (C 18:3)

Docosahexaenoic acid (DHA; C 22:6)

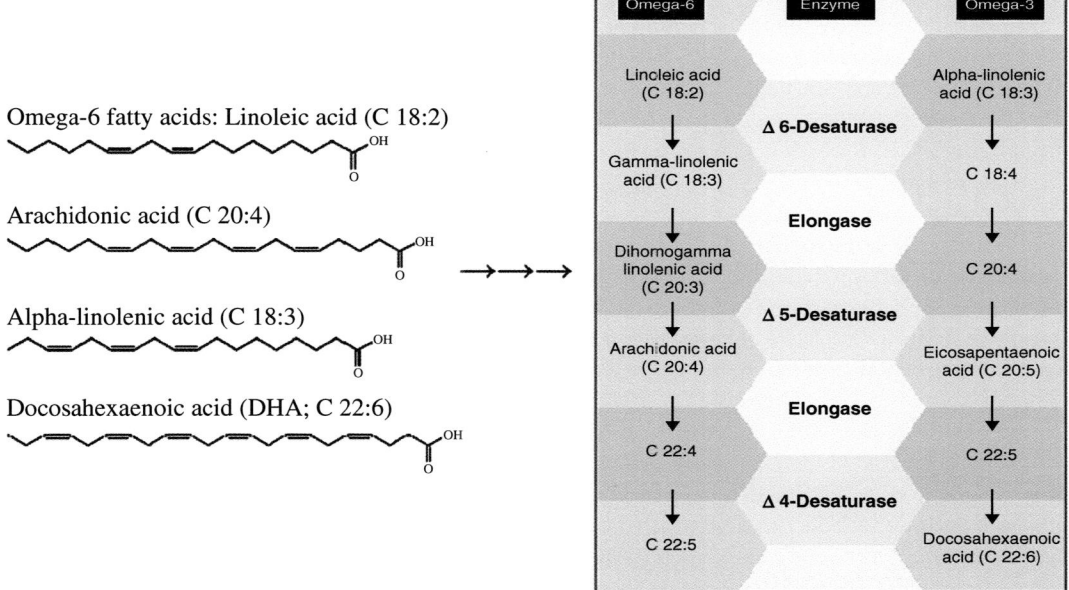

Figure 8.7 Polyunsaturated fatty acid pathway.

Synthesis of the Main Actions of Omega-6 Fatty Acids

Series 1 prostaglandins derive directly from DGLA. The conversion of DGLA into AA in humans is very slow and this testifies to the importance of PG1 in many tissues, such as the platelets, the immune system, the kidneys and the brain. In particular, PG1 prostaglandins possess a number of actions that make the biological availability of gamma-linolenic acid, and thus of DGLA, extremely important:

- vasodilation and reduction of arterial pressure
- inhibition of thrombosis
- increase of levels of cyclic AMP
- activation of the gamma lymphocytes for the prevention of liver damage by ethanol
- inhibition of abnormal proliferation

A blockage of the conversion from linoleic to gamma-linolenic acid causes a reduction in the synthesis of PG1. The reasons are the same as those described for the omega-3 fatty acids, as delta-5 desaturasis is common. When the formation of gamma-linolenic acid is reduced, it is possible to restore production of PG1 by administering this fatty acid directly. Arachidonic acid produces PG2 prostaglandins directly through the action of cyclo-oxigenasis. These have an important role in the process of platelet aggregation for the aggregating action of thromboxane

A1 (TXA2) and prostacyclin I2 (PGI2) with its anti-aggregating action. The leukotrienes are also formed from arachidonic acid through the activity of 5-lipooxigenase. These substances perform a bronco-constricting action and have characteristics similar to those that are triggered during the anaphylactic process, particularly SRSA (Slow Reacting Substance of Anaphylaxis). In inflammatory processes there are high levels of free arachidonic acid and prostaglandins of the series 2. PG1 with hydroxy acid that is formed from DGLA and vitamin E perform a prevalently anti-inflammatory action. In line with what has been said about the main families of polyunsaturated fatty acids, the exogenous (dietetic) and endogenous (metabolic and hormonal) conditioning factors need to be considered very carefully, especially when the lipid supplementation concerns persons under conditions of severe metabolic stress [28,29,32].

Omega-3 Integration

As concerns omega-3 and cellulite therapy, their integration may be a great way to reduce the inflammatory state of subcutaneous fatty tissue and at the same time bring an overall improvement of body conditions.

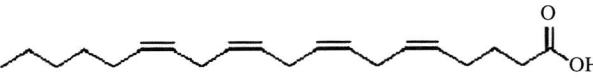

Arachidonic acid: three dimensional representation, top; chemical structure diagram, bottom. The molecule is a long chain of CH and CH2 units, terminated by the acid unit (COOH). There are 20 carbons in a linear chain that is folded as indicated in the 3-D respresentation

Figure 8.8 Stoichiometric structure of Arachidonic Acid.

Table 8.4 The effects of a diet poor in omega-3 fatty acids

Poor omega-3 intake increase:
production of arachidonic acid
platelet aggregation and the formation of thromboxane
macrophage function
formation of type 4 leukotrienes
the production of PAF (platelet activating factor)
production of interleukin 1; production of PDGF (platelet derived growth factor);
an increase in LDL, VLDL, triglycerides, fibrinogen and hematic viscosity.

The omega-3 is a powerful anti-inflammatory and can work on several levels, for example, it can cancel the transcription activity of nucleus like NFkappaB, or can reduce cytokines production like TNF-α (even if some researchers don't agree on this particle) and IL-1β [77].

Besides this omega-3 inhibits IL-6 which is a molecule involved in the inflammatory state of subcutaneous fatty tissue [78].

Supplementation of omega-3 in obese women during weight loss increases the postprandial surfeit sense and this is very important in compliance with the dietary process [79].

As concerns supplementation the recommended dose is 2.5 g per day – considering that 0.5 is the daily quantity taken with food. This value can be considered nominal as it's not valid for every subject.

In fact, in some inflammation cases with a high degree of intensity we can think to increase omega-3 quantity as well as decrease it in case of healthy weight women with a slender build (e.g. h 162 cm 48 kg). Omega-3 optimum intake can be evaluated by the fatty acids composition of blood; obtaining an AA/EPA ratio we can understand the inflammatory state of the patient. Omega-3 ideal result value is near three. Today the massive quantity of omega-3 supplements disarms both patient and doctor who has to prescribe them; in general molecular distillation, EPA and DPA quantity and fatty acids oxidation are good parameters for omega-3 evaluation.

Vitamin C

As concerns cellulite, considering all the assumptions which assert that it is related to an inflammatory state and also to adipose tissue storage level, may result in a very interesting correlation between vitamin C and fat tissue. It has been proved that vitamin C helps to reduce both inflammation and adipose tissue [80].

On a system level vitamin C facilitates iron absorption, chelating it or maintaining its level low (Fe 2+).

This effect can be achieved only if food contains vitamin C but the same meal could also contain iron absorption inhibitors such as phytates and pholiphenols [81–83].

Due to a major iron need during the menstrual period we can assume that an implementation of vitamin C in the woman can be useful both in inflammatory and overweight case that results in cellulite.

Besides that the association between bioflavionoidis and vitamin C is fundamental as in nature it has its better results in synergy with these phytocomplexes together with a good measure of vitamin E which helps to gain a great antioxidizing cover that reduces cell tissue lipoperoxidation and keeps inflammation processes under control.

Glycine Propionyl-L-Carnitine

Dietary supplementation with the naturally occurring nutrient L-carnitine has been extensively studied as an aid to improve fatty acid metabolism and aerobic exercise capacity, to provide antioxidant benefits, and to enhance blood flow to active tissues.

While multiple forms of carnitine have been the focus of ongoing scientific study over the past several decades, and several are currently available for retail sale, propionyl-L-carnitine (PLC) has been shown to provide an optimal vasodilatory effect to blood vessels, and to support healthy heart and skeletal muscle function.

Those affected by cellulite can benefit from use of GPLC to improve pathological conditions.

GPLC has significant effects on the organism and its integration as concerns subjects who practice sport, can fix the levels of acyl camitine in the muscle tissue and this brings fatty acids to optimization by mitochondria which can be very useful in a weight loss process accompanied by physical activity [84].

Carnitine is critical for the transport of activated long-chain fatty acids into the mitochondria of the cell. Increased fatty acid metabolism would result in the increased "burning" of fat as an energy source, leading to improvements in blood triglycerides, body fat, and energy levels. This is particularly true for individuals who may have problems in these specific areas, like women with cellulite disease.

GPLC stimulates blood flow in active muscles on a circulatory level and this is probably caused by the production of nitric oxide which acts in blood vessel dilation, allowing for enhanced blood flow. This flow augmentation brings about a decrease of the lipid oxydase [84].

This is of particular importance for individuals with compromised blood flow due to cardiovascular disease, as well as for athletes seeking to enhance blood flow to aid oxygen and nutrient delivery to working skeletal muscles during and following acute bouts of exercise, and also for the woman who wants to improve the cardiovascular flux in the adipose tissue [84].

Conclusion

As has already been described broadly, cellulite derives from genetic causes, but at the same time there are many environmental factors that let this pathology develop.

Actual studies show that the subcutaneous adipose tissue can not only increase in volume, break the optimal connection with the connective tissue and suffer an edema status, but it is also a tissue able to become inflamed and therefore subject to all those phenomena related to the irritation.

Nowadays the adipose tissue is called adipose organ, since it not only stores triglycerides, but it is also able to communicate with the outside through hormones and cytokines.

Recent studies have shown for instance that 1/3 of the IL-6 circulating comes from the adipose tissue, therefore the level is proportional to the quantity of available adipose tissue [6].

To plan a good medical therapy with the purpose of improving the pathological condition of the cellulite, means to act on different factors.

Of course the first important step that the patient should accomplish is a right diet.

Until a few years ago, but in some cases still nowadays, it was thought that a correct diet should be a low-calorie diet, and the primary goal was not a status of optimal health, but there was a disposition to create a caloric disequilibrium able to "to dry up" triglycerides from the adipose tissue.

Nowadays it is seen that in the majority of cases all this led up to a yo-yo effect, that subsequently damages the connective tissue, and at the same time it doesn't change the inflammatory state of the subcutaneous adipose tissue.

An evident example of this behavior is the use, by women who want to become thin, of crackers made of rice, a kind of food accounted as light, but at the same time with a very high glycemic index, therefore not able to manage the inflammation.

Table 8.5 Nutrition Tips

The goals of right nutrition are:

To introduce the subject to a correct diet, able to be maintained through the years
To choose food able to manage the inflammation
To manage the carbohydrates according to the glycemic index and to the load
To have 5 meals a day to better manage the insulin feedback
To introduce the right protein amount to avoid loss of thin mass
To daily introduce more vegetables and fruits
To introduce monounsaturated fat as olive oil, almonds, green olives, walnuts

---

Following a good diet means also managing to the best all the cases of malabsorption or intolerance, that attentively have to be monitored in the management of the diet of the patient.

The following step is to see if the subject needs integration and since the first factor to deal with is the inflammation, the integration with omega-3 is the first therapy to plan.

Afterwards we will consider an integration with bioflavonoides, the vitamin C and the glycine propionil-L-carnitine, according to the case, and to the needs of the patient.

In conclusion as it regards cellulite the medical therapy is behavioral to 70%, and integrative to 30 %.

With this we want to insist on the fact that to fight cellulite, as with any other chronic illness, we need to act on environmental factors such as the sedentary job, stress, physical activity, an appropriate diet, and then, on the integration that lately has been very important, since pollution and extreme urbanization are leading to food impoverishment and to a great presence of detrimental substances in all the things that we breathe or eat.

BIBLIOGRAPHY

1. LE Braverman, RD Utiger. The Thyroid. A Fundamental and Clinical Text. Eighth Edition. Lippincott Williams & Wilkins.
2. FS Greespan, DG Gardner. Basic & Clinical Endocrinology, 7 Edition, McGraw-Hill Medical.
3. F Distante, PA Bacci, M Carrera. Efficacy of a multifunctional plant complex in the treatment of the so-called 'cellulite': clinical and instrumental evaluation. Int J Cosmet Sci 28(3):191–206, Jun 2006.
4. TL Nielsen, C Hagen, K Wraae et al. Visceral and subcutaneous adipose tissue assessed by magnetic resonance imaging in relation to circulating androgens, sex hormone-binding globulin, and luteinizing hormone in young men. J Clin Endocrinol Metab 92(7):2696–705, Jul 2007. Epub 2007 Apr 10.
5. L Lionetti, MP Mollica, A Lombardi et al. From chronic overnutrition to insulin resistance: The role of fat-storing capacity and inflammation. Nutr Metab Cardiovasc Dis 24 Jan 2009.
6. V Mohamed-Ali, S Goodrick, A Rawesh et al. Interleukin-6 regulates pancreatic alpha-cell mass expansion. Proc Natl Acad Sci USA 2;105(35):13163–8, Sep 2008. Epub 2008 Aug 21.
7. H Ellingsgaard, JA Ehses, EB Hammar et al. Interleukin-6 regulates pancreatic alpha-cell mass expansion. Proc Natl Acad Sci USA 105(35):13163–8, 2 Sep 2008. Epub 2008 Aug 21.
8. BK Pedersen, M Febbraio. Muscle-derived interleukin-6—a possible link between skeletal muscle, adipose tissue, liver, and brain. Brain Behav Immun 19(5):371–6, Sep 2005.
9. MH Fonseca-Alaniz, J Takada, MI Alonso-Vale et al. Adipose tissue as an endocrine organ: from theory to practice. J Pediatr (Rio J) 83(5Suppl):S192–203, Nov 2007. Epub 2007 Nov 8.
10. A Green, SB D3obias, DJ Walters et al. Tumor necrosis factor increases the rate of lipolysis in primary cultures of adipocytes without altering levels of hormone-sensitive lipase. Endocrinology. 134:2581–88, 1994.
11. C Grunfeld, KR Feingold. Tumor necrosis factor, interleukin, and interferon induced changes in lipid metabolism as part of host defense. Proc Soc Exp Biol Med 200:224–27, 1992.
12. P Peraldi, GS Hotamisligil, WA Buurman et al. Tumor necrosis factor (TNF)-alpha inhibits insulin signaling through stimulation of the p55 TNF receptor and activation of sphingomyelinase. J Biol Chem 271:13018–22, 1996.
13. H Ruan, N Hacohen, TR Golub et al. Tumor necrosis factor-alpha suppresses adipocyte-specific genes and activates expression of preadipocyte genes in 3T3–L1 adipocytes: nuclear factorkappaB activation by TNF-alpha is obligatory. Diabetes 51:1319–36, 2002.
14. S Buscemi, R Manneri, A Dia Noto et al. Valutazione della composizione corporea in gruppi di soggetti con differente taglia corporea. Confronto tra metodica plicometrica ed impedeziometrica. Ann Ital Med Int 9:223, 1994.
15. SM Shetterly, JA Marshall, J Baxter et al. Waist-hip ratio measurement location influence association with measures of glucose and lipid metabolism. Ann Epidemiol 3:295, 1993.
16. FE Johnston, TA Wadden, AJ Stunkard. Body fat deposition in adult obese women. Pattern of fat distribution. Am J Clin Nutr 47:225, 1988.
17. M Rebuffè, Scrive, B Anderson, L Olbe et al. Metabolism of adipose tissue in intraabdominal depots in severely obese men and women. Metabolism 39:1021, 1990.
18. CM Rotella, V Ricca, E Mannucci. L'Obesità- Manuale per la diagnosi e la terapia. SEE-Firenze.
19. RF Kunshner, DA Schoeller. Estimation of total body water by bioelectrical impedance analysis. Am J Clin Nutr 44:417, 1986.
20. MS Westerterp-Plantenga, MP Lejeune, I Nijs et al. High protein intake sustains weight maintenance after body weight loss in humans. Int J Obes Relat Metab Disord 28(1):57–64, Jan 2004.
21. KJ Acheson, E Ravussin, J Wahren. Thermic effect of glucose in man. J Clin Invest 74:11, 1572, 1984.
22. AD D'Alessio, EC Kavle, KJ Smalley. Thermic effect of food in lean and obese men. J Clin Invest 81:6, 1781, 1988.
23. F Contaldo, M Mancini. Nutrizione Clinica. Gnocchi (ed.) 1995.
24. ME Valera Mora, A Scarfone, M Calvani et al. Insulin clearance in obesity. J Am Coll Nutr 22(6):487–93, Dec 2003.
25. JP Felber, KJ Acheson, L Tappy. From obesity to diabetes. J Wiley and Sons, Chichester, England; 1993.
26. L Pirola, AM Johnston, E Van Obberghen. Modulators of insulin action and their role in insulin resistance. Int J Obes Relat Metab Disord 27(Suppl 3):S61–4, Dec 2003.
27. RA Hegazi, K Sutton-Tyrrell, RW Evans et al. Relationship of adiposity to subclinical atherosclerosis in obese patients with type 2 diabetes. Obes Res 11(12):1597–605, Dec 2003.

28. H Xu, GT Barnes, Q Yang et al. Chronic inflammation in fat plays a crucial role in the development of obesity-related insulin resistance. J Clin Invest 112(12):1821–30, Dec 2003.

29. JR Sowers. Obesity as a cardiovascular risk factor. Am J Med 8;115(Suppl 8A):37S–41S, Dec 2003.

30. RW Nesto. The relation of insulin resistance syndromes to risk of cardiovascular disease. Rev Cardiovasc Med 4(Suppl 6): S11–8, 2003.

31. GM Reaven. The role of insulin resistance in human disease. Diabetes 37:1595, 1988.

32. WA Hsueh, TA Buchanan. Obesity and hypertension. Endocrinol Metab Clin North Am 23:405, 1994.

33. WA Hsueh, TA Buchanan. Obesity and hypertension. Endocrinol Metab Clin North Am 23:405, 1994.

34. GA Bray, CM Champagne. Obesity and the metabolic syndrome: Implications for dietetics practitioners. J Am Diet Assoc 104(1):86–9, Jan 2004.

35. C Turkoglu, BS Duman, D Gunay et al. Effect of abdominal obesity on insulin resistance and the components of the metabolic syndrome: evidence supporting obesity as the central feature. Obes Surg 13(5):699–705, Oct 2003.

36. M Baltali, A Gokcel, HT Kiziltan et al. Association between the metabolic syndrome and newly diagnosed coronary artery disease. Diabetes Nutr Metab 16(3):169–75, Jun 2003.

37. TL McLaughlin. Insulin resistance syndrome and obesity. Endocr Pract 9(Suppl 2):58–62, Sep-Oct 2003.

38. H Oflaz, N Ozbey, F Mantar et al. Determination of endothelial function and early atherosclerotic changes in healthy obese women. Diabetes Nutr Metab 16(3):176–81, Jun 2003.

39. MB Yilmaz, SF Biyikoglu, Y Akin et al. Obesity is associated with impaired coronary collateral vessel development. Int J Obes Relat Metab Disord 27(12):1541–5, Dec 2003.

40. MF White. Insulin signaling in health and disease. Science 302(5651):1710–1, 5 Dec 2003.

41. BV Howard, G Ruotolo, DC Robbins. Obesity and dyslipidemia. Endocrinol Metab Clin North Am 32(4):855–67, Dec 2003.

42. KE Watson, BN Horowitz, G Matson. Lipid abnormalities in insulin resistant states. Rev Cardiovasc Med 4(4): 228–36, Fall 2003.

43. AE Caballero. Endothelial dysfunction in obesity and insulin resistance: a road to diabetes and heart disease. Obes Res 11(11):1278–89, Nov 2003.

44. C Rattarasarn, R Leelawattana, S Soonthornpun et al. Regional abdominal fat distribution in lean and obese Thai type 2 diabetic women: relationships with insulin sensitivity and cardiovascular risk factors. Metabolism 52(11):1444–7, Nov 2003.

45. S Novak, LM Stapleton, JR Litaker et al. A confirmatory factor analysis evaluation of the coronary heart disease risk factors of metabolic syndrome with emphasis on the insulin resistance factor. Diabetes Obes Metab 5(6):388–96, Nov 2003.

46. GS Hotamisligil. Inflammatory pathways and insulin action. Int J Obes Relat Metab Disord 27(Suppl 3):S53–5, Dec 2003.

47. A Marette. Molecular mechanisms of inflammation in obesity-linked insulin resistance. Int J Obes Relat Metab Disord 27(Suppl 3):S46–8, Dec 2003.

48. P Dandona, A Aljada, A Bandyopadhyay. Inflammation: the link between insulin resistance, obesity and diabetes. Trends Immunol 25(1):4–7, Jan 2004.

49. L Di Renzo, A Bertoli, M Bigioni et al. Body composition and -174G/C interleukin-6 promoter gene polymorphism: association with progression of insulin resistance in normal weight obese syndrome. Curr Pharm Des 14(26):2699–706, 2008.

50. T McLaughlin, A Deng, O Gonzales et al. Insulin resistance is associated with a modest increase in inflammation in subcutaneous adipose tissue of moderately obese women. Diabetologia 51(12):2303–8, Dec 2008. Epub 2008 Sep 30.

51. T McLaughlin, A Deng, O Gonzales et al. Insulin resistance is associated with a modest increase in inflammation in subcutaneous adipose tissue of moderately obese women. Diabetologia 51(12):2303–8, Dec 2008. Epub 2008 Sep 30.

52. T You, BJ Nicklas. Chronic inflammation: role of adipose tissue and modulation by weight loss. Curr Diabetes Rev 2(1):29–37, Feb 2006.

53. Walter Willett, Meir Stampfer: Nuova piramide alimentare americana (Articolo tratto da FLORILEGIUM n° 5 - Attualità in tema di Prevenzione Nutrizionale delle Malattie Cardiovascolari); 2003.

54. R Pagano, C La Vecchia. Overweight and obesità in Italy 1990–1991. Int J Obesità 18:665,1994.

55. M Cairella, M Fumarola, G Marchini. Obesità e metabolismo energetico. Società ed. Universo, Roma; 1992.

56. CA Davis, P Britten, EF Myers. (USDA, Center for Nutrition Policy and Promotion, Alexandria, VA 22302, USA): Past, present, and future of the Food Guide Pyramid. J Am Diet Assoc 101(8):881–5, Aug 2001.

57. WC Willett, MJ Stampfer. Rebuilding the food pyramid. Sci Am 288(1):64–71, Jan 2003.

58. JM Kinney. The US Department of Agriculture Food Pyramid; the birth and aging of an idea. Curr Opin Clin Nutr Metab Care 6(1):9–13, Jan 2003.

59. MA Hess. Food guide pyramid stimulates debate. J Am Diet Assoc 95(3):297–8, Mar 1995.

60. C Willett Walter, M.D., Eat Drink and Be Healty, Simon & Schuster Source; 2001.

61. EL Fox, RW Bower, ML Fos. Nutrizione, esercizio e controllo del peso. Pensiero scientifico ed. Roma; 1995.

62. Kent HayGlass in "First Main Lecture of Vancouver 2003 World Allergy Congress".

63. H Sampson, Update on food allergy. J Allergy Clin Immunol 113(5):805–19, May 2004; quiz 820.

64. FD Finkelman. Anaphylaxis: lessons from mouse models. J Allergy Clin Immunol 120:506–15, 2007.

65. A Speciani. Le allergie. Cause, diagnosi e terapie. 2^ edizione, Tecniche Nuove ed., Milano; 2008.

66. A Speciani. e Speciani L., Diete di segnale e Dieta GIFT. Rizzoli ed. Milano; 2009.

67. M Zeyda, D Farmer, J Todoric et al. Human adipose tissue macrophages are of an anti-inflammatory phenotype but capable of excessive pro inflammatory mediator production. Int J Obes (Lond) 31(9):1420–8, Sep 2007. Epub 2007 Jun 26.

68. CH Larramendi, M Martin Esteban, C Pascual Marcos et al. Possible consequences of elimination diets in asymptomatic

immediate hypersensitivity to fish. JM Allergy, 47(5):490–4, Oct 1992.

69. J Barnes, LA Anderson, JD Phillipson. Herbal Medicine, A guide for healthcare professional, 2nd edition, Pharmaceutical Press; 2002.

70. CC Miller, W Tang, VA Ziboh, MP Fletcher. Dietary supplementation with ethyl ester concentrates of fish oil (n23) and borage oil (n26) polyunsaturated fatty acids induces epidermal generation of local putative antiinflammatory metabolites. J Invest Dermatol 96:98–103, 1991.

71. CC Miller, VA Ziboh, T Wong, MP Fletcher. Dietary supplementation with n23 and n26 enriched oils influences in vivo levels of epidermal lipoxygenase products. J Nutr 120:36–44, 1990.

72. CA Erdelmeier, J Cinatl, H Rabenau et al. Antiviral and antiphlogistic activities of Hamamelis virginiana bark. Planta Med 62:241–45, 1996.

73. SJ Taussig, SJ Batkin. Bromelain, the enzyme complex of pineapple (Ananas comosus) and its clinical application. An update. Ethnopharmacol 22(2):191–203, Feb-Mar 1988.

74. E Bouskela, FZ Cyrino, G Marcelon. Effect of Ruscus extract on the internal diameter of arterioles and venules of the hamster cheek pouch microcirculation. J Cardiovasc Pharmacol 22:221–24, 1993.

75. AB Rossi, AL Vergnanini. Cellulite: a review. J Eur Acad Dermatol Venereol 14(4):251–62, Jul 2000.

76. MF Linton, S Fazio. Macrophages, inflammation, and atherosclerosis. Int J Obes Relat Metab Disord 27(Suppl 3):S35–40, Dec 2003.

77. JX Kang, KH Weylandt. Modulation of inflammatory cytokines by omega-3 fatty acids. Subcell Biochem 49:133–43, 2008.

78. I Vedin, T Cederholm, Y Freund Levi et al. Effects of docosahexaenoic acid-rich n-3 fatty acid supplementation on cytokine release from blood mononuclear leukocytes: the OmegAD study. Am J Clin Nutr 87(6):1616–22, Jun 2008.

79. D Parra, A Ramel, N Bandarra et al. A diet rich in long chain omega-3 fatty acids modulates satiety in overweight and obese volunteers during weight loss. Appetite 51(3):676–80, Nov 2008. Epub 2008 Jun 14.

80. J Campión, FI Milagro, D Fernández et al. Vitamin C supplementation influences body fat mass and steroidogenesis-related genes when fed a high-fat diet. Int J Vitam Nutr Res 78(2):87–95, Mar 2008.

81. L Hallberg, M Brune, L Rossander-Hulthen. Is there a physiological role of vitamin C in iron absorption. Annals of the New York Academy of Sciences 498:324–32, 1987.

82. L Hallberg, L Rossander, H Persson, E Svahn. Deleterious effects of prolonged warming of meals on ascorbic acid content and iron absorption. Am J Clin Nutr 36(5):846–50, Nov 1982.

83. L Hallberg. Wheat fiber, phytates and iron absorption. Scandinavian Journal of Gastroenterology 129(Suppl.): S73–S79, 1987.

84. WA Smith, AC Fry, LC Tschume et al. Effect of glycine propionyl-L-carnitine on aerobic and anaerobic exercise performance. Int J Sport Nutr Exerc Metab 18(1):19–36, Feb 2008.

9 Topical Management of Cellulite

Doris Hexsel, Débora Zechmeister do Prado, and Mitchel P Goldman

Introduction

Cellulite is the unsightly skin dimpling that is frequently found on the thighs and buttocks of women. Approximately 85% of post-adolescent women have some degree of cellulite [1–3]. Many allegedly successful cosmetic and medical treatments show little effect in improving cellulite, and none have been shown to lead to its complete disappearance.

This chapter describes the role of topical agents to reduce the appearance of cellulite. Also, the effect of supplementary aids, such as occlusive garments, will be addressed. As the various therapies are presented, there will be a focus on how the therapy addresses current concepts of the origin and nature of cellulite.

Definition and Nature of Cellulite

The term "cellulite" is used in modern times to describe the dimpled or puckered skin of the posterior and lateral thighs and buttocks seen in many trim and overweight women. The appearance is often described to resemble the surface of an orange peel or that of cottage cheese. The condition is best described by Goldman as a normal physiologic state in post-adolescent women which maximizes adipose retention to ensure adequate caloric availability for pregnancy and lactation [4]. Adipose tissue is also essential for nutrition, energy, support, protection, and thermal insulation [5].

At the histological level, cellulite is the result of localized adipose deposits and edema within the subcutaneous tissue. In women, fascial bands of connective tissue are oriented longitudinally and extend from the dermis to the deep fascia. These bands form fibrous septa which segregate fat into channels resembling a down quilt or mattress, and the subcutaneous fat is projected superficially into the reticular and papillary dermis. As the fat layer expands, the perpendicular connective tissue remains fixed and anchored to the underlying tissue, creating a superficial puckered appearance of the skin [5–8]. Fatty acids are then believed to be modified through peroxidation by free radicals. These events are thought to contribute to the worsening of local microcirculation by disrupting venous and lymphatic drainage.

This skin phenomena is rarely found in men as the connective tissue in males is not normally arranged vertically, but rather in a criss-crossing pattern that is gender-typical for the skin of the thighs and buttocks [5,7].

Pathophysiologic Mechanisms of Cellulite

Hormones, specifically estrogens and androgens, are thought to influence the formation of cellulite. Estrogen is known to stimulate lipogenesis and inhibit lipolysis, resulting in adipocyte hypertrophy [9]. This may explain the onset of cellulite at puberty, the condition being more prevalent in females, and the exacerbation of cellulite with pregnancy, nursing, menstruation and estrogen therapy (oral contraceptive use and hormone replacement) [9]. The opposite seems true for men. From the limited number of studies involving men, it is hypothesized that the combination of gender-specific soft tissue histology at the cellulite-prone anatomic sites, with a relatively lower circulating estrogen level, may be responsible for the lower incidence of cellulite in males [10,11]. Although not proven, it is possible that circulating androgens may have an inhibitory effect on cellulite development by contributing to a different pattern of adipose tissue storage (that is, more truncal than on the buttocks and thighs).

Adipose tissue is vascular, leading to the theory that cellulite may worsen in predisposed areas where circulation and lymphatic drainage have been decreased, possibly due to local injury or inflammation. In response to impairment of microvascular circulation, there is increased microedema within the subcutaneous fat layer, causing further stress on surrounding connective tissue fibers and accentuation of skin irregularities [2,4]. Many of the currently accepted cellulite therapies target deficiencies in lymphatic drainage and microvascular circulation. The lipids within adipocytes are derived from plasma-circulating lipoproteins. In a dynamic process, the stored fat is hydrolyzed and eliminated again to the plasma as free fatty acids and glycerol. Various enzymes, including insulin and cyclic AMP participate in this process. In particular, triglyceride lipase is very important in the promotion of lipolysis. This enzyme is activated by adenylyl cyclase stimulation by means of an antagonist effect. This inhibitory process causes triacylglycerol hydrolysis and releases free fatty acids and glycerol into the interstitial space and plasma.

The surface of adipocytes have receptors that promote the storage of fat and lipogenesis, such as neuropeptide Y and peptide YY. Conversely, other surface receptors promote the elimination of fat and lipolysis, such as $\beta1$ and $\beta2$. Manipulation of these surface enzymes by topical medications is a new mechanism by which to control cellulite development.

Topical Management

When using topical treatments to reduce the appearance of cellulite, the concentration and pharmacokinetics of the active ingredients must be considered, as well as the nature of the vehicle. Vehicles can be in the form of gels, ointments, foams, creams and lotions, all of which aim to efficiently deliver active product to the skin layers and subcutaneous tissue. Factors that affect the clinical response to treatment are: 1) the interaction of the drug with the vehicle and the skin, 2) the method which the drug is applied, and 3) other biological and environmental factors [12–14]. Percutaneous absorption is a complex biological process, as skin is a multilayered biomembrane [15]. The main barrier to drug penetration is the stratum corneum, the cornified outermost layer of the epidermis.

Topical drugs may use two diffusion routes to penetrate normal intact skin: the appendageal route, that comprises transport via the sweat glands and the hair follicles, and the transepidermal route in which molecules cross the intact horny layer. The transepidermal route is composed by 2 micro-routes of entry, the transcellular (or intracellular) and the intercellular. The principal pathway taken by a drug is decided mainly by the partition coefficient (log K). Hydrophilic drugs partition preferentially into the intracellular domains, whereas lipophilic agents traverse the stratum corneum via the intercellular route. Most molecules pass the stratum corneum by both routes. However, the intercellular pathway is widely considered to provide the principal route and major barrier to the permeation of most drugs [16].

Formulations for topical use may include drug delivery systems or "skin enhancers", which significantly increase cutaneous penetration when included in the formulation. Skin enhancers can be chemical and physical promoters and also trandermal and vesicular systems. Chemical promoters such as common solvents (water, alcohol, methyl alkyl sulphoxide) or surfactants, causes modifications in the lipid bilayer structure and alteration of the vehicle/skin partitioning coefficient. Physical promoters such as massage, eletroporation, phonophoresis and iontophoresis are useful for ionic molecules, large molecular weight actives and substances with low potency. Transdermal systems have the ability to facilitate the administration of the exact dosage of active drugs in the site of action. Transdermal patchs tested in vitro showed adequated absorption of caffeine, theobromine and paulinea cupeana extract [17]. Skin enhancers may also be vesicular systems or colloidal carriers, such as liposomes, nanoemulsions, and solid-lipid nanoparticles, which, when attached to the active drug, increase their lipid solubility. Multivesicular emulsion systems involve the creation of a 2-phase, oil-in-water emulsion system that produces concentric multilamellar spheres of oil and water. By this novel percutaneous delivery system, active ingredients can be controlled-released from their respective layers upon application to the skin [18].

Topical anti-cellulite preparations can be divided into four major groups according to their proposed mechanism of action (See *Table 9.1*).

1. Agents that increase microvascular flow
   This includes most of the active ingredients in cellulite treatments. They are included to increase microvascular flow and lymphatic drainage, which is thought to play a role in cellulite pathogenesis.
2. Agents that reduce lipogenesis and promote lipolysis
   With the goal of reducing the size and volume of adipocytes, decreased tension on surrounding connective tissue is thought to decrease the clinical appearance of puckering.
3. Agents that restore the normal structure of the dermal and subcutaneous tissue
   By thickening the dermis or preventing fat herniation into superficial tissue, the appearance of cellulite may be reduced.
4. Agents that prevent or destroy free-radical formation
   It is believed that free radicals modify free fatty acids by peroxidation, contributing to the availability of lipids for cellulite formation. Free radicals may also damage elements of the microcirculation further assisting cellulite development.

The following discussion summarizes the current knowledge of individual and combination topical therapies used to reduce cellulite.

Table 9.1 Topical therapies for cellulite, based on proposed mechanism of action

Agents that increase microvascular flow
Ivy
Indian or horse chestnut (*Aesculus hippocastanum*)
Ginkgo biloba
Rutin
Pentoxyphilline
Butcher's broom (*Ruscus aculeatus*)
Asiatic centella
Silicum
Chofitol or artichoke (*Cynara scolimus*)
Common ivy (*Hedera helix*)
Ground ivy (*Glechoma hederaceae*)
Sweet clover (*Melilotus officinalis*)
Red grapes (*Vitis vinifera*)
Papaya (*Carica papaya*)
Pineapple (*Ananas sativus, Ananas comosus*)

Agents that reduce lipogenesis and promote lipolysis
Methylxanthines (theobromine, caffeine, aminophylline, theophylline)
Beta-adrenergic agonists (isoproterenol, adrenaline)
Alpha-adrenergic antagonists (yohimbine, piperoxan, phentolamine, dihydroergotamine)

Agents that restore the normal structure of the dermal and subcutaneous tissue
Retinol (vitamin A)
Ascorbic Acid (vitamin C)
Bladderwrack (*Fuccus vesiculosus*)

Agents that prevent or destroy free-radical formation
Alpha-tocopherol (vitamin E)
Ascorbic Acid (vitamin C)
Ginkgo biloba
Red grapes (*Vitis vinifera*)

Agents that Increase Microvascular Flow

Drugs which act on the microcirculation of the skin include the ivy and Indian chestnut vegetable extracts, which are rich in saponines, ginkgo biloba and rutin, which contain bioflavonoids. These compounds decrease capillary hyperpermeability and increase venous tone by stimulation of proline hydroxylase and inhibition of prostaglandin E$_2$ (PGE$_2$). These agents also decrease platelet aggregation, thereby inhibiting microthrombus formation. Studies using oscillometry, Duplex ultrasound, hemodynamic methods and capillaroscopy have demonstrated that ginkgo biloba extract is anti-edematous and improves venous return and arterial circulation [19,20]. This is accomplished by decreasing capillary hyperpermeability, and is employed as an active agent in many topical anti-cellulite formulations.

Ginkgo biloba is a member of the Ginkgoaceae family. The leaf extracts contain substances such as flavonoids (quercetin, campherol epicathecol derivates, etc.), biflavons (ginkgetin) and terpenes (ginkgolide B) among others [21]. *Ginkgo biloba* is used in the treatment of cellulite due to its several effects on peripheral circulation, such as reducing blood viscosity. The terpenes, especially ginkgolide B, inhibit the platelet-activating factor. They increase red blood cell deformability, diminish vascular permeability and improve vascular wall tone. These actions improve microcirculation.

The methylxanthine pentoxyphylline improves microcirculatory perfusion through its effect on hematological factors such as erythrocyte shape, platelet aggregation, and plasma fibrinogen concentration. It also has immunomodulatory activity. It has been utilized for peripheral vascular disease treatment with significant benefit. For the treatment of cellulite [22], it has been used transdermally together with other drugs, making its evaluation difficult.

Butcher's Broom (*Ruscus aculeatus*) is a potent venous vasoconstrictor and has the ability to diminish edema. It acts as an alpha-adrenergic receptor agonist of the smooth muscle of veins and therefore reduces vascular permeability. The main active ingredients are saponins, ruscogenin and neororuscogenina [23].

Asiatic centella extract both topically and systemically has been used for treating cellulite, demonstrating an effect on the microcirculation through capillaroscopy in patients with chronic venous insufficiency who were treated for venous ulcers [24]. Consisting of 40% asiaticosideo, 30% madecassic acid and 30% asiatic acid, topical and systemic asiatic centella has been shown to be harmless by toxicity tests. The compound also acts in vitro on fibroblasts, stimulating collagen and mucopolysaccharide synthesis. Asiatic centella also acts as an anti-inflammatory agent, which may be beneficial in protecting dermal and subcutaneous structures from inflammatory cell injury [21].

Silicum is a structural element of connective tissue which regulates and normalizes cellular metabolism and cellular division. In the microcirculation, it modifies venous capillary and lymphatic permeability and, in the fatty tissue it stimulates cAMP synthesis as well as triglyceride hydrolysis, likely activating adenyl cyclase in the cellular membrane [25].

Chofitol or artichoke (*Cynara scolimus*) is a member of Arteraceae family. Its principal active chemical constituents are numerous enzymes, cynarin, ascorbic acid, caffeoylquinic acid derivates and flavonoids. It has an anti-edema and diuretic effect, as well as a stimulating effect on the circulation [21].

Common ivy (*Hedera helix*) is a phytomedicine that grows in places with rich soil, sun or shade. The parts of the plant used are dried leaves and stems. The leaves have flavonoids, such as rutosid and rutinosid, and saponines, such as hederin, hederacosid and hederagenin [21,26]. The fruits have saponines, especially hederin, and the trunk has gomoresins and saponines. All saponins improve venous and lymphatic drainage and reduce edema. One of these compounds, hederin, also has an analgesic and anti-inflammatory effect. It has vasoconstrictor and antiexudative proprieties, and can also reduce capillary permeability. It increases circulation, and reduces inflammation.

Ground ivy (*Glechoma hederaceae*) contains flavonoids, triterpenoids and phenolic acids. It grows in moist soil in Europe, especially the Caucasus, and in North America [21].

Indian or horse chestnut (*Aesculus hippocastanum*) belongs to the Hippocastanaceae family. The seeds and the shells are used in the elaboration of the standard extract [27]. The active ingredients contained in the seeds are triterpenoid saponines, such as escin and aesculin, and flavones, coumarins, and tannins [27], with anti-inflammatory and anti-edema properties [28]. Escin is the principal component of horse chestnut, and it has the capacity to reduce lysosomatic enzyme activity by up to 30%, probably by stabilizing the cholesterol content of the lysosome membranes, thus reducing enzyme release and capillary permeability. The recommended concentration is 1–3%.

Sweet clover (*Melilotus officinalis*) is a plant from the Fabaceae family. The active ingredient is contained in the flowers and leaves. One of the components of this botanical extract is coumarin, which reduces lymphatic edema and diminishes capillary permeability [29]. It is usually recommended to patients with chronic venous insufficiency and lymphatic congestion, conditions. The recommended concentration is 2–5% [29].

Red grapes (*Vitis vinifera*) have procianidins that increase the permeability of lymphatic and micro-arterial vessels [29]. In topical products, the essential oil is used at a concentration of 2–7% [29].

The fruits and leaves of papaya (*Carica papaya)* and pineapple (*Ananas sativus, Ananas comosus*) have anti-inflammatory and anti-edema effects [30]. They contain the proteolytic enzymes papain and bromelain, respectively. These plants are originally from tropical America and were introduced to southern Florida. The recommended concentration is 2–5%.

Extracts from the fruits and leaves of pineapple (*Ananas sativus, Ananas comosus*) also stimulate lymphatic flow [31].

Two well known Brazillian plants, catuba (*Meliaceae*) and marapuama (*Olacaceae*) contain the bioflavonoid, rutin and tannins, saponins, alkaloids, behenic acid, and aromatic oils lupeol and flavalignans. It is believed that the synergistic effect acts as an antioxidant and stimulates the microcirculation to reduce the appearance of cellulite [32–37]. Forty-three women with moderate cellulite used this product for 60 days. There was a statistically significant reduction in waist, abdomen, upper thigh and leg circumference but not lower or medial thigh [38].

Agents that Reduce Lipogenesis and Promote Lipolysis

Drugs that have a lipolytic effect on adipose tissue include the methylxanthines (theobromine, caffeine, aminophylline and theophylline). These act through phosphodiesterase inhibition and are the most common active ingredients in commercial anti-cellulite formulations [39]. The most useful and safest methylxanthine is caffeine, normally used at a concentration of 1–2%. It offers good skin penetration, and is therefore rapidly absorbed with rapid action. Caffeine acts directly on adipocytes, promoting lipolysis, through the inhibition of phosphodiesterase by augmentation of cyclic adenosine monophosphate (cAMP) [40]. Methylxanthines all activate the enzyme triglyceride lipase and transform triglycerides into free acids and glycerol. Caffeine also has a stimulating effect on the cutaneous microcirculation. *Table 9.1* lists botanical sources of methylxanthines, extracts of which are very common in anti-cellulite agents.

Lupi et al. have published a clinical study using a 7% caffeine solution (Elancyl® ChronoActive) on 134 women with cellulite of which 99 completed the study [41]. Patients applied the medication for 30 days to one leg (thigh and hip) twice a day with the other leg serving as a control. Patients thigh circumference were measured. Patients were also evaluated with orthogonal polarization spectral imaging (OPS) to evaluate functional capillary density (FCD) that increases in proportion to the reduction in interstitial edema, the measurement of the diameter of dermal papilla (DPD) which decreases when edema decreases and capillary diameter (CD) which also increases with reduction in edema. There was no statistically significant difference in any of the OPS measurements but the circumferential measurements of the thigh showed a mean reduction of 2.1 cm in over 80% of treated patients.

This outcome may suggest that a 30 day treatment while showing a modest improvement in thigh diameter is not adequate to effect a significant change in intercellular edema and microcirculation.

A histological evaluation was performed on 20 Wistar female mice to determine the effect caffeine and siloxanetriol (a caffeine derivative [SAC]) on fatty tissue [42]. Mice were either treated with an emulsion or gel formulation of caffeine 4% or caffeine 4% + sodium benzoate 4% or SAC 6% for 21 days. Caffeine emulsion caused a 17% reduction of adiposity cell diameter. Caffeine + sodium benzoate emulsion did not produce any cell diameter differences. The SAC emulsion reduced adipocit diameter by 16% and reduced adipocit number by 32%. Thus, in the mice adipocit model, caffeine and a caffeine derivative (SAC) demonstrate a histologic effect on fat cell diameter and number which may explain some of the clinically beneficial effects of topical cellulite therapy which contain caffeine.

Beta-adrenergic agonists such as isoproterenol and adrenaline, and alpha-adrenergic antagonists such as yohimbine, piperoxan, phentolamine and dihydroergotamine have also shown the ability to cause lipolysis. In vitro studies have shown that both the methylxanthines and beta-adrenergic agonists stimulate lipolysis and a reduction in adipocyte size through an increase in cAMP inhibition of phosphodiesterase [43,44].

Greenway and Bray demonstrated a statistically significant reduction in the anthropometric measurement of the medial thigh by a double-blind placebo-controlled study which utilized topical isoproterenol (a beta-adrenergic agonist), aminophylline (a methylxanthine with phosphodiesterase inhibitory properties), and yohimbine (an alpha-adrenergic antagonist) [45]. The reduction in thigh measurement was greatest when all active drugs were used together, three to five times a week for four weeks' duration. Of the three agents used separately, the best results were obtained by aminophylline.

The effects of methylxanthines can be enhanced by coenzyme A and the amino acid L-carnitine [25]. These agents work by stimulating the mobilization and destruction of free fatty acids and inducing their active transport through the membranes of mitochondria. This is important as free fatty acids may cause saturation of the system, leading to negative feedback of lipolysis. Also, the mobilization and destruction process of free fatty acids generates adenosine triphosphate (ATP), which increases lipase activity, enhancing hydrolytic breakdown of triglycerides.

Yohimbe (Corynanth yohimbe, Pausinystalia yohimbe and Rauwolfia serpentine) and alpha-yohimbe are alkaloid derivatives extracted from the leaves, shell and roots of Rubiaceas and Apocynaceas [21]. They are adrenergic blockers, capable of stimulating the catabolism of fat, due to the presence of alkaloids that act directly on the fat cells [21].

Agents that Restore the Normal Structure of the Dermal and Subcutaneous Tissue

Retinol (vitamin A) and the retinoids have been evaluated for their effectiveness in the treatment of cellulite. Topical retinoic acid and related vitamin A derivatives have been used to stimulate circulation, decrease the size of adipocytes, and increase collagen deposition in the dermis [9,46]. Based on the capacity of all-trans-retinoic acid (tretinoin) to promote the synthesis of glycosaminoglycans in normal skin and increase the deposition

of collagen in the photodamaged dermis, Kligman et al. proposed the use of topical retinol to improve cellulite [46]. The premise for its use in cellulite treatment is to increase the thickness and firmness of the dermis, minimizing the herniation of superficial fat. Retinol was proposed instead of tretinoin due to its better tolerability and evidence that retinol is metabolized to retinoic acid in the skin. In Kligman's study, 19 patients completed a study of retinol 0.3% versus placebo applied to opposite lateral thighs twice daily for six months duration. Twelve of the 19 patients demonstrated greater clinical improvement on the actively treated side by clinical evaluation and laser Doppler velocimetry.

Pierard-Franchimont et al. demonstrated that topical retinol treatment may improve the tensile properties of skin in a beneficial way for cellulite [47]. In a randomized, placebo-controlled study combining retinol with gentle massage, skin elasticity was increased by 10.7% while viscosity was decreased by 15.8% at retinol-treated sites. The main retinol-related change consisted of a two- to five-fold increase in the number of factor XIIIa+ dendrocytes both in the dermis and fibrous strands of the hypodermis. This indicates increased skin firmness and smoothened appearance of the surface. In addition, vitamin C may help by stabilizing collagen and/or stimulating collagen deposition [3,4,9].

Bladderwrack (Fuccus vesiculosus) is a brown marine algae that contains sulfated polysaccharides, iodine compounds and alginic acid. It is reported to produce contraction of the dermal connective tissue through the increased expression of integrin molecules [21]. Increased dermal density is the likely mechanism by which this agent improves cellulite. It also has a stimulating effect on vascular flow.

Agents that Prevent or Destroy Free-Radical Formation

Vitamins such as ascorbic acid and vitamin E may work as antioxidants, protecting dermal and subcutaneous cell membranes from free radical toxicity. This in turn may prevent and allow for repair of fat herniation. Also, certain vitamins may improve microcirculation.

Ginkgo biloba also has flavonoids which act as antioxidant and anti-inflammatory agents [21].

Red grapes (Vitis vinifera) are rich in tannins, that are antioxidants that diminish lipid peroxidation [29].

Combination Agents

Most topical cellulite therapy consists of agents that contain multiple active ingredients. In addition to providing different mechanisms of action directed to the same goal of reducing cellulite, the different constituents may work synergistically to yield results better than each component alone. Unfortunately, there are very few good studies in the literature that document the use of these combination products.

Bertin et al. performed a double-blind evaluation of an anticellulite product, and showed it to be more effective than placebo in reducing cellulite [48]. This product combines retinol with a microencapsulated time release mechanism to treat cellulite. The compound also contains caffeine to stimulate the lipolysis and prevent fat accumulation, esculoside to improve local microcirculation, asiatic centella as an anti-inflammatory, and L-carnitine to stimulate free fatty acid transport and breakdown. Efficacy parameters included cellulite appearance before and after treatment, histology, cutaneous flowmetry and skin mechanical characteristics. As mentioned, retinol has been shown to increase dermal thickness. The product also contains ruscogenine, which inhibits elastase activity, allowing recovery of extracellular matrix integrity that contributes to thickening of the dermis and masking of cellulite.

In a multicenter, randomized, placebo-control trial testing a combination anti-cellulite cream, subjects applied cream on a nightly basis with occlusion on one posterolateral thigh. Overall, 62% (21/34) noticed an improvement in their cellulite, with 62% (13/21) reporting greater improvement in the thigh that received active product. The average measured decrease in thigh circumference was 1.9 cm (range: 0.1 – 4.5) with active product, and 1.3 cm (range: 0.1 – 3.0) with placebo. Upon review of the pre- and post-study photographs, dermatologist evaluators found thighs treated with active product to show greater improvement than thighs treated with placebo in 68% of subjects. This product contained several active ingredients, including caffeine, green tea extract, black pepper seed extract, citrus extract, ginger root extract, cinnamon bark extract and capsicum annum resin [49].

A novel agent named *Bio-actif* consists of a compound containing neuropeptide Y and peptide YY [50]. These agents are known to participate in the metabolism of fat with lipogenic effects on adipocytes. *Bio-actif* is a topical gel of these neuropeptides, combined with green tea, ivy, aloe vera, wheat protein and other agents, and was shown to decrease fat herniation responsible for the appearance of cellulite.

External Aids to Topical Therapy

Supplemental techniques such as massage and warmth have been shown to assist in topical medication delivery into the skin and further reduce the appearance of cellulite [47]. Goldman describes the use of a synthetic bioceramic-coated neoprene garment to stimulate lymphatic and vascular flow that assisted to improve cellulite [51]. This is depicted in Fig. 9.1.

A double-blinded randomized placebo-controlled trial examined the effect of this same garment for the treatment of cellulite [52]. In this study, 17 subjects were evaluated for cellulite reduction using an anti-cellulite cream and occlusive garment on only one thigh. Four weeks later, 76% of subjects noticed an improvement in their cellulite, with 54% reporting greater improvement in the thigh that received garment occlusion. Average thigh circumference reduction was 1.3 cm in the occluded thigh, and 1.1 cm in the non-occluded thigh. Dermatologist evaluators found an overall improvement in cellulite in 65% of treated legs with occlusion and 59% of treated legs without occlusion. Furthermore, the evaluators found the occluded thighs to show greater improvement than the non-occluded thighs in 65% of subjects. This study demonstrated that although modest, occlusion by compression garments is beneficial in assisting topical agents to improve cellulite. In addition to potentiating topical drug delivery through occlusion, the warmth created by the garment likely improves microcirculation, which may be an etiological factor in cellulite development.

Adverse Events

Physicians need to be informed about the great range in efficacy among purported treatments for cellulite, if for no other reason than to avoid untested products. Sainio et al. investigated 32 anti-cellulite products, mostly botanicals and emollients, each

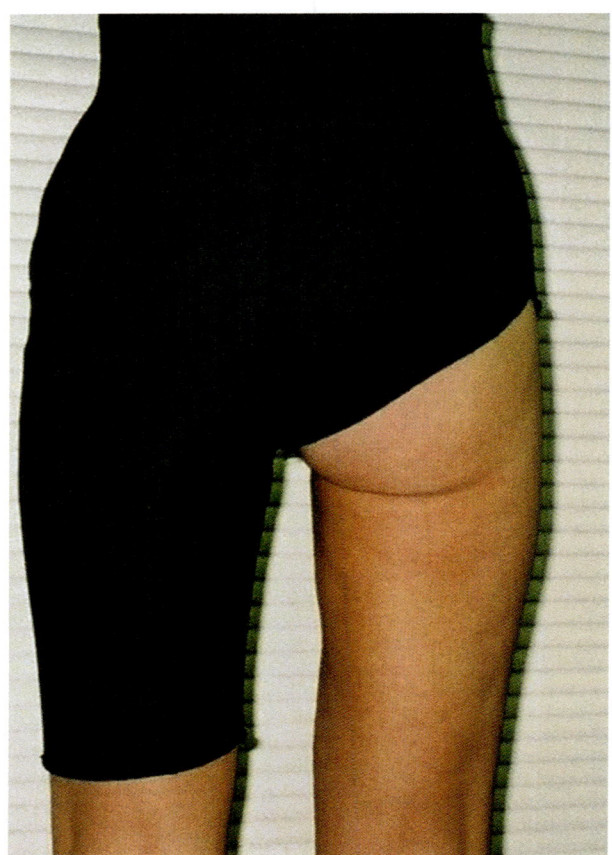

Figure 9.1 Bioceramic-coated neoprene shorts, worn after topical application of an anti-cellulite product to the posterior and lateral thighs to provide greater penetration into the skin by occlusion.

containing an average of 22 ingredients [3]. It was found that one fourth of the substances used have been shown to cause allergy, including isothiazolinones and dibromoglutaronitril. This indicates that despite the fact that most topical cellulite therapies are acceptably safe to many consumers, the risk of adverse events should be taken into account.

There are some reports in the literature of cases of hypersensitivity to ginkgo contained in anti-cellulite products [3]. There are also citings of allergic reactions in patients that used topical products containing ivy [3]. The leaves of this plant are considered poisonous when ingested, as they contain arsenic oxide. Hypersensitivity has been reported in users of products containing escin, the principal component of horse chestnut [53]. Cases of contact dermatitis on the hands have been reported, resulting from squeezing the fruit to obtain juice, which contains several acids such as oxalic, malic, tartaric and racemic [31].

Conclusion

The multifactorial etiology and nature of cellulite makes it a particularly difficult condition to treat. To better serve patients, the search for a complete cure to cellulite should be avoided. Rather, the aim of treatment should be to minimize the physical aspects of cellulite and prevent its progression by safe, cost-effective means. Topical treatments may improve the appearance of cellulite and represent a reasonable, affordable modality to reduce the severity of this unwanted condition. It is also reasonable to speculate that many of these products may have a role as a preventive measure. The supplemental use of external aids such as compressive bandages or garments to combine the effects of compression and enhanced penetration of topical agents has shown to be useful.

REFERENCES

1. ZD Draelos, KD Marenus. Cellulite – etiology and purported treatment. Dermatol Surg 23:1177–81, 1997.
2. Cellulite meltdown. Harv Health Pub Group 5:7, 1998.
3. EL Sainio, T Rantanen, L Kanerva. Ingredients and safety of cellulite creams. Europ J Derm 10:596–603, 2000.
4. MP Goldman. Cellulite: A review of current treatments. Cosmet Derm 15:17–20, 2002.
5. B Querleux, C Cornillon, O Jolivet et al. Anatomy and physiology of subcutaneous adipose tissue by in vivo magnetic resonance imaging and spectroscopy: relationships with sex and presence of cellulite. Skin Res Technol 8:118–24, 2002.
6. Another cellulite remedy. Harv Health Pub Group 6:7, 1999.
7. GE Pierard, JL Nizet, C Pierard-Franchimont. Cellulite: from standing fat herniation to hypodermal stretch marks. Am J Dermatopathol 22:34–47, 2000.
8. F Pellicier, P Andre, S Schnebert. The adipocyte in the history of slimming agents. Pathol Biol 51:244–47, 2003.
9. ABR Rossi, AL Vergnanini. Cellulite: a review. J Eur Acad Dermatol Venereal 14:251–62, 2000.
10. F Nürnberger, G Müller. So-called cellulite: an invented disease. J Dermatol Surg Oncol 4:221–29, 1978.
11. M Rosenbaum, V Prieto, J Hellmer et al. An exploratory investigation of the morphology and biochemistry of cellulite. Plast Reconstr Surg 101:1934–39, 1998.
12. WJ Addicks, ND Weiner, RL Curl et al. Drug delivery from topical formulations: theoretical prediction and experimental assessment. In: J Hadgraft, RH Guy, editors. Transdermal drug delivery: developmental issues and research initiatives. Marcel Dekkar, New York; 1989: 221–24.
13. J Hadgraft. Skin penetration enhancement. In: J Hadgraft, KA Walters, editors. Predication of percutaneous penetration. Marcel Dekkar, New York; 1993: 138–48.
14. JE Riviere. Biological factors in absorption and permeation. In: JL Zatz. Skin permeation: fundamentals and application. Allured Publishing Corporation, Wheaton; 1993: 113–25.
15. R Wester, HI Maibach. Cosmetic percutaneous absorption. In: R Baran, HI Maibach. Textbook of Cosmetic Dermatology. 3rd ed. Taylor&Francis, United Kingdom; 2006: 41–47.
16. R Daniels. Strategies for Skin Penetration Enhancement. Skin Care Forum 37;2004: In: www.scf-online.com, accessed on: 22th Dec, 2008.
17. CM Heard, S Johnson, G Moss et al. In vitro transdermal delivery of caffeine, theobromine, theophylline and catechin from extract of Guarana, Paullinia Cupana. Int J Pharm 6;317(1):26–31, Jul 2006.
18. J Bikowski, B Shroot. Multivesicular emulsion: a novel, controlled-release delivery system for topical dermatological agents. J Drugs Dermatol 5(10):942–6, 2006.
19. M August, F Clostre. Effects of an extract of ginkgo biloba and diverse substances on the phasic and tonic components of the contraction of an isolated rabbit aorta. Gen Pharmac 14:277–85, 1983.
20. U Bauer. Six-month double-blind randomized clinical trial of ginkgo biloba extract versus placebo in two parallel groups in patients suffering from peripheral arterial insufficiency. Arznein Forsch 34:716–23, 1984.
21. FS Amelio. Botanicals: A Phytocosmetic Desk Reference. CRC Press, Boca Raton, London, New York, Washington, DC, 1999.
22. CP Samlaska, EA Winfield. Pentoxifylline. J Am Acad Dermatol 30:603–21, 1994.
23. G Rubanyi, G Marcelon, PM Vanhoutte. Effect of temperature on the responsiveness of cutaneous elicited by Ruscus aculeatus. Gen Pharmacol 15(5):431–4, 1984.
24. JC Lawrence. The morphological and pharmacological effects of asiaticoside upon skin in vitro and in vivo. J C Europ J Pharmacol 1:414–24, 1967.
25. RM di Salvo. Controlling the appearance of cellulite: surveying the cellulite reduction effectiveness of xanthines, silanes, CoA, L-carnitine and herbal extracts. Cosm Toil 110:50–59, 1995.
26. M Carini, FR Maffei, A Brambills et al. Anti-hyaluronidase and anti-elastase activity of saponins from Hedera helix, Aesculus hippocastanum and Ruscus aculeatus: an explanation of their efficacy in the cosmetic treatment of liposclerosis. Phyto Pharm 36:613–23, 1998.
27. H Fluck. Medicinal plants, W. Foulsham & Co, New York; 1988.
28. RF Weiss. Herbal Medicine. Lehrbuch der Phytotherapie by A.R. Meuss, 6th German edition. The Bath Press, London; 1986.
29. Manufacture information - Croda (Crodarom S.A.), Croda International Ilc, Yorkshire, UK; 2002.
30. K Van Rietschoten. Plants with anti-inflammatory action. The British Journal of Aromatherapy Vol. 1. Autumn/Winter 1990.
31. PN Behl, RM Capitanin, BMS Bedi et al. Skin irritant sensitizing plants found in India. P. N. Behl, New Delhi; 1966.
32. A Rolim, T Oishi, CPM Maciel et al. Total flavonoids quantification from O/W emulsion with extract of Brazilian plants. Int J Pharm 308:107–14, 2006.
33. AR Baby, CPM Maciel, TM Kaneko et al. UV spectrophotometric determination of bioflavonoids from a semisolid pharmaceutical dosage form containing *Trichilia catigua* Adr. Juss (and) *Ptychopetalum olacoides* Bentham standardized extract: analytical method validation and statistical procedures. J AOAC Int 89:1532–37, 2006.
34. LA Souza, IS Moscheta, KSM Mourão et al. Morphology and anatomy of the flowers of *Trichilia catigua* A Juss, *T elegans*, A Juss and *T. pallid* Sw (Meliaceae). Braz Arch Biol Technol 44:383–94, 2001.
35. SE Drewes, J George, F Khan. Recent findings on natural products with erectile-dysfunction activity. Phytochemistry 62:1019–25, 2003.
36. IR Siqueira, C Fochesatto, AL Silva et al. *Ptychopetalum olacoides*, a traditional Amazon "nerve tonic", possesses anticholinesterase activity. Pharmacol, Biochem Behav 75: 645–50, 2003.
37. AR Baby, KF Migliato, CPM Maciel et al. Accelerated chemical stability data of O/W fluid emulsion containing the

extract of Trichilia catigua Adr. Juss (and) Ptychopetalum olacoides Bentham. Rev Bras Cienc Farm 43:405–12, 2007.

38. Anticellulite efficacy of an exotic botanical extract:Anthropometric measurements and statistical procedures. J Cosme Dermatol 2009 (in press).

39. N Collis, LA Elliot, C Sharpe et al. Cellulite treatment: a myth of reality: a prospective randomized, controlled trial of two therapies, Endermologie and aminophylline cream. Plast Reconstr Surg 104:1110–14, 1999.

40. G Potard, C Laugel, A Baillet et al. Quantitative HPLC analysis of sunscreens and caffeine during in vitro percutaneous penetration studies. Int J Pharm 5;189(2):249–60, 1999.

41. O Lupi, IJ Semenovitch, C Treu et al. Evaluation of the effects of caffeine in the microcirculation and edema on the thighs and buttocks using the orthogonal polarization spectral imaging and clinical parameters. J Cosm Dermatol 6:102–07, 2007.

42. MV Velasco, CT Tano, GM Machado-Santelli et al. Effects of caffeine and siloxanetriol alginate caffeine, as anticellulite agents, on fatty tissue: histological evaluation. J Cosmet Dermatol 7(1):23–9, 2008.

43. U Smith, J Hammersten, P Bjorntorp et al. Regional differences and effect of weight reduction on human fat cell metabolism. Eur J Clin Invest 9:327–32, 1979.

44. HJ Motulsky, RA Insel. Adrenergic receptors in man: direct identification, physiologic regulation and clinical alterations. New Engl J Med 308:18–29, 1982.

45. FL Greenway, GA Bray. Regional fat loss from the thigh in obese women after adrenergic modulation. Clin Therap 9: 663–69, 1987.

46. AM Kligman, A Pagnoni, T Stoudemayer. Topical retinol improves cellulite. J Dermatol Treat 10:119–25, 1999.

47. C Pierard-Franchimont, GE Pierard, F Henry et al. A randomized, placebo-controlled trial of topical retinol in the treatment of cellulite. Am J Clin Dermatol 1:369–74, 2000.

48. C Bertin, H Zunino, JC Pittet et al. A double-blind evaluation of the activity of an anti-cellulite product containing retinol, caffeine, and ruscogenine by a combination of several non-invasive methods. J Cosmet Sci 52:199–210, 2001.

49. J Rao, MH Gold, MP Goldman. A two-center, double-blinded, randomized trial testing the tolerability and efficacy of a novel therapeutic agent for cellulite reduction. Am J Cosm Surg 4:93–102, 2005.

50. E Hernández-Pérez, M Aristimuno, M Lemm, JA Cortes: The Bio-actif a/Y in the treatment of cellulite Am J Cosm Surg 19:117–121, 2002.

51. MP Goldman. Cellulite: A review of current treatments. Cosm Dermatol 15:17–20, 2002.

52. J Rao, KE Paabo, MP Goldman. A double-blinded randomized trial testing the tolerability and efficacy of a novel topical agent with and without occlusion for the treatment of cellulite: A study and review of the literature. J Drugs Dermatol 3:417–25, 2004.

53. JS Comaish, PJ Kersey. Contact dermatitis to extract of horse chestnut (esculin). Cont Derm 6:150–1, 1980.

10 Golden Lift® in the Management of Cellulite
A New Member from the Golden Peel® Family

José Enrique Hernández-Pérez, Mauricio Hernández-Pérez, and Enrique Hernández-Pérez

Abstract
Treatment of cellulite constitutes a challenge for dermatologists. We are showing good results for this condition in 30 women after only five sessions of Golden Lift®, which is a modification of Golden Peel Plus® (Jessner's solution plus 53% resorcin and 10% glycolic acid). Assessment was made through subjective evaluation, photographs, circumferencial measurements, and ultrasonographic evaluation. "T" Test in before and after cases showed a statistically significant improvement: $P < 0.01$

Introduction
Cellulite is synonymous with edematous panniculopathy, fibrosclerosis and genetic lipodystrophy. It is seen especially in females and very rarely in males. The areas most commonly affected are the outer thighs and gluteal region [1,2]. "Orange peel aspect" of the skin is the term most commonly used by patients to describe cellulite. Its diagnosis is easy, but treatment is difficult and often disappointing. A number of local and non-surgical treatments have been used, among them caffeine, theophylline, aminophylline, lactic acid, tretinoin, botanic extract mixtures, neuropeptide Y and peptide YY, as well as bio-actif alpha and Y, either alone or in combination, with variable results [4–6]. Cellulite does not respond easily to body weight loss [7]. Massage and skin kneading known as endermologie, open surgery and superficial liposuction have also been used, with uneven results [3–7]. Subcision, a procedure popularized worldwide by Doris Hexsel, has also been used with very good results. It is fully explained in other chapters of this book.

The Golden Peel® Family
For many years we have been using the formulas developed by us known as Golden Peel® [8–12]. The basic ones are composed of 24% resorcinol (the soft one) and 53% resorcinol (the strong one). They were used with good results in problems related to photoaging and scars, mostly secondary to acne. The results obtained were dependent upon resorcin concentration and the contact time with the skin [8,10,12]. In an attempt to increase its penetration, decreasing at the same time its skin contact time, we made some modifications: by applying Jessner's solution before the strong formulation, we achieved our aim. This modality was named Golden Peel Plus®; the last one had very nice results with shorter application time. Used this way the penetration of the peel reaches to the upper reticular dermis, becoming a medium-depth chemical peel [9]. Later on we made another modification: by adding 5% tretinoin to the strong formula, and using it as described for the Golden Peel Plus®, we developed a formulation very effective in the treatment of striae distensae (Golden Stretch®) [12]. Finally, when instead of tretinoin we added 10% glycolic acid to the strong formula, we have a lifting effect which is very useful in the treatment of cellulite (Golden Lift®), as well as in the breasts and buttocks lifting [12]. The treatment of cellulite through the use of Golden Lift®, will be the purpose of this chapter.

The Active Principle and Mode of Action
Resorcin, resorcinol, or m-dihydroxi-benzene is a phenol derivative possessing keratolytic properties, precipitating cutaneous proteins [8]. It is soluble in water, alcohol, ether, and oil, having great affinity for oxygen, and acts as an effective reducing agent [8,9]. Resorcin is a solid colorless water-soluble agent, with a slightly acidic reaction. It is a mild reducing agent, being obtained from the phenyl m-disulphonic ($C^5 H^4 (SO^3 H)^2$ blending with caustic sodium. It is also obtained by distillation of natural resins—that is the origin from its name—with potassium carbonate of pernambucan Brazilian tree extracts (Pau Brazil) [8,12].

When topically applied, it separates the stratum corneum and the most superficial layers of the epidermis from the deeper ones; such a split seems to occur in the stratum granulosum [9]. A deep inflammatory reaction, histologically noticeable, is associated with vasodilation, visible six hours following its application. Findings one week later consist of increased mitosis in the stratum germinativum, prolonged vasodilation of dermal vessels, proliferation of fibroblasts, a thickened papillary dermal band, and a higher concentration of elastic fibers in the deep dermis. With the exception of vasodilation, dermal changes are still visible four months later [9,10]. The nature and intensity of these changes will depend on the concentration of resorcin applied as well as on the time in which this preparation is left on the skin [12].

Histolopathologic examination shows improvement in the epidermal thickness, as well as reduction in atrophy, keratinous plugs, loss of polarity, and basal cell degeneration. Decrease in elastosis, edema, and telangiectasias are also observed. The morphology of connective tissue is greatly improved after Golden Peels, showing much more normal staining features which explain the enhancement reached in cellulite or breasts and buttocks lifting [13,14]. According to the depth of the biological changes (wounding) induced by this combination of peeling agents (papillary dermis and upper part of the reticular dermis), it must be considered a medium-depth peel [9].

Application Technique
Application of Golden Lift® is very easy, but every step must be carefully followed in order to get the best results: cleansing with astringents (rose water, acetone) and scrubbing with polyethylene granules [9,12]. Then the Jessner solution is applied in several passes up to the point of frosting, on average 1–3 minutes. The Golden

Peel® medium paste (53% resorcin plus 10% glycolic acid) is then applied and left on the skin for 2 minutes at the first session. The time may subsequently be increased according to the patient´s skin tolerance, with a burning sensation indicating termination. On average the paste is left for 2–5 minutes. The skin where the paste is removed becomes white in the center and edematous and congestive in the periphery. During the next two to three days the skin changes from congestive, red, and swollen, to brown and sometimes deep brown. After four to five days desquamation occurs [10,12]. Benefits of this treatment modality are noted after the first session, but they are enhanced after subsequent ones. For the purposes of this study, we performed just five sessions, but in the practice we usually offer packages of six to 10 sessions looking for the best results.

Complications

When using these formulations, we have never seen any case of hypopigmentation, milia, or unsightly scars as is commonly observed after deeper peelings [15,16].

Serious complications related to resorcin absorption [15–17] can be avoided if we take the appropriate precautions concerning the time of contact on the skin and do not apply them over several anatomical regions (or large areas) in the same session. On the back, for instance, the procedure must be performed focally. The same precautions may be followed when used for cellulite.

In only four cases have we observed mild and transitory dizziness when the patient stands up immediately after the peeling. In all of these cases, resorcin paste had been applied at the same time on dorsum of the hands, forearms, and V-line of the neck. No changes in blood pressure or cardiac rhythm were noted, and patients recovered after drinking a cup of coffee and reclining for 10 minutes in the Trendelenburg position [8].

After more than three decades using resorcin peels we have noted only two cases of what seemed to be an authentic allergic contact dermatitis to resorcin. The patients experienced the rapid onset of pruritus and burning, and the skin became erythematous, edematous, and showed multiple small vesicles. The condition was treated with oral antihistamines and topical corticoids, and improved rapidly.

The most common complication has been mild to moderate grades of hyperpigmentation that disappeared spontaneously, most of our cases have been Fitzpatrick III or IV [8].

Materials and Methods

Thirty randomly selected Hispanic females whose ages varied between 15 to 54 years (average 32), weighing from 47 to 87.7 kg (average 65.6) and having heights of 1.42 to 1.68 meters (average 1.54) were included in the study. Pregnant and lactating females, those with allergies, having systemic infections and those who had received treatment for weight loss in the last three months, and patients having kidney impairment, were excluded from the study. No patient had lost weight in the previous three months. Eighty per cent of the patients were of Fitzpatrick skin type III or IV. Informed consent was required prior to the study from all patients.

The severity of cellulite was classified according to Amad, Cordero, and Cordero scale [17]:

01 Not seen not felt
02 Not seen but felt

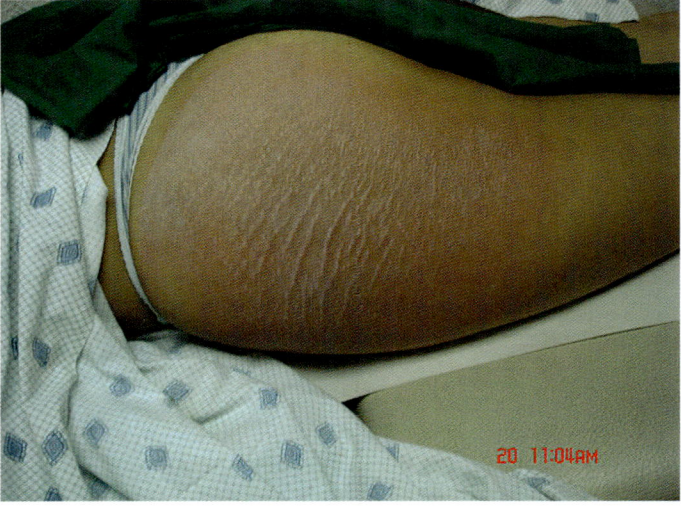

Figure 10.1 Golden Peels are highly selective. Note the specificity on these striae distensae.

03 Seen and felt
04 Macronodules

There was no patient of type 1 severity; type 2: three cases; type 3: eight cases; and type 4: four cases. The areas included in the study were the outer thighs and gluteal region. Subjective evaluation of cellulite was done by three observers: one physician, one nurse (always the same) and the patient herself with a range of 0 to +++, with +++ being excellent. Photographs were taken before and after completion of the study, as well as six months later. Evaluation of cellulite was also carried out using circumferential thigh measurements in centimeters before and after treatment, and diagnostic ultrasound in millimeters pre- and post-treatment. Circumferential measurements were made with a metric band from the root of the thighs at the inguinal fold.

Results

Circumference of thighs decreased on the right side from 60.4 cm (average) to 57.9 cm (average), and on the left side from 60.4 cm (average) to 57.5 cm (average) (Figs. 10.1–10.4). Ultrasonic measurements in millimeters improved from 27.9 mm

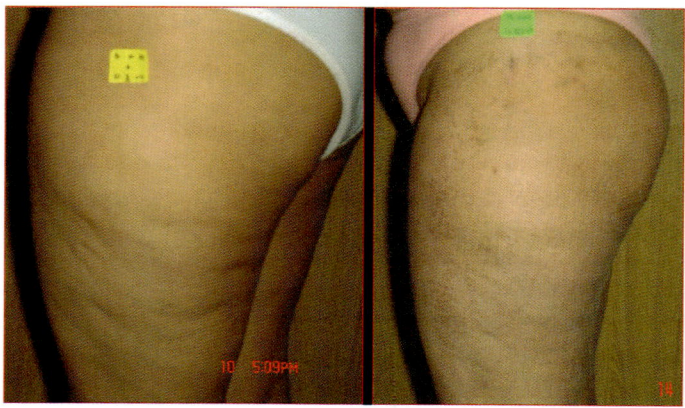

Figure 10.2 Cellulite. Before and after only 5 sessions of Golden Lift®.

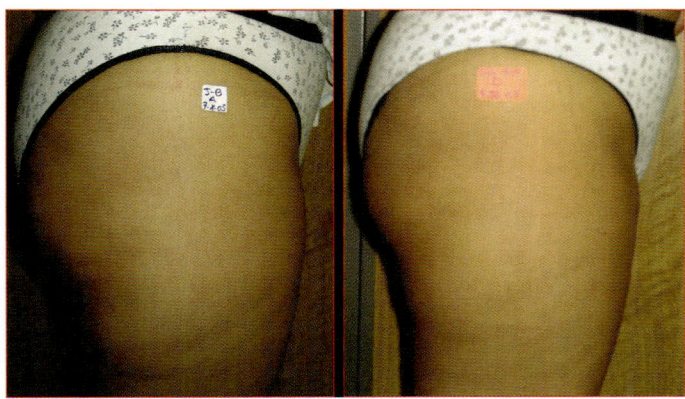

Figure 10.3 Note the changes in before (left) and after (right).

(average) to 22.6 mm (average) on the right side, and from 28.4 mm (average) to 23.8 mm (average) on the left side (Figs. 10.5, 10.6).

Regarding side effects, mild and self-limited post-inflammatory pigmentation was noted in two out of 15 cases (13%). Eczematous contact dermatitis was not noted in any case.

A statistically significant difference was noted in the improvement of the thighs ($p < 0.01$).

Discussion

Etiologically, cellulite can be related to genetic factors, abundance of female hormones, or it can be a manifestation of a secondary sexual character [1,2,7,8,17].

Neuro-vegetative, circulatory and other factors have been postulated as etiological factors [2,8,9]. In the case of multiple lipomas, some authors suggest that they are inherited as a dominant genetically transmitted disease [9,18–20]. For others the cause of the disorder included an abnormal blood supply [9,18–20] or a neurogenic factor should be looked for in view of the unusual number of nerve sizes sometimes found [18,20]. Aggravating factors leading to cellulite are stress, sedentary lifestyle, fried foods, as well as orthopaedic and veno-lymphatic disturbances. In areas of cellulite, there is predominance of alpha 2 insulin receptors (anti-lipolytics, and stimulants of lipogenesis) [7,8,17,21]. The

areas most commonly affected are the outer thighs and gluteal region; however, the inner thighs, inner knees, lower abdomen below the umbilicus, and upper arms are other areas which can be affected. Histologically, fat is deposited in the dermis in the form of loculi separated by fibrous septa, giving the characteristic nodular appearance of cellulite [1,2,7,8].

Cellulite (or a similar deformity) can also take place as a result of very superficial liposuction especially in the outer thighs with an incorrect technique. With cannula tunnels leading up to the dermis, post-operative compression can result in deeper fat being pushed upwards into the dermis resulting in cellulite [6,9,22]. It can also take place in cases of fat transfer, if the injected fat is deposited in loculi very superficially in the upper dermis [22].

There are important differences in the organization of fat in hips, thighs, breasts and abdomen in men and women. These differences explain herniation of adipocyte lobules by hypertrophy and hyperplasia within structural connective tissue compartments in women, whereas in men adipose tissue is placed in hypertrophic distribution either caudally or cephalically without developing cellulite [21]. In the trochanteric areas, thighs, hips, buttocks and femoral areas of women, there is a strong predominance of anti-lipolytic alpha-2 receptors, in addition to a number of insulin receptors. These are anti-lipolytic and favour lipogenesis, which increases the deposition of adipose tissue in these zones and results in cellulite [21,22].

The skin tightening effect of Golden Peel Plus® has been well known to dermatologists for several years [8,10,12]. The addition of 10% glycolic acid increases this property. Recently, we have also demonstrated improvement in breast flaccidity and breast lift using Golden Peel Plus® [11]. The gluteal lift effect of the Golden Peel Plus® is desirable in a number of ways. It leads to improvement of sagging skin, leading to a more youthful appearance of the buttocks, with enhancement of self-esteem. All these effects are improved using the new modifications [11,12]. As the complications are minimal or none, in our opinion, this is a very good and minimally invasive way of improving cellulite.

Golden Peel Plus® is safe, simple, inexpensive and effective. Nice results are obtained using Golden Peel® in photodamage, upper limbs, V-line of the neck, striae distensae, and in breast flaccidity [10,12]. It leads to an increase in epidermal and dermal thickness and decreases dermal elastosis. As it reaches the papillary and upper reticular dermis, it is a medium deep peel [8,9]. All depends upon the time that the chemical substance is left on the skin. Improvement can take place as a result of re-orientation of collagen fibers, breakage of fat loculi as a result of epidermolysis, as well as on the formation of proteinaceous precipitates consisting of necrotic epidermis and keratin. Golden Peel® also results in higher vascularity in the epidermis and dermis, with an increase in metabolic activity [8]. This could also result in clearing of excess superficial fat. When 10% glycolic acid is added to the classical formula (Golden Lift®), the effect on the skin tightening is greatly enhanced. This improvement has been proven clinically, ultrasonographically, and statistically in the management of cellulite.

Phenol peel may be cardiotoxic. However, the members of the Golden Peel® family, though made up of resorcin, a phenol derivative, are free of its toxic effects [10–12].

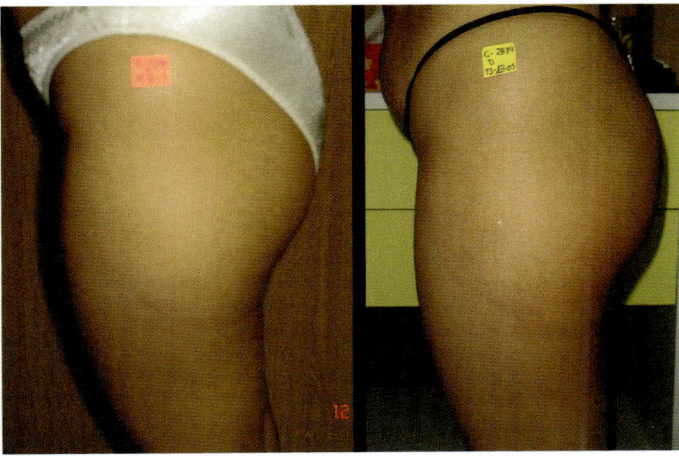

Figure 10.4 In the lower trochanteric area there is noticeable difference between before and after Golden Lift®.

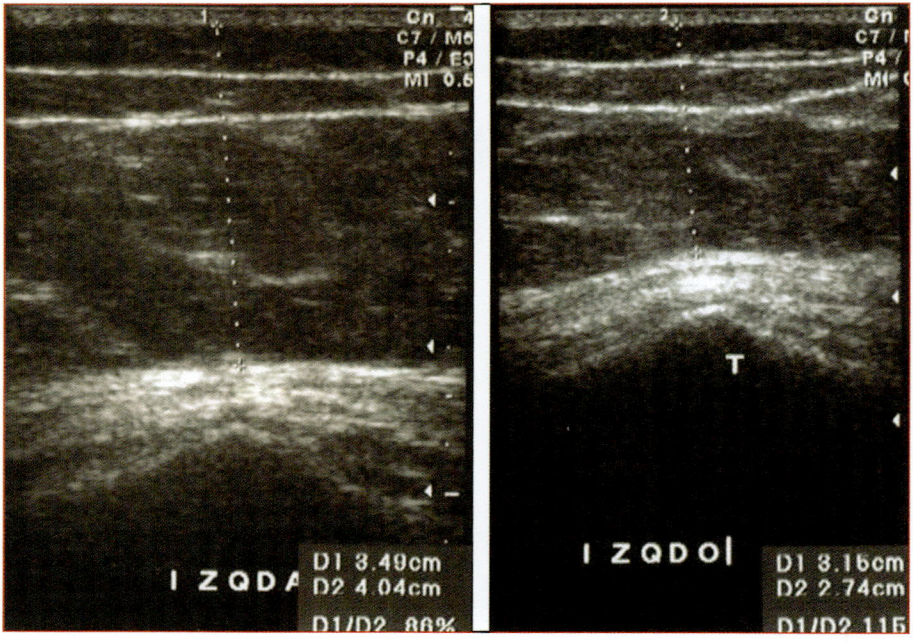

Figure 10.5 Ultrasonographic changes before and after 5 sessions of Golden Lift®. There are noticeable differences in the fat thickness.

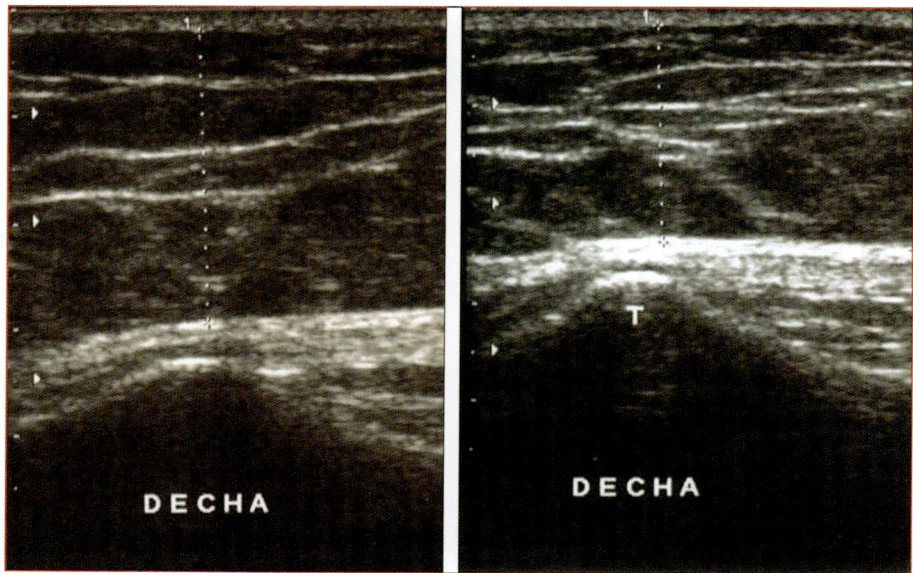

Figure 10.6 There is decrease in the adipose tissue in these before and after pictures.

Conclusion

Golden Lift® is highly recommendable in cellulite treatment. Its efficacy has been proven clinically, ultrasonographically, and statistically. Adverse effects are practically nil. Furthermore it is inexpensive with no "down time" period. For the increased satisfaction of the patient it might be convenient to perform a bigger number of peelings or combine with other medical modalities at home.

Acknowledgments

Statistical analysis was performed by Manuel Gavidia, MD, Professor of Biostatistics, Evangelic University of El Salvador.

Golden Peels are produced and were very kindly donated by Manuel Machón, Pharmacist, Director of Pharmator Laboratories, San Salvador. The authors of this chapter do not have any other relationship with these products.

REFERENCES

1. G Leibaschoff. Cellulite (lipoesclerosis): Etiology and treatment. Am J Cosm Surg 14:395–401, 1997.
2. ZD Draelos. Purported cellulite treatments. Dermatol Surg 23:1177–81, 1997.
3. E Hernández-Pérez, M Aristimuño, M Lemm, JA Seijo Cortes. The Bio-actif alpha/Y in the treatment of cellulite. Am J Cosm Surg 19:117–21, 2002.

4. R Farina, R Baroudi, B Golcman, R de Castro. Lipodistrofia pelvi-trocanterica tipo calca de montaria (lipomatose trocanterica), Hospital 57:717– 21, 1960.

5. I Pitanguy. Surgical reduction of the abdomen, thighs and buttocks. Surg Clin North Am 51:479, 1971.

6. EH Courtiss. Aesthetic Surgery. Trouble—How to avoid it and how to treat it. Saint Louis, Missouri, CV Mosby; 1978: pp 223–31.

7. S Lopez-Velasco, E Hernández-Pérez. Metabolismo del tejido graso: una síntesis para el cirujano dermatólogo. Act Terap Dermatol 18:365–70, 1995.

8. E Hernández-Pérez. Different grades of chemical peels. Am J Cosm Surg 7:67–70, 1990.

9. HA Khawaja, E Hernández-Pérez. Lipomatose formation after fat transfer: A report of 2 cases. Int J Cosm Surg 6:144–45, 1998.

10. E Hernández-Pérez. Resorcinol Peel as a part of a facial rejuvenation program. Am J Cosm Surg 14:35–40, 1997.

11. E Hernández-Pérez, JA Seijo-Cortes, HA Khawaja. Golden Peel Plus® for the treatment of breast flaccidity: A clinical, histological, and statistical study. Cosm Dermatol 19:425–27, 2006.

12. E Hernández-Pérez, HA Khawaja. The Golden Peel®. In: MA Shiffman, SJ Mirrafati, SM Lam, CG Cueteaux: Simplified Facial Rejuvenetion. Springer 1ˢᵗ Ed, Berlin; 2008: pp 119–24.

13. E Hernández-Pérez, E Carpio. Resorcinol peels: Gross and microscopic study. Am J Cosm Surg 12:337–40, 1995.

14. SB Hopping. Chemical peeling in 1996: what have we learned? J Int Aesth Restor Surg 4:73–80, 1996.

15. W Coleman. Dermatologic cosmetic surgery. J Dermatol Surg Oncol 16:170–76, 1990.

16. E Hernández-Pérez, V Jáurez-Arce. Gross and microscopic findings with a combination of Jessner´s solution plus 53% resorcinol paste in chemical peels. Am J Cosmet Surg 17: 85–89, 2000.

17. AD Amad, A Cordero, AA Cordero. Celulitis y adiposidad localizada. Act Terap Dermatol 21:64–74, 1998.

18. G Enzi. Multiple symmetric lipomatosis: An update clinical report. Medicine (Baltimore) 63:56–64, 1984.

19. SR Uhlin. Benign symmetric lipomatosis. Arch Dermatol 115:94–95, 1979.

20. N Mohar. Familial multiple lipomatosis. Acta Dermato Venereol (Stockh) 60:509–13, 1980.

21. M Berlan, J Galitzky, M Lafontan. Heterogeneite fonctionelle du tissu adipeux: Recepteurs adrenergiques et lipomobilisation. J Med Esth Chir Derm 19:7–15, 1992.

22. HA Khawaja, E Hernández-Pérez. Fat transfer review: Controversies, complications, their prevention and treatment. Int J Cosm Surg Aesth Dermatol 4:131–38, 2002.

11 Injection Lipolysis for Body Sculpting and Cellulite Reduction
Martin Braun

Introduction

Injection lipolysis is an injection into adipose tissue to dissolve fat. This treatment slowly breaks down fatty deposits with subcutaneous injections of an adipocyte-dissolving formula. It is also known by the trademarked name lipodissolve. It has been practiced in Europe and South America for over a decade, and in North America since 2003. Despite the fact that practitioners of injection lipolysis outside the United States tout the benefits, based on their favorable experiences, there exists a considerable amount of healthy skepticism in the American cosmetic medical community concerning this procedure. However, an abundance of scientific literature demonstrating the histopathology, mechanism of action, and detailed measurable clinical results is now available and will be reviewed.

Injection lipolysis is suitable for non-obese patients with localized fat accumulation which cannot be reduced with appropriate diet or sincere efforts at exercise. This fat accumulation on the hips and thighs is associated with a worsening appearance of cellulite. One can improve the appearance of cellulite by diminishing the underlying subcutaneous fat and reducing the girth of the thigh. Injection lipolysis does not result in weight loss; injection lipolysis modifies body contours. The ideal patient has a normal body mass index of less than 25 (normal BMI 18–25). Injection lipolysis is not a substitute for liposuction. Injection lipolysis is an alternative to liposuction for areas of fat accumulation in a patient who prefers a less invasive non-surgical procedure. Liposuction is a more cost-effective and efficient procedure than injection lipolysis for larger fatty deposits which can be removed with one procedure. However, liposuction rarely improves the appearance of cellulite, whereas injection lipolysis does improve the appearance of the skin overlying the fat.

The active ingredient of injection lipolysis is a mixture of phosphatidylcholine (PC), a natural substance derived from soy bean lecithin, and deoxycholate (DC), a bile salt. Aventis Pharma (part of the Sanofi-Aventis Group, Paris, France, the third largest pharmaceutical company in the world), markets phosphatiylcholine/deoxycholate preparations under the trade names Lipostabil and Essentiale in Europe (primarily Germany and Italy), Russia, South America, and South Africa. Lipostabil contains 5% PC (50 mg/ml) and 4.75% DC (47.5 mg/ml) with 0.9% benzoyl alcohol, vitamin E, and saline. Lipostabil is not sold in the USA or Canada.

Review of Scientific Literature on Injection Lipolysis

Phosphatidylcholine (PC) is an essential phospholipid which comprises 40% of the human cell membrane. PC is commonly known as lecithin, and the commercial preparations of purified PC are derived from soy bean lecithin, rather than egg yolk. PC is composed of choline, phosphate, and two fatty acids. (See Fig. 11.1). One end is polar; the other non-polar. This is the primary constituent of the bilipid cell membrane. The length of the two fatty acid chains varies amongst different PC commercial preparations, affecting its solubility.

PC is involved in the regulation of lipid metabolism [1,2] and is marketed by Aventis as an injectable intravenous infusion to lower cholesterol and triglycerides called Lipostabil. Lipostabil has also been used in the treatment of hepatitis [3,4,5], and cardiovascular atheromatous diseases in Europe and Russia [2]. It is also a common constituent of chelation formulas.

The known ability of oral and intravenous PC to reduce systemic triglycerides and cholesterol eventually led to its use as a subcutaneous injection in an attempt to decrease fatty deposits. The first published trial using Lipostabil in a subcutaneous injection was by the Italian physician Sergio Maggiori to treat xanthelasma in 1988 [6].

Subsequently, Lipostabil was reported as a successful office-based procedure for fat dissolution of the "buffalo hump" at an AIDS lipodystrophy meeting at an HIV symposium in Athens, Greece, in 2001 by Brazilian dermatologist Marcio Serra. He described the substantial reduction of buffalo humps in two HIV patients injected on five occasions every two weeks with 200 mg of PC. Local side effects of erythema and edema were reported to resolve over three to four days [7].

In 1999 Brazilian dermatologist Patricia Rittes reported the injection of PC into the small fat pads of the lower eyelid area at the 54th Brazilian Dermatology Congress [8]. The first paper published in an English peer-reviewed journal describing this use of PC for localized fat dissolution was by Rittes in 2001 [8]. Rittes has performed this office procedure thousands of times since 1999. Rittes' paper in *Dermatologic Surgery* describes the injection of 30 patients (22 females, eight males, ages 30–70) up to four times in each of the three infraorbital fat pads at 15 day intervals [8]. Cosmetic improvement was reported in all patients, with local side effects of erythema and edema for up to three days. Follow-up was for two years with no recurrences. This paper gives the total dose of PC per infraorbital fat pad (PC 20 mg), but does not report the exact technique. Dr. Rittes has described her injection technique at many medical meetings, and it is shown in Figure 4. Rittes injected the three infraorbital fat pads with a total dose of PC 20 mg.

Her work was reproduced by American dermatologists Ablon and Rotunda in 2003 [9]. Ten patients (seven women and three men aged 42–71) were injected at 14-day intervals up to five times using the Rittes' technique. Immediate local side effects were mild burning, erythema and edema. Dr. Rotunda reported that 6/10 patients had moderate to significant improvement with no significant side effects during a six- to 10-month period of follow-up [9]. Treacy and Goldberg found similar efficacy in their study of 21 patients on infraorbital fat [20].

Rittes published a second article describing injections of PC 40 mg per injection site into areas of fatty accumulation other

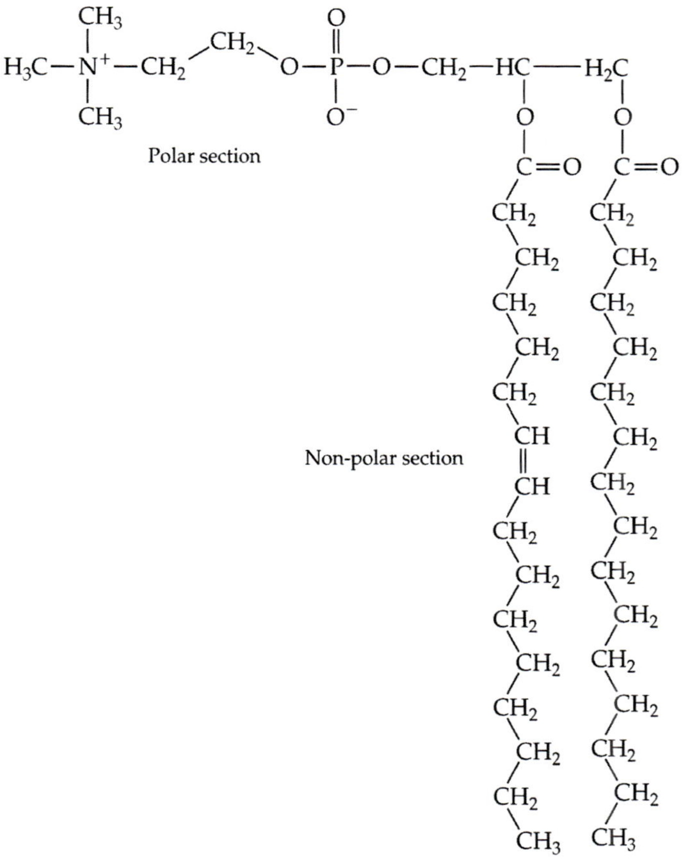

Figure 11.1 Phosphatidylcholine (PC).

Figure 11.3 Note each injection point is equidistant. The injection pattern should resemble the 5 side of a die. Each point represents 20 mg of PC injected to a depth of 13 mm.

30 days are mentioned. No lipoatrophy occurred. Rittes reported the treatment safe and effective [10].

Brazilian dermatologists Hexsel and Serra reported injections of PC 10 mg per injection point in 213 patients up to five times every 15 days [11]. PC 10 mg was injected every 2 cm using a 30 G 1 inch needle at a depth of 1–2 cm. A maximum of 500 mg of PC was injected at any one session. The 213 patient group included eight HIV patients who were treated for buffalo humps at 30 day intervals. By the fifth session, 80–100% remission or "considerable improvement" was reported. Local side effects included transitory pain at the site of injection, erythema and edema. No systemic adverse reactions were observed. Thirteen patients underwent pre and post liver and renal function testing. There were no significant alterations in laboratory parameters. Hexsel and Serra reported the treatment safe, effective, low cost, as well as much simpler compared to surgical liposuction.

Unfortunately, these were all open label clinical studies. Due to the immediate erythema and edema which occurs following injection of PC/DC, it would be virtually impossible to design a double-blind study. The studies also have not shown any histopathology concerning the mechanism of action of the PC/DC. Measurements are lacking, although some very good before and after photographs are shown in the papers discussed. Only Hexsel and Serra reported any lab data in 13/213 patients [11].

Rose and Morgan were the first to report histological findings following an injection of PC/DC into a human patient. Biopsies taken at one and two weeks after treatment with PC/DC showed a normal epithelium and dermis, with mixed septal and lobular panniculitis. The fat lobules were infiltrated by increased numbers of lymphocytes and macrophages. The macrophages consisted of conventional forms, foam cells, and multinucleated fat-containing giant cells. The inflammation was associated with serous atrophy [12].

Schuller-Petrovic et al. subsequently performed histology on a human volunteer and rats, and found that PC/DC dose-dependent

than infraorbital fat pads in 50 patients (40 female and 10 male, aged 25–60) up to four times every 15 days [10]. PC 40 mg was injected every 2–3 cm using a 30 G 1/2 inch needle into the fatty deposit. A total dose of PC 250 mg was injected uniformly over an 80 sq cm area. Various areas of the body with fatty accumulation were chosen. Before and after photographs were taken, but no measurements. Cosmetic improvement was reported in all patients, with fat reduction and improvement in body contour with the loss of a roll of fat. In the discussion, Dr. Rittes reports no return of fat in four years of follow-up, but exact numbers are not given. Local side effects of burning pain, erythema, and edema are again described. Subcutaneous nodules which disappeared within

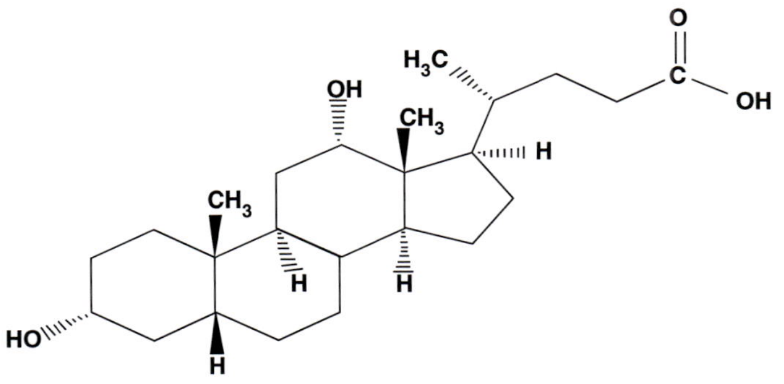

Deoxycholic Acid (deoxycholate)

Figure 11.2 Deoxycholic Acid (DC).

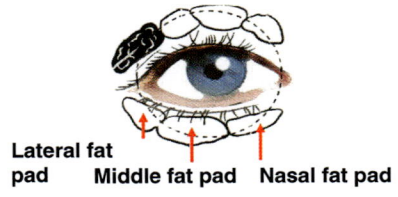

Lateral fat pad **Middle fat pad** **Nasal fat pad**

Figure 11.4 Location of periorbital fat pads.

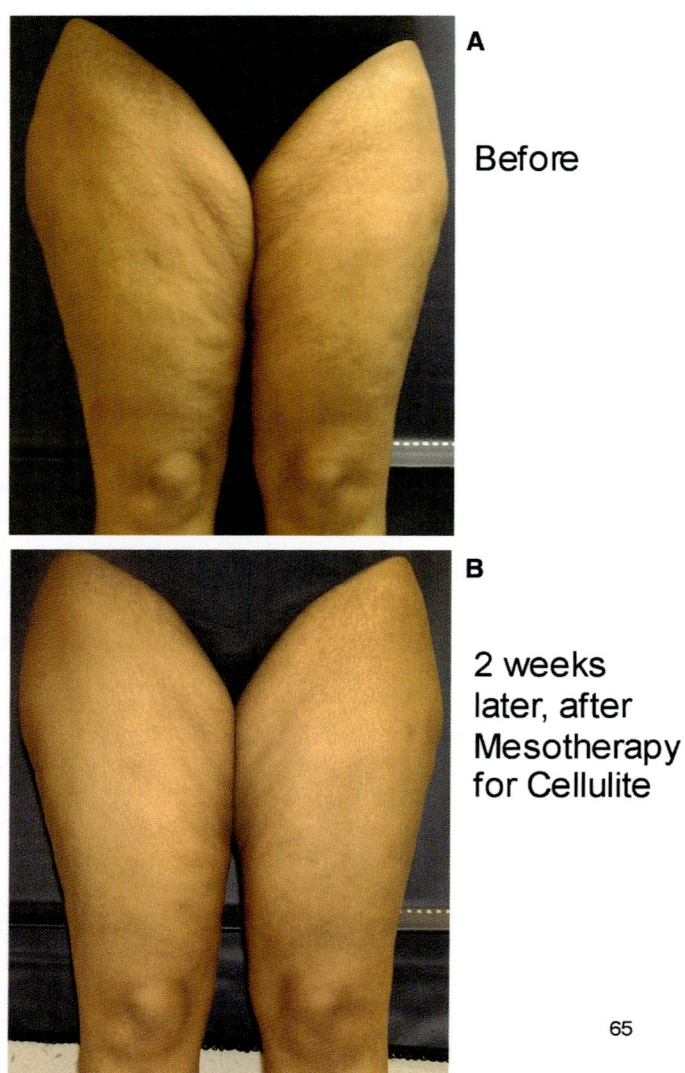

A

Before

B

2 weeks later, after Mesotherapy for Cellulite

65

Figure 11.5 (A) Before and (B) two weeks after mesotherapy for cellulite (by permission of Dr Charles Mok).

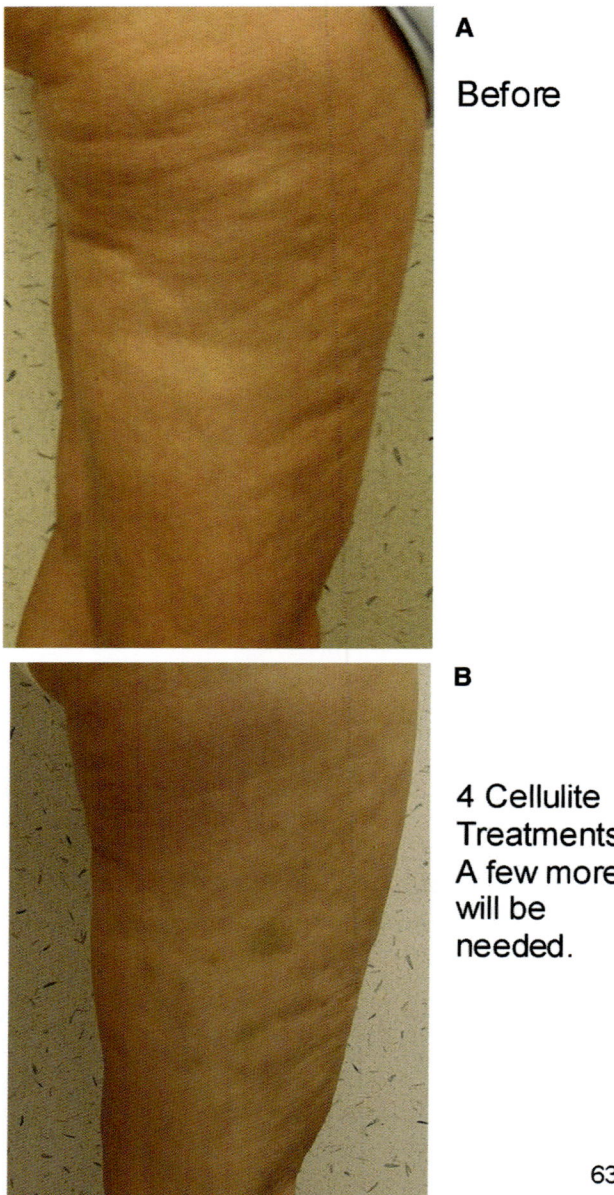

A

Before

B

4 Cellulite Treatments A few more will be needed.

63

Figure 11.6 (A) Before and (B) after four cellulite treatments (a few further treatments will be needed) (by permission of Dr Charles Mok).

reduced membrane integrity and cell viability. Histologic alterations induced by PC/DC included fibroplasia, bandlike fibrosis in the region of the cutaneous muscle, and partial muscle loss if injected into rat muscle [13]. It is critical to only inject PC/DC into adipose tissue, and not muscle [13,16].

Bechara et al. performed sequential histology on lipomas following injections of Lipostabil brand PC/DC. Between four and 48 hours after injection, histology shows a lobular neutrophilic infiltrate with partially destroyed fat cells. At day 10 the inflammatory process is accompanied by an infiltration of T-lymphocytes. After 60 days, formation of macrophages with foam cells are visible, accompanied by thickened septa and capsula [14]. Bechara et al. also demonstrated an average reduction in size of 46% in 30 lipomas (10 patients) injected with PC/DC on four occasions [15]. These and other studies have conclusively demonstrated the loss of adiposite viability following PC/DC injections into fat. However, could it be possible that the active ingredient in PC/DC is DC?

Deoxycholate (Deoxycholic acid)

Deoxycholate (DC) is a bile acid found in human bile. DC has a primary detergent effect to emulsify fats in our diet (Fig. 11.2).

DC is also widely used as a laboratory reagent to solubilize cell membrane proteins due to its detergent effects. Detergents have had various uses in medications for many years, especially as sclerosing agents for sclerotherapy injections. A specific example of deoxycholate as a detergent is to solubilize amphotericin B. Amphotericin B is insoluble in water; presence of sodium deoxycholate in the formulation solubilizes amphotericin B during reconstitution with sterile water providing a colloidal dispersion of the drug for intravenous injection.

Rotunda et al. published their findings in *Dermatologic Surgery* in 2004 [16] describing a loss of cell viability with cell membrane lysis and disruption of fat and muscle architecture in porcine cell

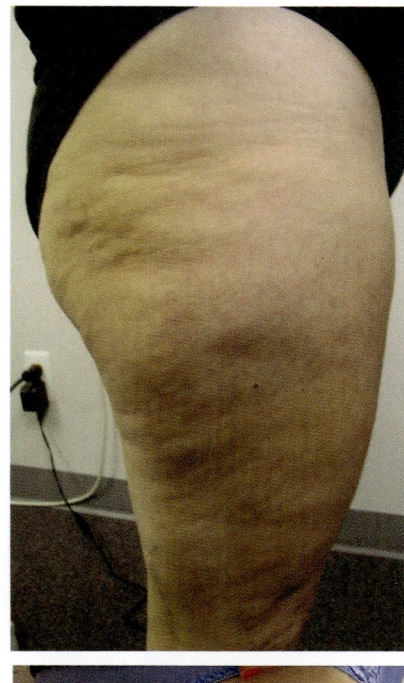

A
Before

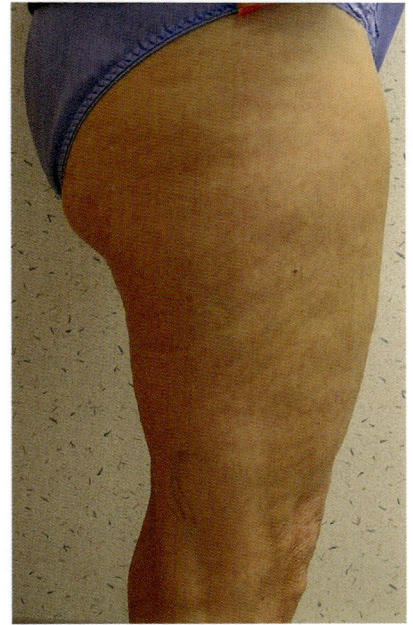

B

After 5
Mesotherapy
cellulite
treatments

Figure 11.7 (A) Before and (B) after five mesotherapy cellulite treatments (by permission of Dr Charles Mok).

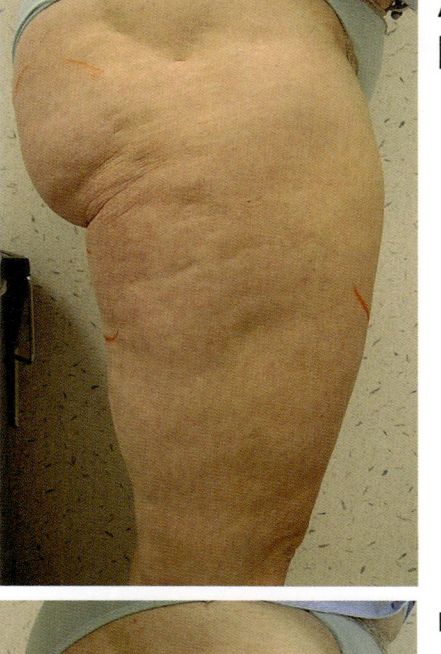

A
Before

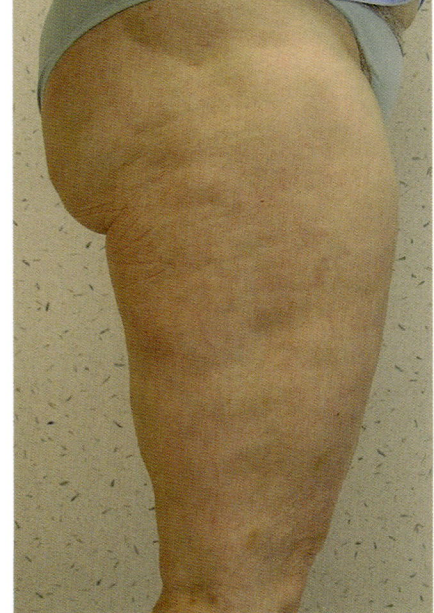

B

6
Treatments
Later

51

Figure 11.8 (A) Before and (B) after six treatments (by permission of Dr Charles Mok).

cultures and tissue specimens treated with PC/DC and DC alone. As mentioned previously, DC is a detergent that is used to emulsify and solubilize compounds that are insoluble in water, such as injectable amphotericin. Rotunda et al. showed that injecting the deoxycholate alone produced similar effects as the combination PC/DC Libostabil formulation, suggesting that DC is an active ingredient. They were unable to test PC in isolation, as PC is not soluble in aqueous saline solution by itself. The DC is used to increase the solubility of PC in the PC/DC formulation.

Histology of the porcine skin did not show any changes of the epidermis, dermis or adenexal structures after injection of PC/DC. This finding shows that one can treat the adiposity of cellulite without affecting the structures of the skin, as long as the

injection of PC/DC is at least 6 mm from the epidermis. There was a concentration dependent increase in cell lysis in both the PC/DC and DC treated cell cultures. Muscle cell viability was also compromised with injections into porcine muscle, indicating the critical importance of limiting PC injections to adipose tissue, and avoiding any underlying muscle. Rotunda summarized the effect of the PC/DC formula as a detergent action causing nonspecific lysis of cell membranes, with a brisk inflammatory response, and subsequent adipocyte necrosis.

These findings were confirmed by several other investigators: Yagima et al. injected pure DC 10 mg/ml, 25 mg/ml or placebo on four occasions in 30 volunteers. Clinical, hematologic, and ultrasonographic evaluations were performed for three months and histology at three and six months. Both concentrations of DC induced an inflammatory response at the injection site, with

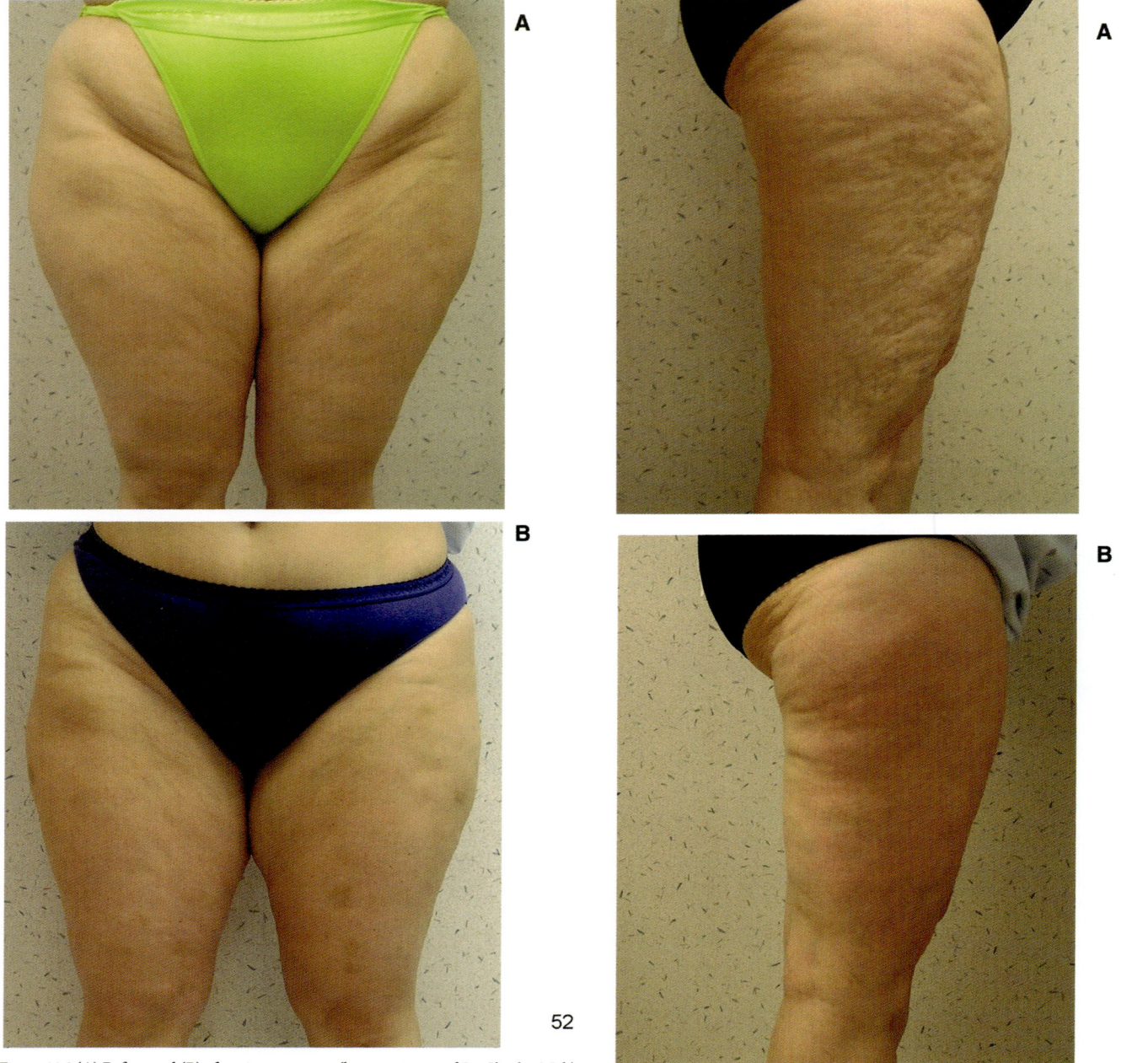

Figure 11.9 (A) Before and (B) after six treatments (by permission of Dr Charles Mok).

Figure 11.10 (A) Before and (B) after six treatments (by permission of Dr Charles Mok).

dose-dependent adipocyte lysis. Patients reported mild, localized heat, erythema, swelling, and intense pain. Microscopic evaluation revealed necrosis of adipose tissue with adipocyte lysis, fat dissolution, acute lymphomononuclear inflammatory reaction, and intense phagocytosis of fat cells by macrophages. Fibrosis was observed only at the six-month biopsy. Nodules at the injection sites, compatible with areas of inflammation, were detected by ultrasonography two weeks after the first injection. Placebo injections induced no histologic changes [17].

Rotunda and Ablon also demonstrated that DC alone was effective in the dissolution of lipomas. A total of six patients with 12 lipomas were treated with injections of sodium deoxycholate (1.0%, 2.5%, and 5.0%) at intervals of two to 20 weeks. Tumor size, cutaneous reactions, and patients' subjective responses were recorded before and after treatment. All lipomas decreased in size

(mean area reduction, 75%; range, 37%–100%) as determined by clinical measurement (with ultrasound confirmation in one lipoma) after an average of 2.2 treatments. Several lipomas fragmented or became softer in addition to decreasing in volume. Adverse effects, including transient burning, erythema, and local swelling, were associated with higher deoxycholate concentrations but resolved without intervention. There was no clear association between deoxycholate concentration and efficacy [18].

In order to resolve the question of the active ingredient in the PC/DC mixture, Salti et al. performed a double-blind study comparing PC/DC to DC. Thirty-seven consecutive female patients were studied for the treatment of localized fat in gynoid lipodystrophy. Each patient received injections of a PC/DC on one side and DC on the contralateral side, each single patient being

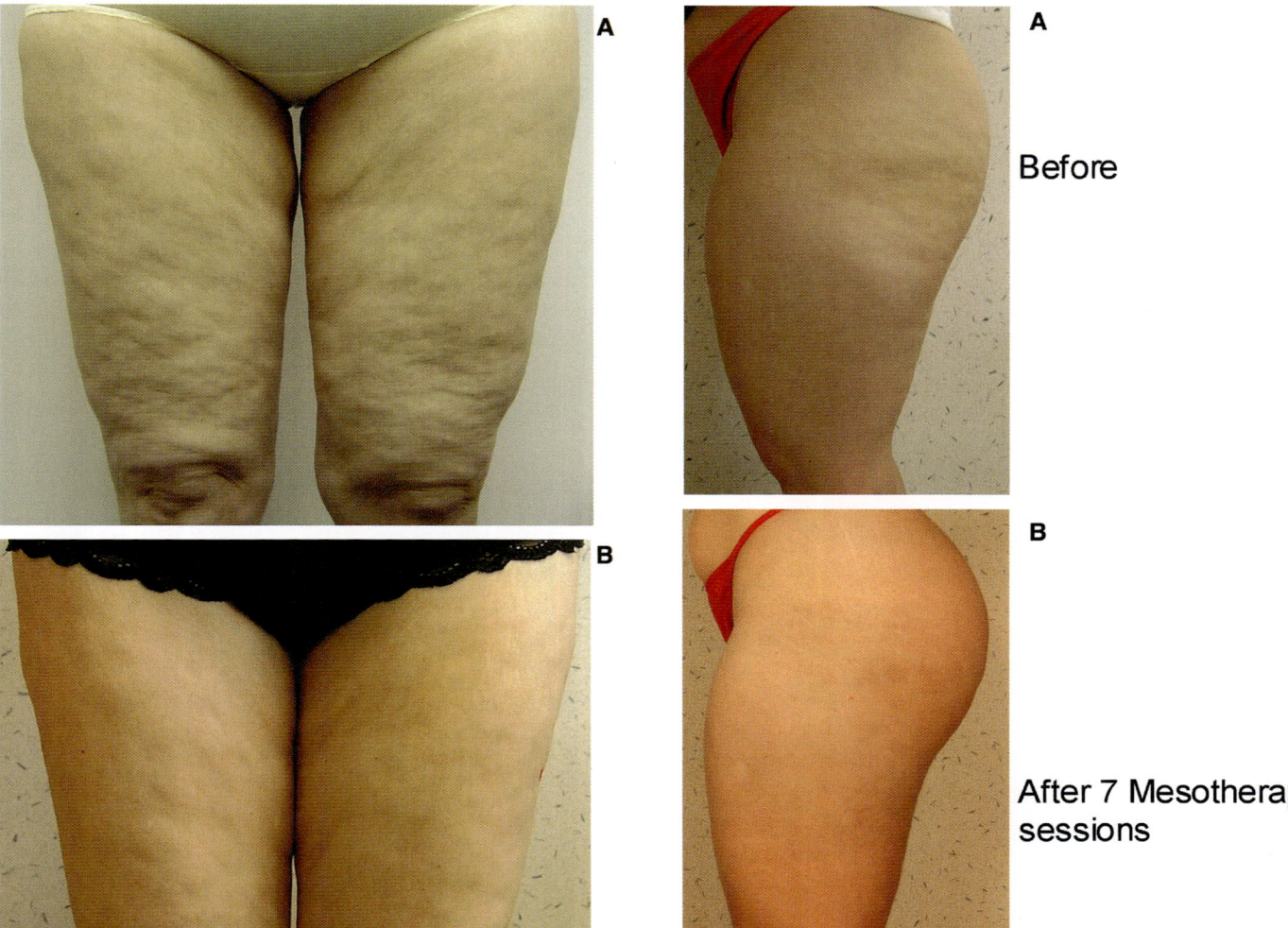

Figure 11.11 (A) Before and (B) after six treatments (by permission of Dr Charles Mok).

Figure 11.12 (A) Before and (B) after seven mesotherapy sessions (by permission of Dr Charles Mok).

herself the control. Four treatments were carried out every eight weeks in a double-blind, randomized fashion. Metric circumferential evaluations and photographic and ultrasonographic measurements were done. An overall reduction of local fat was obtained in 92% of the patients without statistically significant differences between the treated sides. Reduction values on the PC/DC treated sides are in the order of 6.5% metrically and 36.9% ultrasonographically, whereas on the DC treated sides they are in the order of 6.8% metrically and 36% ultrasonographically. Both treatments, at the dose used in the study, proved safe in the short term. The most common side effects were local and few, but were more pronounced on the deoxycholate-treated sides [19].

Clinical Safety of Phosphadidylcholine/Deoxycholate Injections

The preceding studies did not report a single, serious adverse effect. Palmer et al. reported a retrospective review of 10,581 injection lipolysis treatments performed by 39 physicians in the UK in 2006.

Three-quarters of the patients were satisfied or very satisfied with their treatments, and there was not a single, serious adverse side effect. Fifteen of 10,581 treatments (0.14%) had associated pain or swelling that was rated as "unusually severe or prolonged beyond two weeks" [21]. Duncan and Chubaty reported on a retrospective clinical safety data survey sent to 75 physicians from 17 countries who collectively performed 56,320 injection lipolysis sessions on 17,376 patients. There was not a single serious adverse effect as defined by death, hospitalization, skin ulceration, infection, or chronic skin irritation [22]. Hasengschwandtner et al. reported no serious adverse effects in over 80,000 treatments in data collected by Network Lipolysis, a European-based organization that teaches injection techniques and pools data from its members [23].

There have been isolated reports of mycoplasma infections following injection lipolysis, probably related to violations of aseptic technique and/or dubious sources of injectable solutions [24–26]. One case that is widely quoted by critics of injection lipolysis resulted from an unidentified quack injecting unknown substances into the fat of unsuspecting Virginians in their kitchens [27]. This is not the standard practice of safe medicine,

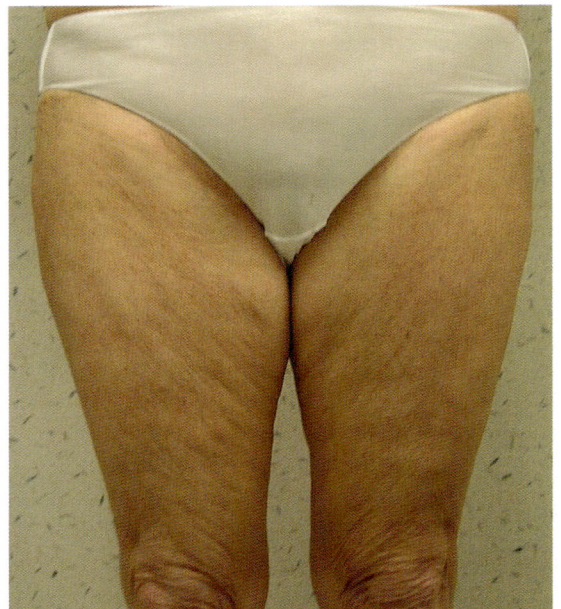

A

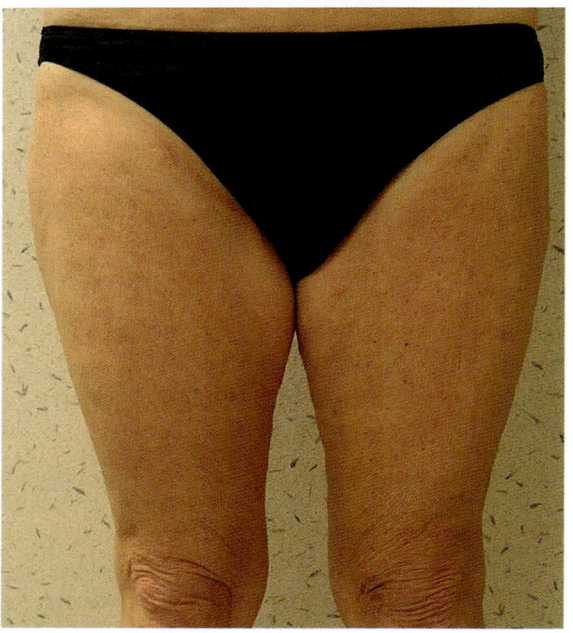

B

62

Figure 11.13 (A) Before and (B) after eight treatments (by permission of Dr Charles Mok).

and this incident should not reflect poorly on injections done by a competent doctor in a sterile enviroment. Lee and Chang reported a case of fat necrosis from Korea following multiple injections of dextrose and water into abdominal fat which healed with scarring following treatment with oral minocycline and prednisone [28]. It is well known that water will cause massive necrosis when injected into fat, and this article simply shows that this known fact will occur. It has nothing to do with the safe practice of injection lipolysis using PC/DC or DC alone. Yet this article is quoted as an example of "mesotherapy," when no proper mesotherapy was done.

Dr. Diane Duncan, an American plastic surgeon, has published an excellent paper detailing the need for a standard of practice for this promising therapy [29].

Availability of Lipostabil in the United States and Canada
Unfortunately, Aventis has no plans to market Lipostabil in the United States or Canada (personal communication with the manufacturer). Thus, it has not gone through the FDA regulatory process, and its use is therefore illegal in the United States. In a letter written to warn a U.S. importer of Libostabil, an official of the FDA wrote,

> "If a drug is marketed as an injectable product, it does not qualify as a dietary supplement since it is not intended for ingestion as set forth in section 210(ff)(2)(A)(i) of the Federal Food, Drug, and Cosmetic Act (the Act).
>
> Based on the route of administration (i.e., injectable) of this product and the claims made for the product to affect the structure or function of the body, it is a "drug" within the meaning of section 201(g) of the Act. Moreover, the product is a "new drug" [section 201(p) of the Act] because there is no substantial evidence that the product is generally recognized as safe and effective for its intended use.
>
> Since the product is a "new drug" it may not be marketed in the United States without an approved new drug application [section 505(a) of the Act]. In addition, in accordance with section 503(b)(1) of the Act, injectables other than insulin may not be sold directly to consumers." [30]

However, since the principle constituents of Lipostabil are phosphadylcholine derived from soy bean lecithin, and the bile salt deoxycholate, the ingredients are readily available to compounding pharmacies in the United States and Canada. Therefore a physician can order these substances to be mixed to any specification. Since the route of administration is parenteral, and claims are being made that these substances will dissolve fat, the FDA would consider the entire process to be the practice of medicine with the simple administration of a drug falling under the duties of responsibility and judgement of the physician.

In view of the fact that injectables cannot be sold directly to consumers (other than insulin), a licensed physician can write a prescription instructing a compounding pharmacy to make the formula to dissolve fat. This physician takes the responsibility for the administration and safety of the prescribed treatment, as is the case with any other medical treatment. It is the author's hope that these rules will prevent non-medical personnel from injecting PC/DC formulations as previously occurred in Brazil. Due to the widespread popularity of Lipostabil in Brazil, this formula was being injected in beauty salons, gymnasiums, and spas by non-medical individuals, which alarmed Aventis Pharma.

Aventis notified the Brazilian health authority, the Brazilian National Agency of Sanitary Monitoring (Anvisa). Aventis Pharma Brazil issued a notice stating that it does not market the product in Brazil and has no plans to do so. When Anvisa investigated the widespread unauthorized use of Aventis' Lipostabil (fosfatidilcolina) to reduce fat, it found two Internet companies had been distributing Lipostabil in Brazil. This led to the banning of Lipostabil at the national level in Brazil in January 2003 with the intent that non-medical people would have difficulty purchasing and administering it outside a physician's direct control. Many North American physicians have quoted the

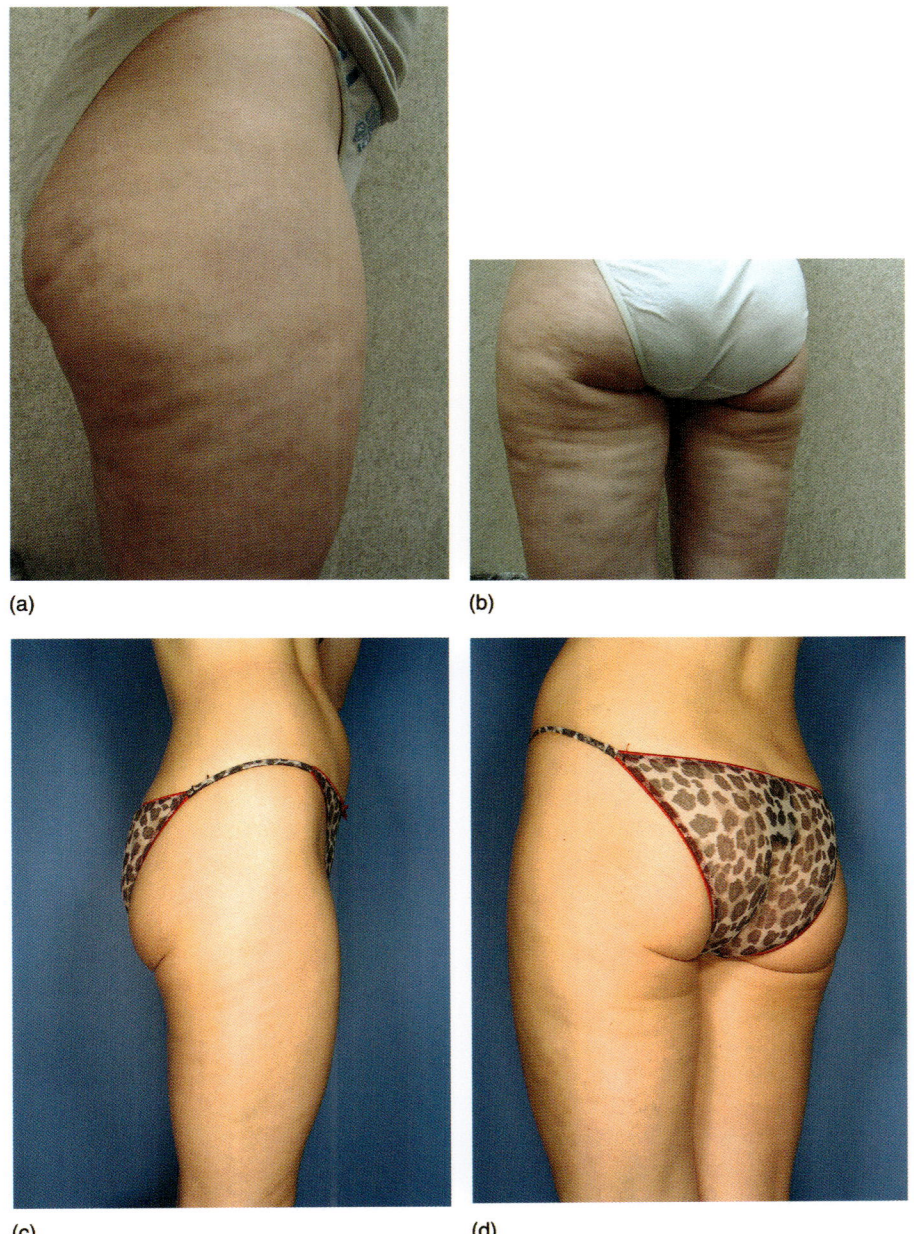

(a)

(b)

(c)

(d)

Figure 11.14 (a, b) Before and (c, d) after ten treatments.

banning of Lipostabil in Brazil as "evidence" that Lipostabil must be inherently unsafe, without understanding the true background that led to the ban.

UCLA Harborview has obtained a US patent for the use of deoxycholate and any other bile salt for the purposes of fat dissolution. Kythera Biopharmaceuticals Inc. has finished Phase 2 trials enrolling 157 patients demonstrating the efficacy of deoxyxholate for submental fat reduciton in order to obtain FDA approval for the use of deoxycholate for fat dissolution [31].

Contraindications for Injection lipolysis Injections

1. Pregnancy and breast-feeding
2. Minors
3. Serious obesity
4. Allergy to any ingredients, especially soy
5. Unrealistic expectations

Local Side Effects (in the injected area)

For a few days:

1. Pain 100%
2. Swelling 100%
3. Sensitivity to touch 100%
4. Pruritis 100%
5. Erythema 100%
6. Ecchymosis occasionally
7. Hematoma rarely

For a few weeks:

8. Nodules and "dents" which will eventually disappear

Systemic Side Effects (Cholinergic - more common with higher dose)

1. Nausea
2. Perspiration
3. Diarrhea
4. Altered Taste Sensation/Salivation
5. Cardiac arrythmia has been reported with intravenous PC

Dosages and Techniques for Injection Lipolysis Injections

Toxicity studies have been done with PC (*International Journal of Toxicology* 2001). The maximum non-lethal subcutaneous dose of PC for mouse, rat and rabbit was 10,000, 4000, and 1000 mg/kg respectively [15]. Different doses of PC to dissolve localized fat are used by various experts:

Dr. Franz Hasengschwandtner (Founder and Director of Network-Lipolysis at www.network-injection lipolysis.com and Chairman of the Austrian Society for Injection lipolysis) uses a maximum of 2500 mg PC per session. He spaces his sessions four to six weeks apart. He injects 0.4 ml of 50 mg/ml Lipostabil per injection site (20 mg of PC) approximately 2 cm apart to a depth of 13 mm into fatty pads.

Dr. Patricia Rittes (world's foremost specialist on injection lipolysis with over 26,000 cases in Brazil, www.prittes.com.br) injects 0.8 ml of 50 mg/ml PC per injection site (40 mg of PC) approximately, 4–6 cm apart to a depth of 13 mm. A typical injection pattern would involve six injections of 0.8 ml each in an area of about 80 sq cm. This area corresponds roughly to a 4 × 4 inch gauze (10 × 10 cm) and would require about 250 mg of PC. Rittes limits her total injection dose to 500 mg per session.

Therefore, Dr. Hasengschwandtner is performing more injections closer together using half the PC that Dr. Rittes uses for each injection site. Her injection technique involves injecting more PC into each site, but using fewer injections that are spaced farther apart. It may be that there is less pronounced nodulation with smaller amounts injected into more sites.

The nodulation following PC injection is a direct result of fat necrosis, and it makes intuitive sense to limit the volume of injection into any one point, although the optimal amount to inject in any one point is unclear. The author uses 20 mg of PC injected into one point. The author also limits his initial total dose of PC to 1000 mg to observe patient response and to minimize the chance of any systemic side effects. This is an office-based elective cosmetic procedure, and patients choosing this treatment do not want any "downtime" with excessive pain, swelling, or complications.

Pre-Treatment Considerations for Injection Lipolysis

Firstly, a proper medical history should be taken to determine if the patient has any contraindications or unrealistic expectations. The ideal patient for injection lipolysis therapy is an individual who does not wish to pursue surgical liposuction because they have relatively small fat deposits. A patient with smaller areas of fat accumulation would very likely have a Body Mass Index less than 27.

Following the consultation, measurements should be made with standard reference points. For example, if the plan is to treat the "love handles" at the sides of the waist, take a measurement with a tape at this area. Measure the distance from the simphysis pubis or umbilicus so that the identical measurement can be taken

weeks later. The loss of fat is gradual, and other than looser fitting clothing, the patient may not notice. It is invaluable to show the patients that they lost several centimeters in their standard measurement at a subsequent visit. It is not absolutely necessary to have the patient's height and weight, but it can be useful to demonstrate a body contour improvement to a patient without the loss of any weight. Furthermore, if a patient gains weight they will lose the body contour improvement, similar to gaining weight after liposuction. The remaining adipocytes simply swell as they store more fat, and the fatty deposit reappears. A pre-treatment weight can therefore be useful to defend the effectiveness of the therapy.

Photograph patients using a tripod, standard positions, and neutral background. Some areas are difficult to measure with a tape, so good photographs can be invaluable.

Disinfect the skin prior to any injections and after the injections to spread the material while massaging the skin. A potential complication is mycobacterium infection, and this is obviously related to good aseptic technique [24,26].

Have the patient stand to mark the injection sites with a surgical marking pen. Do not inject below the knee due to muscle proximity. Rotunda et al. demonstrated muscle necrosis with PC/DC injections into porcine muscle [12]. There is no need to stop ASA or NSAIDS, although there may be more bruising with the injections.

Consider limiting the first session to 500 mg PC to observe the patient response. This is an outpatient, cosmetic, office-based procedure chosen by a patient who wishes to avoid liposuction. It would be unwise to subject this inexperienced individual to undue pain, swelling, and erythema by injecting multiple sites. By beginning conservatively, the practitioner can gauge this new patient's tolerance for more injections. For future visits, one can then consider the maximum dose of PC = 2500 mg per session spread over multiple areas. Do not use a concentration stronger than PC 50 mg/ml, as all of the published scientific literature has used this concentration of PC [7–11].

Injection sites are marked about 2–3 cm apart (one finger breadth) on skin that has been prepared with a good disinfectant. Inject 20 mg of PC into each location at a depth of 6–13 mm into localized fat using a 30 G needle. Do not inject the exact point marked with the surgical marking pen to avoid tattooing the skin.

Superficial skin ulcerations have been reported when injecting PC more superficially than 6 mm. Therefore, inject at a depth of at least 6 mm.

Sessions should be spaced three to six weeks apart; never closer than two weeks apart. The author routinely waits until any nodulation has disappeared or has markedly diminished before injecting again.

Diet and exercise following this treatment appears to enhance results, but these are not critical to success. However, it makes sense that the body will metabolize the emulsified residue more efficiently if the patient is in a slightly negative or neutral caloric intake, rather than gaining weight. Gaining weight will not enhance the dissolution of any fatty areas or improve body contours, even following liposuction.

Hypothyroidism (may be subclinical) and B-blockers may diminish results. If a patient fails to obtain satisfactory results following injection lipolysis treatments, check their thyroid status.

Repeat injections two to five times in a given area and consider liposuction if the fourth injection session did nothing.

Injection Lipolysis Formula for Fat Pad Dissolution

Most compounding pharmacies in the United States will produce PC at a concentration of 100 mg/ml. The content of DC in the formulation varies considerably with different pharmacies, ranging from 21 mg/ml [16] to 42 mg/ml [17]. The 42 mg/ml concentration of DC is closest to the Lipostabil brand by Aventis which contains DC 47.5 mg/ml.

The following formula assumes one is starting with PC 100 mg/ml concentration and diluting it 50/50 with lidocaine 1%.

Dr. Rittes uses 0.8 ml of 50 mg/ml PC = 40 mg PC per shot
Dr. Hasengschwandtner uses 0.4 ml of 50 mg/ml PC = 20 mg PC per shot

The author has decided to use the Dr. Hasengschwandtner dose, which also necessitates twice the injections closer together than Dr. Rittes.

Maximum PC per session = 2500 mg PC total

At 20 mg PC per shot, the maximum dose that can be given is 2500/20 = 125 maximum shots in one session.

If PC is purchased as 100 mg/ml, then an injection of 0.2 ml (20 mg) of PC is equal to Dr. Hasengschwandtner's dose of PC.

The author injects 0.2 ml of PC in each shot.

Lidocaine

With injections of pure PC 50 mg/ml into the fat, patients report pain on a scale of 8/10 verses 2/10 with the addition of lidocaine (personal clinical experience). Therefore, it appears useful to add lidocaine to the injections. Furthermore, the French have always claimed that lidocaine or procaine enhance the effects of various mesotherapy cocktails used for cellulite reduction.

Maximum safe dose for lidocaine (or marcaine) in an adult is 400 mg according to the package insert. It seems prudent to use 250 mg as the maximum to improve this margin of safety. Alternatively, one can use marcaine 0.5% instead but it is six times the cost of lidocaine.

lidocaine 250 mg/ 125 shots = 2 mg per shot
lidocaine 1% = 10 mg/ml. Therefore, 2 mg of lidocaine 1% = 0.2 ml lidocaine.

The author injects 0.2 ml of lidocaine in each shot.

The author injects a total of 0.4 ml with each injection point which consists of 20 mg PC and 2 mg of lidocaine.

The daily solution for injection is made up by mixing equal volumes of PC 100 mg/ml and lidocaine 1%. This dilutes the PC by 50%, down to 50 mg/ml. Therefore, a 5 ml syringe will contain 250 mg (50 mg/ml x 5 ml) PC. The maximum that should be injected is ten syringes of this solution. It is strongly recommended to start with two to four syringes as a maximum dose (500–1000 mg PC).

Note: If one adds other medications to PC, the solution must be used within 24 hours. It is not known if a mixture of PC with other drugs is stable for longer periods. Many practitioners are routinely adding L-carntine, aminophylline, collagenase, and hyaluronidase to their PC syringes. Thus, an example of an alternative formula mixed in a 5cc syringe for injection:

2 cc	PC 100 mg/ml
1 cc	collagenase 1000u/ml
1 cc	L-carnitine
1 cc	lidocaine 2%

How to Make Injection Lipolysis Solution in the Office

Most compounding pharmacies make up 50 ml bottles of PC 100 mg/ml. One can order only 25 ml of PC in the sterile 50 ml bottle, and then fill the bottle as follows:

PC @ 100 mg/ml (2500 mg) = 25 ml
lidocaine 1% (250 mg) = 25 ml
Total = 50 ml solution

This 50 ml solution can be drawn up into ten 5 ml syringes. This is the maximum amount that any one patient should receive at one session.

This formula was designed so that 0.4 ml can be injected with each injection, which is two lines on a 5 ml BD syringe. One 5 ml syringe will allow the physician to inject 12 points, with a tiny amount left over for a 13th shot.

Some practitioners will prefer a 3 ml syringe based on the size of their hand. If a 3 ml syringe is used there will be 150 mg of PC in each syringe. In this case, a conservative starting dose would be 3 × 3 ml syringes (=450 mg PC).

Procedure for Injecting Injection Lipolysis into Fatty Pads Overlying Cellulite

1. Patient consultation, informed consent signed, pictures and measurements taken.
2. Clean the skin with a good skin disinfectant. The author uses Techni-Care Surgical Scrub as it is gentle on the skin with high efficacy [32]. It can be purchased at http://www.caretechlabs.com.
3. Make up the solution consisting of equal volumes PC 100 mg/ml and lidocaine 1%.
4. Draw up the solution into 3 ml or 5 ml syringes (5 ml = 250 mg PC).
5. Use a surgical marking pen to draw points of injection over the localized fatty deposit. The points should be about 2–3 cm apart.
6. Count the number of points. About 13 points can be injected with one 5 ml syringe with 0.4 ml per injection site. Remember, the most that should ever be injected is 2500 mg of PC in total, or about 130 injection points.
7. Use a 1/2 inch 30 G. needle. Change the needle every one to two syringes as it gets dull. Inject next to the points that are marked to a depth of 13 mm into the fatty deposits to avoid tattooing the skin with ink. A 6 mm needle may also be used.
8. Use a Zimmer cooler or ice or vibration to decrease the pain of injections.
9. Wipe off the skin again with Techni-Care or isopropyl alcohol to remove the surgical marking pen marks and to help spread the PC in the skin.
10. Give the patient instructions and an analgesic prescription if necessary.

Typical Injection Pattern Using Up One 5 ml Syringe

Note each injection point is equidistant. The injection pattern should resemble the five side of a die. Each point represents 20 mg of PC injected to a depth of 13 mm.

Dr. Rittes' technique for injection lipolysis is to inject 0.8 ml of PC 50 mg/ml solution (40 mg PC into each injection point) into six sites spread over about 80 sq. cm.

Injection Lipolysis for Infraorbital Fat Pads (Rittes Technique)
Press gently on the globe of the eye. Observe bulging of the three infraorbital fad pads under the eye. Give three injections to a depth of about 6 mm, perpendicular to the skin into the middle of each infraorbital fat bulge. (See Figure 11.4)

1. Use PC 50 mg/ml. Draw up 0.8 ml (40 mg PC) in a one ml syringe to do both infraorbital fat pads.
2. Use a 1/2 inch 30 G needle. Inject the needle only halfway (about 6 mm) into the fat pad (not the eyeball!) perpendicular to the skin.
3. Use a total of 0.4 ml (20 mg) per eye injected carefully into three sites as in the following pattern (see Fig. 11.4):

Lateral fat pad:	0.1 ml
Middle fat pad:	0.2 ml
Nasal fat pad:	0.1 ml
Total per eye:	0.4 ml

4. Ask the patient to try to avoid ice packs or NSAIDS for eye swelling. Sleep with head elevated on three pillows for two days following treatment to reduce swelling around the eyes.
5. Wait at least two weeks between treatments; skin should tighten.
6. Total two to four injection sessions. It may take six months to achieve optimal results.

Clinical Examples of Injection Lipolysis Therapy
Figs. 11.5–11.14 show improvement of cellulite following injection lipolysis.

Injection Lipolysis Summary: Simple Injections for Fat Reduction
Injection lipolysis is an injectable technique that specifically targets localized fat and indurated cellulite deposits. The ideal patient has a BMI <23. The patient may also have cellulite, stretch marks, and flaccid skin. The treatment slowly dissolves the deposits with injections of a fat-dissolving substance called phosphatidylcholine, a natural substance derived from soy bean lecithin. Phosphatidylcholine makes up 40% of our cell membranes, and is found throughout our bodies. The body naturally eliminates the residue after an injection lipolysis session over the following three to four weeks. Side effects can include mild swelling, bruising, discomfort, or itching.

Treatment typically involves a series of injections, administered in a clinical setting, at the target area(s) over several weeks. On average, one to four treatments, with 14 to 42 day intervals between them, are required to achieve the desired results. No global protocols have been established.

Over the past eight years, physicians have successfully used injection lipolysis on tens of thousands of patients. The areas that respond best to injection lipolysis treatment – in those who are not excessively overweight – are certain stubborn fat deposits that resist further reduction after diet and exercise. These include the lower eyelids, or tear bags, double chins, the abdomen, love handles, backs of arms, thigh saddlebags, knees, and wings (the area on the back, just beside the armpits). Injection lipolysis has also been shown to improve and smooth out the skin, which is a benefit for those with severe cellulite.

In fact, injection lipolysis is now being used to help improve cosmetic irregularities that can occur following liposuction. Furthermore, liposuction does not improve cellulite; only injection lipolysis has been shown to improve the skin texture in cellulite.

Long-term side effects in injection lipolysis applications are unknown at present. However, no long-term adverse effects have been reported from any physicians who have been administering these injections for almost a decade now in areas outside of North America. Injection lipolysis injections should be administered under medical supervision. People who are pregnant, morbidly obese, suffering certain diagnosed illnesses, or allergic to the product should not have injection lipolysis injections.

Further clinical studies must be done to enhance our scientific knowledge of this promising therapy. It should not be discarded simply because the exact mechanism of action or optimal dose are unknown. Allopathic medical practitioners have been injecting cortisone for decades at different depths for a variety of inflammatory conditions, but the exact mechanism of action, optimal dose and interval of injections for a given inflammatory condition in a specific location has never been scientifically proven. This does not mean that cortisone injections should be abandoned; rather caution is advised when using this substance until the careful practitioner gathers clinical experience and confidence with its use. Spending time with a medical practitioner experienced with the use of the injectable substance is invaluable to observe injection technique and clinical practice. The same can be said for injection lipolysis therapy at the present time.

REFERENCES
1. AC Beynen, MB Katan. Lecithin intake and serum cholesterol. Am J Clin Nutr 49(2):266–88, Feb 1989.
2. VI Bobkova, LI Lokachina, BH Korsunsk et al. Metabolic effect of lipostabilforte. Kardiologia; 1989: 29:57.
3. F Kosina, K Budka, Z Kolouch et al. Viral Essential cholinephospholipids in the treatment of hepatitis. Cas Lek Ces 120:957–60, 1981.
4. C Hirayama. M Okamura et al. The effect of polyenephosphatidylcholine in chronic hepatitis in double-blind test. Rinsho you kenkyu 55:194–98, 1978.
5. A Schuller-Perez, FG San Martin. Controlled study using unsaturated phosphatidylcholine in comparison with placebo in the case of alcoholic liver steatosis. Med Welt 72: 717–521, 1985.
6. S Maggiori. Mesotherapy treatment of xanthelasma with polyunsaturated phosphatidylcholine. Presented at the 5th International Conference of Mesotherapy, Paris; 1988.
7. M Serra, FB Pereira. Subcutaneous infiltration with phosphatidylcholine solution for treatment of buffalo hump and fatty pads. Third International Workshop of Adverse Drug Reactions and Lipodystrophy in HIV, Athens, Greece; 2001, abstract P115.
8. PG Rittes. The use of phosphatidylcholine for correction of lower lid bulging due to prominent fat pads. Dermatol Surg 27:391–2, 2001.
9. G Ablon, AM Rotunda. Treatment of lower eyelid fat pads using phosphatidylcholine: clinical trial and review.

Dermatol Surg (United States) 30(3):p422–7, Mar 2004; discussion 428.

10. PG Rittes. The use of phosphatidylcholine for correction of localized fat deposits. Aesthetic Plast Surg 27(4):p315–8, Jul-Aug 2003.

11. D Hexsel, M Serra, R Mazzuco et al. Phosphatidylcholine in the treatment of localized fat. J Drugs Dermatol 2(5):p511–8, Oct 2003.

12. PT Rose, M Morgan. Histological changes associated with mesotherapy for fat dissolution. J Cosmet Laser Ther 7(1): 17–9, Mar 2005.

13. S Schuller-Petrovic, G Wolkart, G Hofler et al. Tissue-toxic effects of phosphatidylcholine/deoxycholate after subcutaneous injection for fat dissolution in rats and a human volunteer Dermatol Surg 34(4):529–42, Apr 2008.

14. FG Bechara, M Sand, K Hoffman et al. Fat tissue after lipolysis of lipomas: a histopathological and immunohistochemical study. J Cutan Pathol 34(7):552–7, Jul 2007.

15. FG Bechara, M Sand, D Sand et al. Lipolysis of lipomas in patients with familial multiple lipomatosis: an ultrasonography-controlled trial. J Cutan Med Surg 10(4):155–9, Jul-Aug 2006.

16. A Rotunda, H Suzuki., R Moy et al. Detergent Effects of Sodium deoxycholate are a major feature of an injectable phosphatidylcholine formulation used for localized fat dissolution. Dermatol Surg 30:1001–08, 2004.

17. ME Yagima Odo, LC Cuce, LM Odo et al. Action of sodium deoxycholate on subcutaneous human tissue: local and systemic effects. Dermatol. Surg 33(2):178–88; discussion 188–9, Feb 2007.

18. AM Rotunda, G Ablon, MS Kolodney. Lipomas treated with subcutaneous deoxycholate injections. J Am Acad Dermatol 53(6):973–8, Dec 2005.

19. G Salti, I Ghersetich, F Tantussi et al. Phosphatidylcholine and sodium deoxycholate in the treatment of localized fat: a double-blind, randomized study. Dermatol Surg 43(1):60–6, Jan 2008.

20. PJ Treacy, DJ Goldberg. Use of phosphatidylcholine for the correction of lower lid buldging due to prominent fat pads. J Cosmet Laser Ther 8(3):129–32, Sep 2006.

21. M Palmer, J Curran, P Bowler. Clinical experience and safety using phosphatidylcholine injections for the localized reduction of subcutaneous fat: a multicentre, retrospective UK study. J Cosmet Dermatol 5(3):218–26, Sep 2006.

22. DI Duncan, R Chubaty. Clinical Safety Data and Standards of Practice for Injection Lipolysis: A Retrospective Study. Aesthetic Surg J 26(5):1–11, Sep 2006.

23. F Hasengschwandtner, F Furtmueller, M Spanbauer, R Silye. Detailed documentation of one lipolysis treatment: blood values, histology, and ultrasonic findings. Aesthetic Surg J 27(2):204–10, Mar 2007.

24. J Marco-Bonnet, M Beylot-Barry, J Texier-Maugein et al. Mycobacterial bovis BCG cutaneous infections following mesotherapy: 2 cases Ann Dermatol Venereol (France), 129(5 Pt 1):p728–32, May 2002.

25. P Rosina, C Chieregato, D Miccolis et al. Psoriasis and side-effects of mesotherapy. Int J Dermatol (United States) 40(9):p581–3, Sep 2001.

26. E Nagore, P Ramos, R Botella-Estrada et al. Cutaneous infection with Mycobacterium fortuitum after localized micro-injections (mesotherapy) treated successfully with a triple drug regimen. Acta Derm Venereol (Norway) 81(4):p291–3, Aug-Sep 2001.

27. W Furlong, BA Cunanan, LA Weymouth et al. Outbreak of mesotherapy-associated skn reactions –District of Columbia February, 2005 MMWR 2005 Nov. 11;54(44): 1127–30.

28. DP Lee, SE Chang. Letter to the Editor: Subcutaneous nodules showing fat necrosis owing to mesotherapy. Dermatol Surg 31:250–51, 2005.

29. D Duncan, M Palmer. Fat reduction using phosphatidylcholine/ sodium deoxycholate injections: standard of practice. Aesthetic Plast Surg 32(6):858–72, Nov 2008.

30. Letter dated July 22, 2003 to Ayoula Dublin from Jerome G. Woyshner, District Director, Public Health Service, FDA, 158–15 Liberty Ave., Jamaca, N.Y. 11433.

31. http://www.kytherabiopharma.com/news.html accessed February 5, 2009.

32. http://www.bene-arzneimittel.de/doc/faqs.htm

12 No-Needle Mesotherapy
Gustavo Leibaschoff

Recently, much interest has been expressed in new devices capable of penetrating ingredients to a useful depth in tissue without the use of conventional injection. Target conditions include cellulite formations, fat masses, photoaging of the face and hyperpigmentation.

Transdermal drug administration has obvious potential advantages over oral, injection, or intravenous drug delivery. Many aesthetic applications seek to deliver ingredient molecules to a specific depth in tissue to rejuvenate photoaged skin, minimize or eliminate hyperpigmentation, smooth tissue areas impacted by cellulite or mobilize localized fat deposits. Conventionally applied topical medications, used for aesthetic treatments, are limited in their ability to penetrate to any significant depth in tissue.

Advantages of transdermal delivery techniques relate to convenience, patient comfort, minimal trauma and possible delegation of treatments to ancillary personnel. Highly localized administration is possible, and delivery can be achieved through absorption by dermal blood supply and distribution via the lymphatic system.

New methods of transdermal delivery focus on techniques that are efficient at delivering molecules to an appropriate treatment site, thus avoiding the risk of a poor outcome. Disruption of the stratum corneum can be achieved by electroporation or the creation of water channels or microconduits. In electroporation, ions and molecules move through the stratum corneum by diffusion and electromotive or electro-osmotic transport [1].

The DermaWave No-Needle Mesotherapy System (DermaWave Company, USA and BTL Industries, Prague, CZ) uses three sequences of electrical waveforms to deliver topical ingredients transdermally. A prescription, conductive, active gel may be used to address the underlying factors contributing to the formation of cellulite, hyperpigmentation, photoaging and fat deposits. Tissue is pretreated with a low-level, non-thermal, dual wavelength laser cluster delivering a combined fluence of approximately 5 joules cm². Specific wavelengths used are 685 nm and 830 nm.

The laser component of the treatment is designed to increase blood flow and cell permeability as a precursor to the delivery of a proprietary mix of ingredients similar to that used in a standard mesotherapy injection dose. Laser application is followed by three phases of electrical stimulation the first of which, using electroporation techniques, delivers the active substances to a chosen depth in tissue. Second and third phase electrical waveforms focus on muscle toning and stimulation of increased blood flow while the third phase enhances lymphatic drainage.

Transdermal drug delivery is critically dependent on molecular size and charge. Electroporation allows the entry of proteins and micrometer-sized particles into cells and across the stratum corneum (SC) [21]. The transport of large macromolecules is hampered by the cross-linked keratin matrix within corneocytes [21]. This method relies on the insertion of aquapores into the skin (aquaphoresis) [22,23] which will create drug penetration routes [24,25] thereby increasing the transdermal delivery of drugs. Lipophyllic drugs passively diffuse across the SC and their absorption is limited by the epidermis and dermis. Therefore electroporation, a physical permeation-enhancing technique for macromolecular transdermal transport, is used to enhance influx of hydrophilic and lipophyllic drugs across the SC [25].

Electroporation is the transitory structural perturbation of lipid bilayer membranes due to the application of high voltage (HV) pulses (>100V). HV pulses are applied for a very short duration to enhance macromolecular transport reversibly by permeabilizing the SC [25]. The skin resistance drops by several orders of magnitude during HV pulsing and is partly reversible [22]. *In vitro* transportation is increased up to four orders of magnitude compared to passive diffusion and the electrical fractional area for small ion transport is approximately 0.1% [22]. Unlike mechanical skin puncture, electroporation itself is self-localizing to the SC, because initial high SC resistance causes most of the transdermal voltages to be concentrated across the SC [21].

Electroporation differs from iontophoresis in the type of electrical waveform used. Electroporation techniques always use pulsed waveforms while iontophoresis current is constant. Constant currents induce tissue accommodation where the body's natural defenses set up a resistance pattern to the stimulus and active penetration depth is minimal. Studies [2] comparing iontophoresis with electroporation show that iontophoresis delivers 100 times *less* drug than injection but provides higher local concentrations than oral administration.

In iontophoresis, the pathways that ingredients take are restricted with the drug permeating the skin via appendageal pores making delivery of actives via iontophoresis inefficient for large tissue areas. Appendageal penetration is slow, so dilution of the medication is a major factor influencing success. In contrast, the number of transdermal pathways available via electroporation is 500 times greater than with iontophoresis [2]. Medication is delivered fast to the treatment site ensuring as much as 90% of the medication strength is maintained.

For example, methylene blue, delivered by electroporation, shows much greater penetration than dye delivered by iontophoresis. Delivery is enhanced by energy in the form of pulses, and even at low electroporation levels delivery of MB was dramatically higher than with iontophoresis [2].

Comparison of no-needle and injection delivery of medication requires an objective determination of the depth delivery potential of the no-needle technique. Radioisotope lymphography is used to establish molecule penetration and retention time in tissue and employs a tagging technique that traces ingredient passage through intact stratum corneum to sites in the extracellular matrix and dermis. The technique monitors the retention of ingredients in tissue at specified times as well as their presence in the lymphatic system.

A small, instrumental study using radioisotope lymphography was carried out to determine the effectiveness of the no-needle

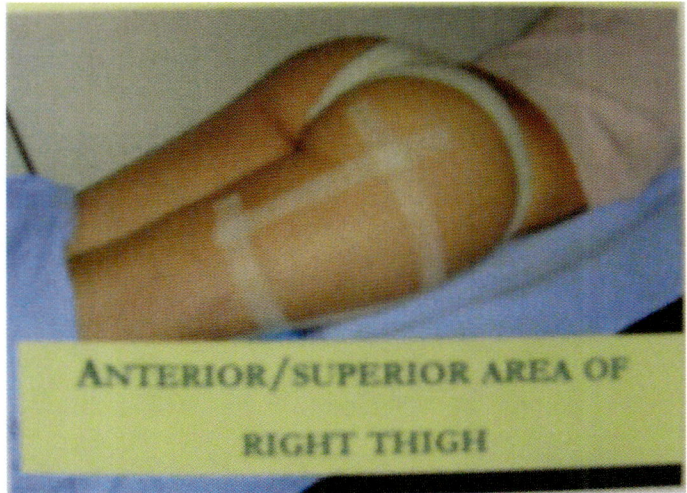

Figure 12.1 Anterior/superior area of right thigh.

technique. The DermaWave device utilizes techniques of molecule delivery called threshold electroporation and aquaphoresis, both of which facilitate transdermal delivery of different topical active ingredients.

The study objective was to monitor absorption of the active ingredients to a specific depth in tissue and to determine if they were present after absorption in the lymphatic system of patients

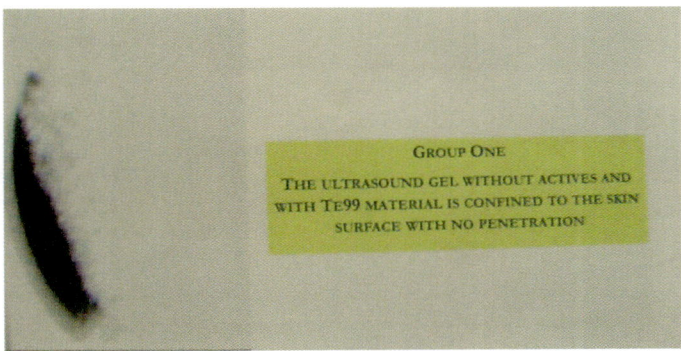

(a)

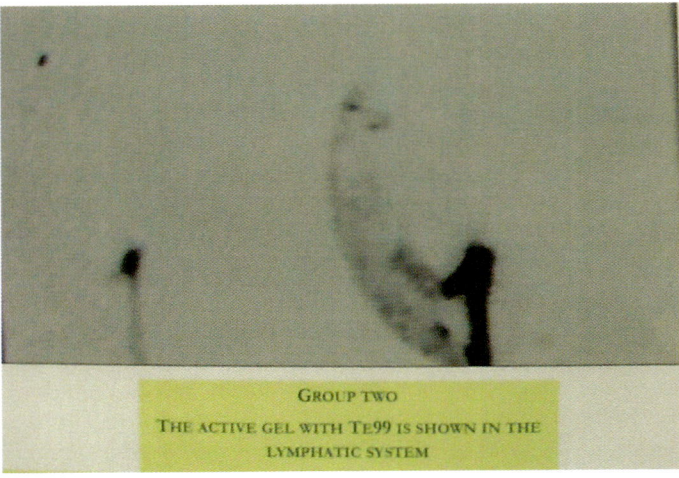

(b)

Figure 12.2 The active gel with 99 mTc is shown in the lymphatic system.

with edematous fibrosclerotic panniculopathy (cellulite). The study also sought to determine if the gel containing the active ingredients was delivered to the required site of action and was present in the lymphatic system at various time intervals after treatment. The presence of the radioactive material in the lymphatic system validates the study hypothesis.

The active ingredients are encapsulated in a standardized, micronized gel specifically designed to be used with the device. Study objectives were to monitor absorption of active ingredients to a specific depth in tissue and to determine if the active ingredients were present after absorption in the lymphatic system of patients with cellulite.

- The study had a prospective, longitudinal, and double-blind design. A total of 10 female patients aged 32 to 45 years were selected.

All patients presented with the same pathology, mild lipodistrophy of the lateral area of the thigh, without skin retraction, lipoedema, lymphoedema or phleboedema.

The patients were divided into two groups—the first group received a regular ultrasound gel not containing active ingredients. The second group received the specially formulated micronized gel containing the active ingredients.

Each of the gels was marked with 10 mCi of 99 mTc tecnesio meta stable, in a mixing technique designed to homogenize the samples. In all cases, the application was on the saddle bag area of the upper right thigh, over a predetermined and perfectly demarcated surface. After delivery of the gels, radioisotope lymphography was used as a non-invasive, instrumental method of tracking the gel through tissue. The test was performed according to standard methods. The radioactive substance used was 99mTc tecnesio meta stable—selected due to the short average life of the material at 6.4 hours at a level of 140Kev. This mix produces substantially less risk of contamination to patients and operator.

One hundred prercent of the group receiving the permeation-enhanced active material showed transdermal penetration through an intact stratum corneum to the extracellular matrix of the dermis in less than 20 minutes and even distribution and retention in tissue up to 24 hours [3].

The images of the bilateral inguinal region and pelvic area under treatment were recorded using a Gamma Planar device with collimator immediately post-treatment and 2–4 and 24 hours after treatment. After 24 hours a sweeping anterior thorax abdominal pelvic scan was added using the anterior superior hip bone as a reference.

Radioisotope lymphography showed that all patients receiving non-active ultrasound gel showed minimal penetration, with most of the tagged material residing in the upper epidermis.

One hundred percent of the lymphography scans of the first group showed no trace of the radioactive substance 99mTc.

The presence of gel with active ingredients: 1,3,7-trimethylxanthine, algesium, allantoin, aloe vera, aminophylline, amino acid complex, antioxidant complex, sodium deoxycholate, grapefruit seed extract, grape seed extract, green tea extract, melilotus, PC, procaine, rutina, silica, trace minerals, xylitol, yohimbine in the lymphatics confirms that transdermal diffusion has occurred.

Most importantly, the connective tissue, comprising the extracellular matrix and lymphatic pre-collector vessels, has absorbed the medication.

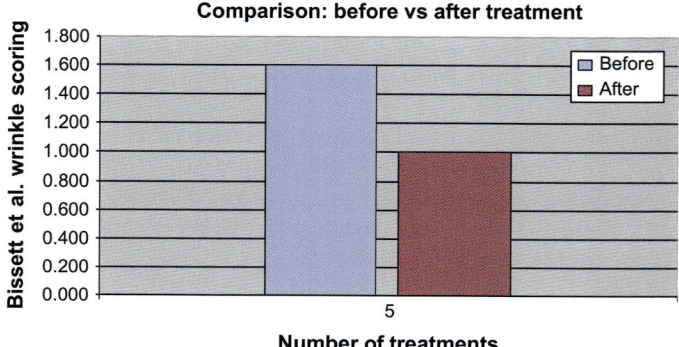

Figure 12.3 Bisset scoring et al. The graph above compares the averages of the before and after five treatments. From the above graph, results showed that there is a significant change in the scores after the treatment.

An *in vivo* study from the University of Pretoria, South Africa, observed the effects of the DermaWave No-Needle Mesotherapy System on facial photoaging.

An *in vivo* study was conducted to observe the effects of the DermaWave on photoaging through transdermal delivery of a combination of agents, i.e. hyaluronic acid, retinoic acid and DMAE. A five-week clinical trial was conducted where 15 volunteers were treated with the DermaWave. All volunteers showed a reduction in photoaging. The system successfully increased transdermal drug delivery and represents a safe, effective alternative to painful needle mesotherapy.

In vitro effects of the combination of agents and individual components on collagen synthesis and cell proliferation in chick embryonic fibroblasts were also studied. Hyaluronic acid, retinoic acid, DMAE and the combination drug reduced the effects of photoaging. Hyaluronic acid, DMAE and the combination drug increased collagen synthesis in chick embryonic fibroblast cultures. *In vitro* retinoic acid inhibited cell proliferation but when topically applied is known to stimulate collagen formation in the upper dermis and accelerate the repair process of photoaged skin. Crystal violet staining showed an increase in fibroblast proliferation when treated with dimethylaminoethanol, and a decrease in cell growth when treated with retinoic acid and hyaluronic acid. Alcian blue staining indicated enhanced collagen synthesis with dimethylaminoethanol, hyaluronic acid and the combination of drugs.

Fifteen volunteers aged between 35 and 50 years with advanced photoaging received facial treatment with the DermaWave system for five sessions. Advanced photoaging is characterized by early wrinkling, sallow complexion with early actinic keratoses. The forehead and periorbital areas were divided into two regions

Table 12.1 Statistical analysis: Percentages of patients with coarse wrinkles in various Bissett et al. scoring groups

Bissett et al. scoring	Control	Treatment*
0	20.0	26.67
1	13.3	53.33
2	53.3	20.0
3	13.3	0

* The treatment is significantly different from the control side p = 0.037, i.e. a greater number of patients entered into the lower wrinkle grade.

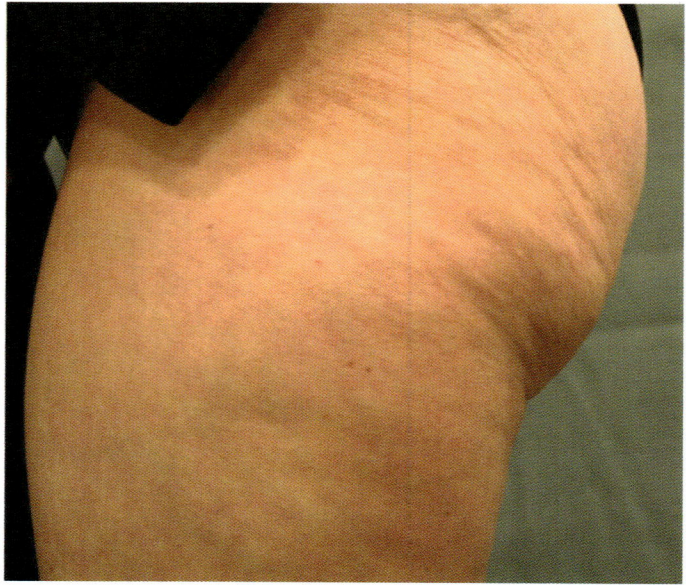

(a)

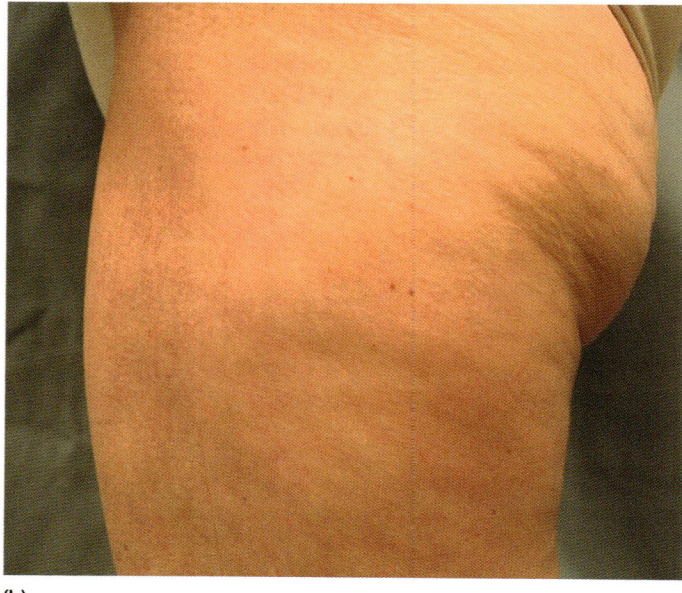

(b)

Figure 12.4 After 6 sessions with DermaWave, courtesy DermaWave.

left and right. Only one side of the facial area was treated with the combination drug containing a combination of: HA, RA and DMAE. In this single blind study sides were randomized and each volunteer was used as their own control. Before treatment photographs were taken and again one week after the fifth treatment. Photographs were rated with the Bissett et al. wrinkle scoring.

This system is a non-thermagenic transdermal drug delivery system that transports the active ingredients in the treatment gel to the mesoderm through aquaphoresis. DermaWave treatments use two specific waveforms (635 nm and 850 nm) of electrical energy to a) create "aquapores" and b) increase metabolic rate by five to seven times, which results in an increased blood flow and subsequent increase in fibroblast activity and collagen deposition.

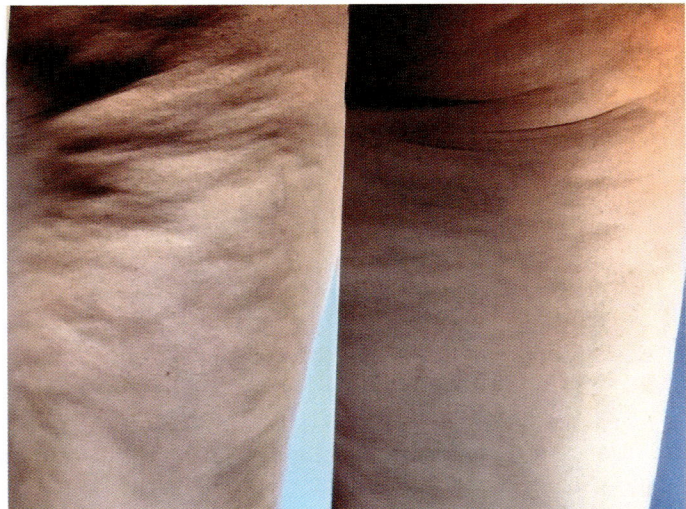

Figure 12.5 Courtesy Dr. Mitch Chasin M.D. New Jersey.

DermaWave applicator with unit dose of medication
The voltage maintained on the forehead was 10V and periorbital 20V. The pain threshold of the volunteers varied from the highest voltage of 30V periorbitally to the lowest 9V.

An *in vitro* model evaluation of active components on fibroblast growth and collagen formation was conducted to verify success of ingredient delivery.

Four-day-old chicken eggs (National Chicks hatchery). Trypsin/ Versene solution (0.25% Trypsin + 0.05% EDTA solution in Ca +2 Mg +2 Free Dulbecco Buffer; HIGHVELD BIOLOGICAL (PTY) LTD), RMPI-1640 medium mixture (medium made up with powder obtained from: SIGMA-ALDRICH-CAT NO R6504-10L) containing 10% fetal calf serum (HI FCS) (Adcock Ingram Scientific, CAT. 14-501AI) and 1% pen/strep mixture (Adcock Ingram Scientific, CAT. 17-602E), PBS (Phosphate Buffered Saline) (Scientific Group), crystal violet (Merck), acetic acid (Holpro), alcian blue (Merck), 2,5% formaldehyde, HA, RA and DMAE. Cell morphology was evaluated using an OLYMPUS 1 × 70 light microscope and the images were acquired under constant power and gain settings using Motic Images software (Multicam 2000).

Chick embryonic fibroblast culturing: four-day-old chicken eggs were incubated for six days at 37, 5-39 °C and 50% humidity. Fibroblasts were isolated from 10-day-old chick embryos by serial enzyme digestion with trypsin. One millilitre fibroblast cell

Table 12.2 Crystal violet and alcian blue staining

Drugs	a) Fibroblast growth (Crystal violet)	b) Collagen synthesis (Alcian blue)
DMAE	+ + +	+ +
Retinoic acid	– –	0
Hyaluronic acid	–	+
Combination	+ + +	+ + +

a) Grading was done visually according to growth of fibroblasts. DMAE and the combination drug increased fibroblast growth, whereas HA and RA decreased the fibroblast growth.
b) Blue stain indicates collagen. DMAE, HA and the combination drug increased collagen synthesis, whereas RA decreased collagen synthesis.

suspension was subcultured in 15 ml RMPI containing 10% FCS supplemented with 1% pen/strep in a 75 cm² tissue culture flask. Cells were incubated in 37 °C 5% CO_2 atmosphere for up to three days. When fibroblasts reached confluency they were trypsinized and counted with a hemocytometer and cultured in a 96-well microplate at a density of 2 × 105 cells cells/ml. Cells at a confluent density were treated with RA (10 ug/ml), HA (00 ug/ml), DMAE (1 ug/ml) and the combination of these agents (10 ug/ml) irrespectively for seven days. Fibroblasts were stained using two other methods: crystal violet staining and alcian blue staining.

Results: *In vitro* model
1a)   b)
c)   d)
e)   f)
g)   h)
2a)   b)
c)   d)
e)   f)
g)   h)

The *in vitro* results clearly show enhanced collagen and fibroblast responses when the cell cultures were exposed to the individual and combination of agents: HA, RA and DMAE.

Results: *In vivo* model
The main outcome of this study was reached. DermaWave™ treatment of the skin using HA, RA and DMAE visually improved the appearance of wrinkles significantly.

Conclusion
DermaWave electroporation of the combination drug containing, DMAE, RA and HA resulted in a significant reduction of coarse wrinkles after five treatments (one treatment per week). This is comparably better than reported results with mesotherapy in literature.

Crystal violet staining of *in vitro* cell cultures showed an increase in fibroblast proliferation when treated with DMAE, and a decrease in cell growth when treated with RA and HA as anticipated. Alcian blue staining indicated increased collagen synthesis with DMAE, HA and the combination drug. Thus the combination drug showed an enhanced effect when compared to its different isolated components.

All volunteers showed a reduction in photoaging. The system successfully increased transdermal delivery and was described as a safe, effective alternative to painful needle mesotherapy [4].

In the case of cellulite formation, it is important to address the visible result of the condition as well as the underlying cause. Cellulite deposits occur as the result of biochemical and metabolic alterations at an interstitial matrix and connective structures level [7-14].

Current strategies for reduction of cellulite are focused on treatments to reduce the external appearance of the disease. Reduction of external dimpling represents only one aspect of cellulite formation and does not address the many underlying causes of the condition. Practitioners employing a single strategy to improve the appearance of dimpled skin may be limited in offering patients a viable long-term solution to their problem.

Transdermal delivery of medications is a major thrust to the world's pharmaceutical companies with upwards of 40% of new drugs being developed for this method. No-Needle Mesotherapy is expected to transition from exclusively aesthetic applications to other areas of interest in medicine [5].

Obviously, downsides for patients undergoing injection mesotherapy are pain, erythema, potential for allergic reaction and the bruising associated with any multiple injection strategy. For the physician, injection techniques require personal involvement and a well practiced technique.

The DermaWave No-Needle Mesotherapy System is a Class II device using a dual wavelength laser, and three complex electrical waveforms, delivered in sequence, to produce an effect called threshold electroporation and aquaphoresis. [15–17]. The two methodologies are delivered via a hand-held applicator and a series of pre-programmed protocols to facilitate transdermal delivery of permeation-enhanced topical ingredients. These ingredients are formulated into a standardized 'cocktail' containing some of the same ingredients used in injection mesotherapy.

The active ingredients are compounded in the form of micromolecules, in a proprietary, permeation enhanced gel [18].

REFERENCES

1. T Kotnik, F Bobanovic, D Miklavic. Sensitivity of transmembrane voltage induced by applied electric fields—a theoretical analysis. Biolectrochem Bioenerg 43:285–91, 1997.
2. PG Johnson, SA Gallo, SW Hui. A Pulsed Electric Field Enhances Cutaneous Delivery of Methylene Blue in Excised Full Thickness Porcine Skin. Journal of Investigative Dermatology 111:457–63, 1998.
3. G Leibaschoff, S Nieto. Navy Hospital Buenos Argentina Preliminary Study to Verify the Transdermal Delivery of a Micronized Gel with Active Ingredients Using DermaWave "No Needle Mesotherapy" (NNM), Lymphatic Foundation. Buenos Aires, Argentina; 2007 (unpublished).
4. EE Visser. DermaWaveTM electroporation: transdermal drug delivery improves photoaged skin.
5. F Albergati, PA Bacci. La matrice extracellulare, Minelli Editore; 2004.
6. D Miklavcic, T Kotnik. Electroporation for electrochemotherapy and gene therapy. In PJ Rosch, MS Markov, Bioelectromagnetic Medicine. Marcel Dekker, New York; 2004: 637–56.
7. C Allegra, G Pollari, V Antonini et al. Pannicolopatia edematofibrosclerotica, Minerva Mesoterapica 1:24–6, 1986.
8. PA Bacci. Il lipolinfedema: riflessioni e osservazioni cliniche, Flebologia Oggi, Torino Minerva Medica 2:10–21, 1997.
9. JF Merlen, SB Curri, AM Sarteel. La cellulite, une mesenchimopatie discuté. Sci Med Lille 96:251–53, 1978.
10. M Binazzi, M Papini. Aspetti clinico istomorfologici. In A Ribuffo, CA Bartoletti, La cellulite. Salus, Rome; 1983:7–15.
11. SB Curri. Liposclerosi e microcircolo. La dermoestetica 1:6–7, 1990.
12. G Leibaschoff. Cellulite: Etiology and treatment. American Journal of Cosmetic Surgery 14(4):395–401, 1997.
13. PA Bacci, G Leibaschoff. Las cellulitis, el protocolo BIMED, Medical Books, Buenos Aires; 2002.
14. F Albergati, L Menegon, Turatello, PA Bacci, Valutazione degli effetti microcircolatori dopo terapia della matrice extracellulare in pazienti con flebolinfedema. Linfologia, Auxilia speciale, Bologna; 2001: 8–11.
15. Robin Bogner. Meghan Wilkosz : Transdermal Drug Delivery, US Pharmacist 28(05):1–9, 2003.
16. SA Freeman, MA Wang. Theory of electroporation of planar bilayer membranes: predictions of the aqueous area, change in capacitance and pore-pore separation Biomembrane Electrochemistry 235:447–70, 1994.
17. R Vanbever, M Leroy, V Preat. Transdermal permeation of neutral molecules by skin electroporation. Journal of Controlled Release 54(3):243–50, 1998.
18. J Horejsova, J Spilka, J Pavlik, et al. No-needle mesotherapy—a review of aquaphoresis technology for cellulite. Institute of Medical Aesthetics, Prague, Czech Republic; September 2005.
19. A Denet, R Vanbever, V Préat. Skin electroporation for transdermal and topical delivery. Advanced Drug Delivery 56(5):659–74, 2004.
20. A Boucaud. Trends in the use of ultrasound mediated tansdermal drug delivery. Drug Discovery Today 9(19):827–28, 2004.
21. BW Barry. Drug delivery routes in skin: a novel approach. Advanced Drug Delivery 54(1):S31–S40, 2002.
22. Mark Prausnitz. Vanu Bose Robert Langer Electroporation of mammalian skin: A mechanism to enhance trasndermal drug delivery. Proc. Natl. Acad. Sci. USA 90:10504–508, November 1993 Medical sciences.
23. T Wong, Y Zhao, A Sen et al. Pilot study of topical delivery of methotrexate by electroporation. British Journal of Dermatology 152(3):524, 2005.

13 Endermologie–LPG Systems® after 15 Years

Pier Antonio Bacci

The treatment Endermologie®, patented by LPG Systems (Valence, France), constitutes a true revolution in the field of physical therapy both for clinical applications and aesthetics [1].

After 15 years of experience, we can certainly affirm this methodology as the most important basic treatment for cellulite. Associated with mesotherapy, it allows us to treat different forms of cellulite offering various solutions, in the area of the aesthetic and functional physiotherapy. It is the basic treatment around which we can rotate other necessary methodologies according to the cases.

This technique represents a revolution both the in the principle and practical application of massage by maximizing the traditional techniques of the physiotherapist. Endermologie® is performed with unique equipment and various protocols for different pathologies.

The equipment consists of a patented tool. The first instrument was named "Cellu M6®" and its use provides various clinical and aesthetic solutions, but it requires training.

After many experiences and studies, LPG produced different versions and today we have the most recent version named "Keymodule 2i®" that allows stretching the skin in various directions (Fig. 13.1). Endermologie® shows a clinical efficacy in cellulite linked with well-documented circulatory, anti-edematous, dermotrophic and lipolytic properties [2–9].

The modern instrument changes the use and the methodology because we have sophisticated control of the different actions, an easy application of treatments and the possibility to choose the best probe for different areas and indications (Fig. 13.2).

The new Keymodule 2i® maintains the same idea of using only compressed air, aiding the performance of various physiotherapeutic maneuvers such as pumping, draining and stimulating the vascular system.

The first maneuver is directed at muscles and tendons, the second is mostly directed at lipodermal tissues. These maneuvers favor emptying of the venous and lymphatic systems with the manual techniques described by Casley–Smith, Foldi and Leduc [10–12].

The fingers of the physiotherapist can perform maneuvers of grazing, pinching, slurring, compression and rotation of the tissues, in additional to the classical "paper-roller" characterized by movements of compression and rotation exploiting the elastic return of the tissue which also stimulates fibroblastic function.

Endermologie® treatment enhances the execution of the same maneuvers and operations performed with the fingers. It's therefore possible to perform stretching and traction at the same time.

The aspiration system of the machine lifts the skin and subcutaneous tissue inside the motorized handpiece as the operator works rolling up and moving the handpiece in the desired directions. The equipment software allows the operator to perform "compression-rotation" or "rhythmic compression-rotation"

maneuvers. This allows the therapist an endless range of therapeutic maneuvers to treat various pathologies or different phases of a complex pathology. Such characteristics increase the indications and fields of application.

To understand the concept and role of this complete and complex medical methodology it is necessary to describe the scientific principles and practical basis of some methods such as massage and lymphatic drainage, focusing on some fundamental principles of anatomy and physiology of the dermo-epidermal tissues.

Anatomy and Physiology

The interstitial matrix

This constitutes and represents the true inside "sea" where all the exchanges and all the vital cellular regulations happen, where life begins and chronic illnesses and degenerative changes such as the processes of aging occur. This is a substance that permeates every space and is found as a solution or gel. The principal cells that constitute it are the fibroblasts and the macrophages because they provide continuous recovery of the tissue and anti-inflammatory action.

Adipose tissue

Adipose tissue is, very probably, the most important tissue in the body. It is a form of connective tissue with energy formation regulatory functions [13–17]. The representative cell of this tissue is the adipocyte whose principal role is to maintain a reserve of fat, in addition to acting as mechanical protection and assisting with thermoregulation.

The quantity of adipocytes varies between individuals and also varies between regions of the body. The variability is based on genetics [18,19]. Above the muscular fascia is a pillow of fat "*parallel fat*", whose principal characteristic is reactivity to the food/caloric intake, constituting an important cause of obesity. Some regions of the body possess subfacial fat that is referred to as "*steatomery.*" It is slightly sensitive to caloric intake and insulin. To be able to lose 1 kg of steatomeric fat one must lose 6 kg of systemic fat. Inside the abdomen another type of fat, "*intravisceral fat*" also responds quickly to caloric intake.

Adipose tissue is connected to the endocrine system through hormones that act on the metabolism of the fats. They are divided into two groups:

1. lipoclastic hormones (catecholamine, adrenaline, glucagons, ACTH, TSH, thyroid hormones)
2. lipogenetic hormones (insulin, sex hormones, in particular estrogens)

Endermologie acts on the skin and subcutaneous tissue, connective tissue, fat tissue and the microcirculation both arteriolar, venous and lymphatics [20,21].

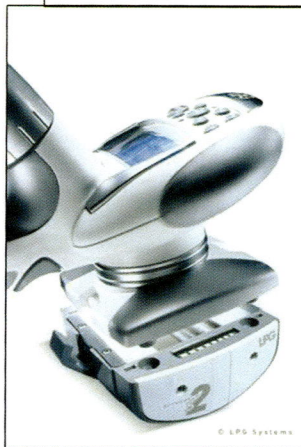

The new instrument "Key Module"

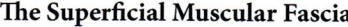

Using this methodology we can have active action for:

- CONNECTIVE TISSUE
- VASCULAR SYSTEM
- METABOLIC FUNCTION
- ADIPOSE TISSUE
- STATUS OF THE SKIN
- COLLAGEN PRODUCTION
- LYMPHATIC DRAINAGE

Figure 13.1 Endermologie® facilitates different activities.

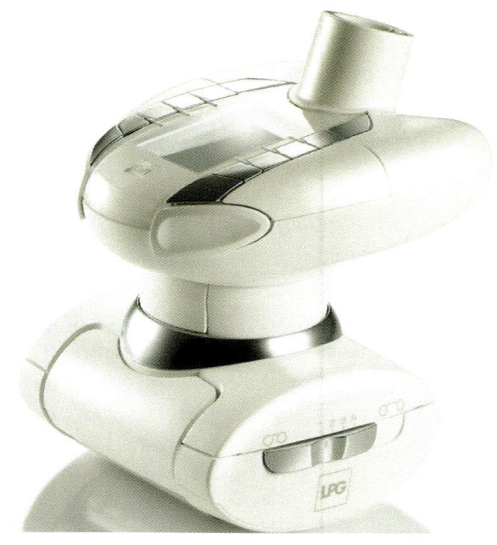

Figure 13.2 New instruments have different probes for different pathologies.

The Superficial Muscular Fascia

Treatment of this fascia is very important to have the best results using Endermologie®.

Surgeons and anatomists have often ignored or denied the importance of the superficial fascia of the body. For example, the anatomical layer on which liposuction or liposculpture occurs is really the superficial fascia, considered sometimes as a systemic bandage: SFS (superficial fascial system). An interesting anatomical and histological examination of the inferior limbs has shown the presence of the "superficial fascia" as responsible for numerous aesthetic alterations of the skin surface [22].

The depressions and elevations of the contour of the body are explained by the anatomy of the superficial fascia and from its relationships with the skin, the fat and the musculo-skeletal system. The study of anatomy and the understanding of physio-pathological exchanges of the superficial bandage system are not only the basis for surgical correction of the silhouette, but above all the basis for recovery in osteopathic therapies.

The Argentineans, Moretti, Schapira and Kaplan have studied 20 patients, 10 males and 10 females withdrawing one 20cm by 4cm "lozenge" in the zone along the side and the knee. Their anatomical study found the presence of a net of connective tissue that extends from the subdermal plane to the muscular aponeurosis [23]. It is really this net that constitutes the true superficial band and it is formed from various horizontal septa of collagen and elastic fibers separated by fat lobules and always crossed vertically by septa-type fibers. At the subdermal level, the presence of the superficial fascia also constitutes a connection with the deep dermis with bigger fibrous septa woven among them in such way to provoke the separation of adipose tissue in small compartments that organize the superficial adipose tissue with the classic structure of a honeycomb of bees.

This structural configuration constitutes the "*bundle-dermal system*", of great functional importance.

Even if anatomically a real plane of separation is not observed among the superficial muscular fascia and the connective fibers of the deep dermis we can deduce that, functionally and histologically, the continuous imbrications of fibers collectively constitute this "*hypodermic superficial fascia*".

In thin patients the superficial band is well delineated and of whitish color. In obese patients the great quantity of adipose tissue stretches the superficial fascia and attenuates the end making it difficult to recognize. The connective and elastic fibers are diluted in the fat fabric and this can explain the error of some studies, ones that put doubts on the existence of this superficial band.

Without doubt, in the facial zone over the iliac crest in men appears as a deep band that is not found in the female sex. In the women, instead, the fibrous band appears with the muscular aponeurosis at a level of the subgluteous that constitutes the base for the adipose tissue situated in this zone. This difference explains the difference in the contour of the gluteus among the two sexes.

The skin, the superficial fascia and the superficial fat must to be considered as a system of protection and functional support. This functional unity constitutes the support of the adipose fabric and helps to prevent the abnormal location of this fabric in other anatomical regions. The traction and stretching of the superficial facial band and the superficial muscular fascia with Endermologie is essential in the treatment.

Massage

Massage is an art, more than a therapeutic action that comprises a feeling between the hand of the operator and the tissues of the patient that must not be traumatized, but instead revascularized, stimulated and cleansed. A well-done massage has to relax the body and the mind to increase the skin temperature with stimulation of the microcirculation which favors intercellular exchange. A global massage of the body can have a sedative action and, at the same time, stimulate the nervous system. But massage doesn't have to be violent or prolonged to avoid provoking lymphatic congestion.

Manual Lymphatic Drainage

Lymphatic drainage is a physical method to reduce the stasis of the lymphatic fluid and the toxic substances in the tissues.

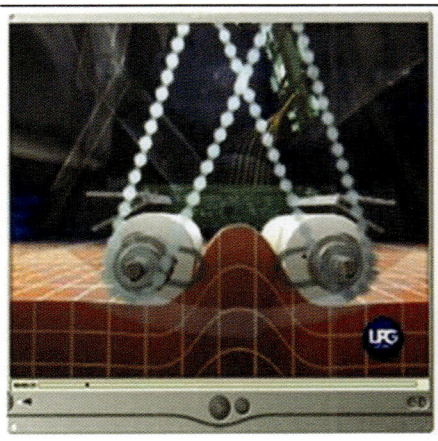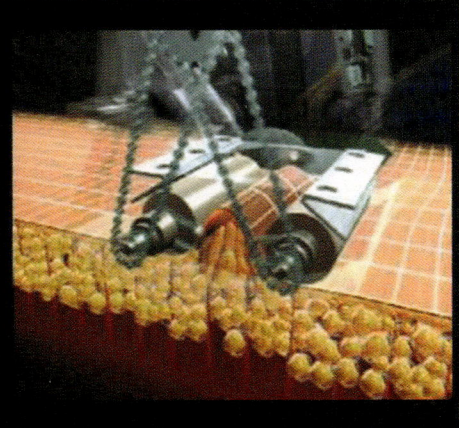

Figure 13.3 Endermologie allows a traction of the skin and connective fibers.

Lymphatic drainage is not traumatic but a gentle massage technique. Manual lymphatic drainage has its scientific basis in the study and teachings of Foldi and Leduc [24,25].

It deals with a series of grazing and compressions on the lymphatic system to improve lymphatic flow. In the Vodder technique, lymphatic drainage becomes less physical and more aesthetic in nature. Periodic cycles of manual lymphatic drainage are recommended according to Vodder, particularly to maintain the tissues free from lymphatic congestion. We believe that manual lymphatic drainage performed with the hands is the only one that can give acceptable results.

The "Endermologie®" Technique
History and principles
Our experience with LPG Systems began in 1993. The French engineer Louis Paul Guitay (LPG) developed a system to help care for the fibrosis he developed as a result of violent trauma. This resembled the movement performed by his therapist's fingers, including additional effects.

Sophisticated software allows for possible phases of continuous and sequential aspiration with mobilization of the tissues, offering the therapist an endless range of possible interventions appropriate for various pathologies. So began a true revolution in physiotherapy. Today scientific research has confirmed the effectiveness of this method [2–9]. This revolution has also given birth to an important professional team formed by the doctor/surgeon and physiotherapist, a union that is important in the fields of the phlebolymphology.

What is Endermologie®?
It is patented equipment that works with two motorized rollers between a vacuum suction with varying programs that lifts the skin reaching the deepest structures (Figs 13.3–13.4).

The hands of the therapist can be helped by the integrated action of this equipment allowing one to make the same physiotherapy maneuvers enriched by stretching the cutaneous tissue to be able to work more deeply. The effect is mainly the stimulation of cellular metabolism (fibroblasts, adipocytes) and the vascularisation with lymphatic drain and a purification through manual lymphatic drainage.

To ensure proper treatment one must have:

1. Correct diagnosis to be able to apply the therapy or the fittest program
2. Qualified personnel

Mechanism of action
Endermologie® possesses five complementary actions that allow treatment of different types of tissue:

1. Mobilization of the tissues that characterize the different structures with consequent activation of the arteriolar microcirculation
2. Traction of the connective tissue with exercise of the skin
3. Activation of the reflected arcs and stimulation of fibrous banding
4. Neurometabolic regulation with metabolic activation
5. Rhythmic compression of the tissues with lymph drainage

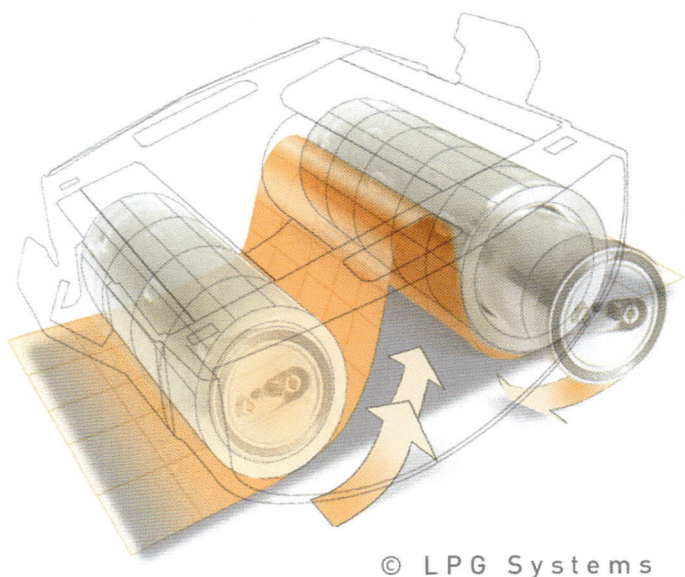

© L P G S y s t e m s

Figure 13.4 Different directions of the rotation facilitates different activities.

Together the stretching and the rhythmic compression of connective tissue activate fat lobules to cause their shrinkage with stretching of the fibrous septae.

The mechanical stimulations act on the mechanoreceptors such as:

1. *Corpuscles of Meissner* are sensitive to the light stimulations with activation of the fibroblasts.
2. *Corpuscles of Water-Pacini*, which are found in the deep dermis and in the lipoderma, are sensitive to deep pressure of the skin and vibration. They stimulate the activity of the fibroblasts.
3. *Corpuscles of the Golgi*, sensitive to the light pressures, stimulate fibroblasts and the regeneration of the collagen and connective tissue.
4. *Corpuscles of Merkel*, situated in the epidermis, are sensitive to vibrations and light pressure. They act on cellular metabolic activity.

The hyperdistension of the subcutaneous tissue will activate the specific receptors to free substances such as the bradychinen, histamine, serotonin and catecholamines. These act on beta adrenergic receptors activating the adenocyclase with an increase of the AMP to increase of tissue AMP, which in turn stimulates protein kinase that activates intra-adipocytic lipase with hydrolytic action on the triglycerides of the fat cells.

To conclude, different methodologies can have different results (Fig. 13.5).

You could hypothesize two principal actions.

The lightest treatment stimulates Golgi complexes to provoke:

1. Vascularisation
2. Stimulation of the receptors = Lipoclasis
3. Stimulation of the fibroblasts = Restructuring connective tissue

Thus stimulation of the beta adrenergic receptors occurs with

1. Lipolytic action
2. Increase tissue AMP
3. Hydrolytic intra-fat action
4. Restructuring of connective tissue

The strongest and deepest treatment, with stimulation of the Pacini corpuscles provokes liberation of bradichinen, histamine, serotonin and catecholamine with:

1. Increase free radicals
2. Alteration matrix
3. Flogosis
4. Fibrosis

Then we have a direct action on cicatrisation rather than toward a restructuring.

Treatment phase

The physician and operator act as a team. The actual procedure can be performed by the physiotherapist or osteopath after the diagnosis is pointed out by the physician specialized in phlebology, in the case of pathologies of the venolymphatic system or from the dermatologist or cosmetic surgeon, in the case of burns or scars that introduce fibrous retractions.

Various phases of application are:

1. Vascularising phase, to reactivate the cutaneous microcirculation
2. Drainage phase, to drain the lymphatic stagnation
3. Stimulation phase, to stimulate the fibroblasts and the interstitial neurophysiologic systems
4. Invigorating phase, to stimulate the skin
5. Exercise phase, in which the patient actively collaborates with isometric contractions pointed out by the operator to produce tissue and muscle tonification
6. Visceral phase, always with the collaboration of the patient along with specific maneuvers to stimulate abdominal visceral activities
7. Lipomassage phase, to increase the metabolism of the fat tissue

Indications

a) Phebolymphology

This treatment enhances the possibilities offered by traditional manual lymphatic drainage overcoming the traditional concept of "emptying of the lymphatic vessels" with the concept of metabolic stimulation.

Unlike the traditional therapies, performing lymphatic drainage with Endermologie® allows one to possibly reduce the necessity for high compression stockings or elastic bandages. This means that the mechanism of action of treatment includes activation of the autonomous nervous system and the interstitial connective tissue [26–29].

b) Plastic and aesthetic surgery

The method here is a natural complement of liposculpture recovering and remodeling the fat tissue decreasing complications

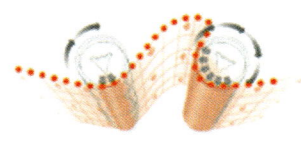 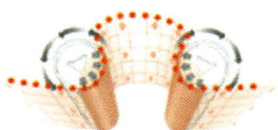 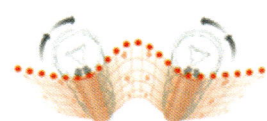

· Plis adapté à la qualité de peau
· Skin fold adapted to the quality of the skin

© copyright LPG 2004

Figure 13.5 Any type of skin can have its best treatment.

(irregularities). In addition, Endermologie® will decrease the incidence of seromas, edemas, alterations of the skin (fibrosis and asymmetries) [30–34].

c) Cellulitic syndromes

As discussed in previous chapters, cellulite is a condition comprised of various pathological expressions of vascular and/or degenerative alterations of the connective tissue or interstitial matrix, often in partnership with lipotrophy of the muscular tissue. Cellulite should not be confused with obesity.

Obesity is when the fat tissue is above 30% of the quantity that can normally be present, while cellulite is a transformation and an alteration of subcutaneous interstitial tissues [35–45].

Endermologie® provides the basic treatment around which many methodologies may be associated for a complete and studied integrated protocol of treatment.

In addition to aesthetic alterations, various subjective symptoms exist including cramps, pain to the touch, heaviness, livedo reticularis, edemas and tiredness. Such symptoms represent important diagnostic signs for the various cellulitic pathologies that are classified in five fundamental groups [46–48].

1) Edematous cellulite

Characterized by orange-peel skin provoked by the stretching of the connective fibers due to an excess of liquid. The principal symptoms are: pain, edematous plasticity, sense of periodic swelling and edema of the ankle.

2) Adipose cellulite

Characterized by the skin stretched by an excess of adipose tissue, with particular increase of the fat "steatomery". There are no imbibitions of interstitial liquid, it is associated with being overweight. Orange-peel skin is caused by the stretching of connective tissue due to an excess of fat tissue. The principal symptoms are no pain, no edema and no sense of periodic swelling.

3) Interstitial cellulite

Characteristic of young subjects is the typical lipoedema which is characterized by the superficial tissue of the thigh imbibed with fluid and superficial adipose tissue. Orange-peel skin is caused by the stretching of connective tissue from edema and fat tissue.

The principal symptoms are pain and edema to the thigh, but not the leg or foot. There is often a sense of swelling to the hands [49–53].

4) Fibrous cellulite

The pathophysiologic point of view is characterized by dehydration of the cutaneous and fibrous connective tissue and fat with the development of nodules of adipose tissue surrounded by a sclerotic capsule. The orange peel appearance of the skin is coarse and caused by the retraction of connective tissue fibers. The principal symptoms are pain without edema.

5) Localized adiposity

They are lipomatosis and localized adiposity in subcutaneous tissue or in the splitting of the superficial fascia. Their anatomic,

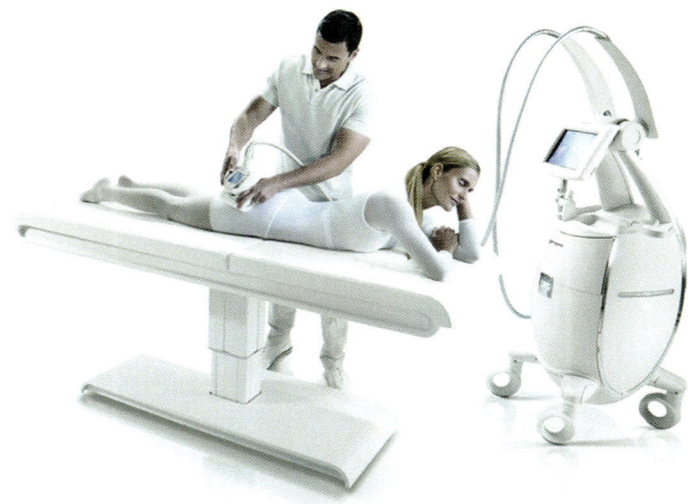

Figure 13.6 Endermologie® treatment may be useful for care or maintenance.

physiologic and pathologic evidence are completely different from the cellulite. The surgeon will proceed to eliminate the localized adiposity through excision or liposculpture.

Today we frequently use a lipolaser with microfibra of 100–200 microns connected by the Eufoton™ laser 940 nanometeres. Using this methodology we can reduce the traumatic action of cannulas and improve the retraction avoiding the irregularities of the skin.

After surgical treatment of liposculpture or mini invasive treatment by lipolaser we can add six to eight sessions of Endermologie® to complete the treatment and to have the best results in short time. The therapist will begin treatments with lymphatic drainage that aids in recovery.

Endermologie® can offer the possibility of good results without surgical treatment in selected patients because we can reduce a fat layer using a particular treatment named Lipomassage. In fact, new LPG Integral stimulates fat tissue increasing its metabolic activity and reducing its quantity with a good aesthetic result.

The method

Endermologie® is ideal in the treatment of the different forms of cellulite but precise protocols of technique are necessary [54,55]. Three fundamental rules provide correct treatment are no pain, no persistent vascularisation and a fluidity of the massage technique from the operator. The therapist doesn't have to provide a strong traction with the rollers; on the contrary, the technique should be like a fluid sliding on the body garment. Another important rule is to position the machinery at the foot of the table on the left.

Positioning LPG Integral in this manner allows the operator to use both hands to massage the patient in a superior-inferior direction (Fig. 13.6).

All the necessary maneuvers are performed, with slow movements in the descending phase, respecting the tissues and favoring the lifting and tonification. The manipulation of the head must be compared to a painter's brush that has to cover the whole surface of the body within every treatment session.

In patients with predominant veno-lymphatic stasis, it is necessary to begin the treatment from the abdomen, treating it in such way as to prepare the lymphatic vessels to drain from the whole body as

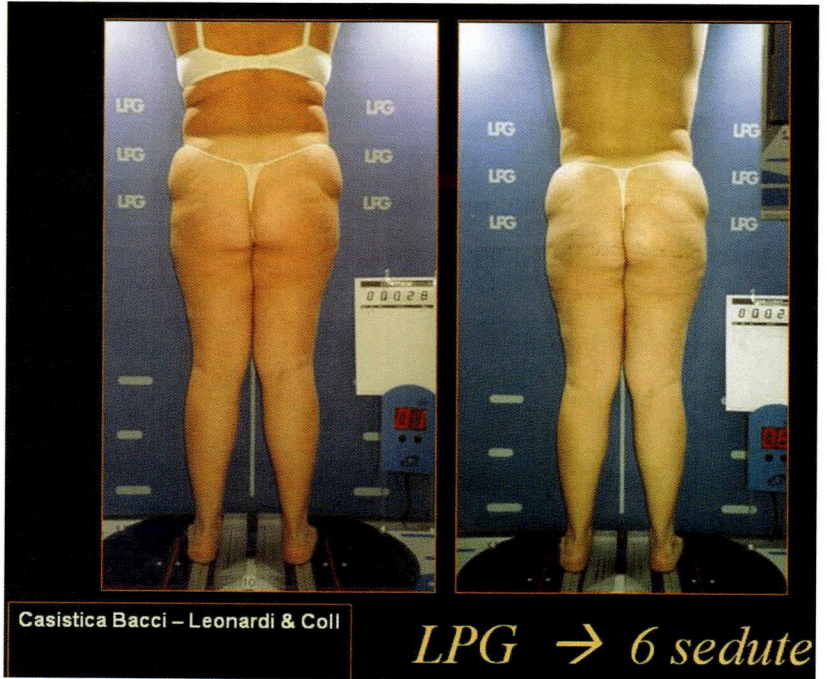

Figure 13.7 We can have good results in local adiposity too.

well as stimulate the muscular fascia, perivisceral fascia (kidney and peritoneum) and the suspensor ligaments of the colon and liver.

The standard time of treatment, applicable to most cases is of 35 minutes. More time may be devoted to subjects notably overweight where it is necessary to work on a single part of the body. Whatever the constitution and problem it is always best to treat the whole body (Fig. 13.7).

If we suggest good nutrition with a reduction of carbohydrates to low stimulation of insulin, our results will be rapidly increased (Fig. 13.8).

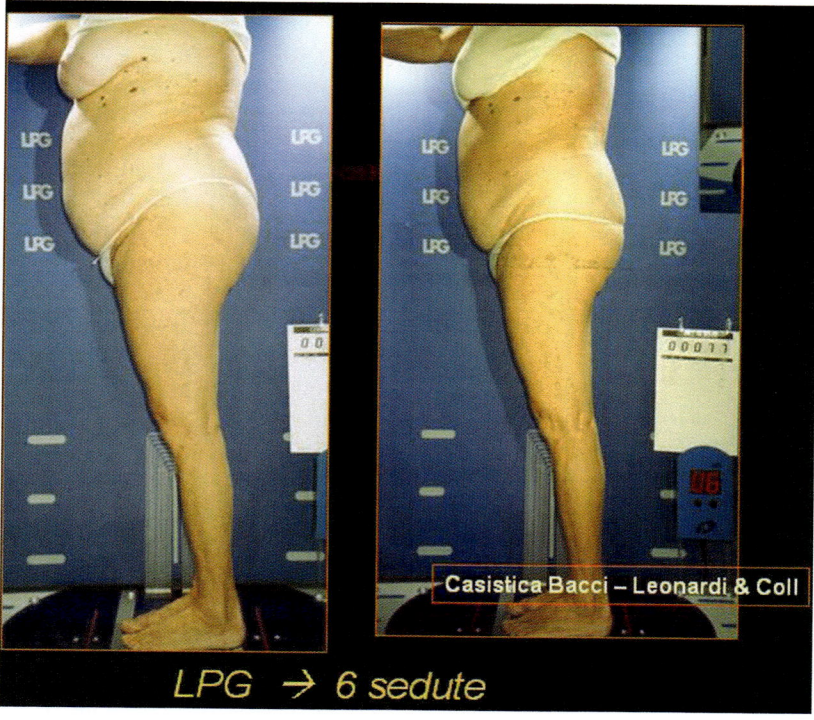

Figure 13.8 The association with protheic nutrition is very interesting.

Endermologie® treatment aims to bring plasticity, elasticity and compactness to the skin and subcutaneous tissue, thanks to the stimulation of connective tissue. The variations of technique follow the clinical indications.

Conclusions

Endermologie–LPG Systems® certainly is not a panacea for all pathologies but it is a real revolution in the field of physical medicine, of physiotherapy and aesthetical physiotherapy [56,57].

The method one doesn't consist of a massage but a real treatment. To massage means to perform a local stimulation with a local result. To make a treatment means to perform a systemic and local stimulation with systemic and local results.

The use of Endermologie® never foresees the execution of a massage or a lymphatic drainage but the execution of a treatment finalized to the metabolic recovery and the stimulation of connective tissue. This aspect represents the revolution and the great difference is in comparison to the manual lymphatic drainage. This is appropriate for cellulitic syndromes.

Endermologie® is a natural complement to cosmetic and plastic surgery in the treatment of lipodistrophy and cellulite as well as various forms of edema and lipolymphedema [58,59]. Endermologie®, for the first time, offers a particularly active treatment in the activation of fibroblasts and the metabolism of the interstitial matrix and, actually, it represents the more important basic treatment for different forms of cellulite.

Particular biopsy shows the possibility of having a new activity in the dermis and subcutaneous layer demonstrated by an improved reticular dermis layer.

All other methodologies can be integrated with Endermologie LPG Integral to have best results and few complications [60–63].

REFERENCES

1. PA Bacci. Il ruolo della metodologia "Endermologie®", in "Le celluliti nel 2004", Minelli Editore, Arezzo; 2004.
2. C Monteux, M Lafontan. Use of the microdialysis technique to assess lipolytic responsiveness of femoral adipose tissue after 12 sessions of mechanical massage technique. JEADV 22:1465–70, 2008.
3. JF Bourgeois. A randomized, prospective study using the LPG Technique in treating radiation-induced skin fibrosis. Clinical and Profilometric analysis. Skin Research and Technology 14:71–76, 2008.
4. AL Moseley. Comparison of the effectiveness of MLD and LPG Technique. Journal of Lymphoedema 2007, Vol 2, No 2, 30–36.
5. JP Ortonne. Treatment of cellulite: Effectiveness and sustained effect at 6 months with Endermologie® demonstrated by several quantitative evaluation methods. Nouv. Dermatol 23:261–69, 2004.
6. D Innocenzi. Evidenza delle modificazioni cutanee indotte dalla tecnica LPG mediante analise d'immagine. DermoCosmetologia Anno II, no 1 – Gennaio/Marzo; 2003: p. 9–15.
7. PA Bacci. Vibroassisted Liposuction and Endermologie® for LipoLymphedema. The European Journal of Lymphology – Vol. X – Nr. 35–36, p16, 2002.
8. D Adcock. Analysis of the effects of deep mechanical massage in the porcine model. Plast. Reconstr Surg 108(1):233–40, Jul 2001.
9. P Lattarulo. Physiological tissue changes after administration of micronized Diosmin/Hesperidin, individually or in association with Endermologie®. International Journal of Aesthetic Cosmetic Beauty Surgery Vol. 1, no 2, p. 25–28, 2001.
10. JR Casley-Smith. Lymph and lymphatic, in "Microcirculation" by G Kaley. and Altura Eds, Vol.I, University Park Press, Baltimore, Maryland; 1977: 423–508.
11. M Foldi. Therapy of secondary lymphoedema, Med. Welt 28(41):669–1670, 1977.
12. A Leduc. Il drenaggio linfatico, Masson Italia editore, Milano; 1982.
13. P Ball, R Knuppen. Interactions between estrogens and cathecolamines. J Clin Endocr 34:736, 1972.
14. P Bjorntorp. The fat cells, a clinical view, Recent advances in II Obesity 1978.
15. P Bjorntorp, L Sjostrom. Number and sizes of adipous tissue fat cells in relation to metabolism in human obesity. Rev Metabolism 1972.
16. J Brunzel. Insulin and adipose tissue, International Journal of obesity 1981.
17. J Vague, P Bjorntorp. Metabolic complications of human obesities, Ph. Vague (Eds). Excerpta Med., Amsterdam; 1985.
18. J Vague. Las obesidades, Cuadernos de medicina estetica, Solal – Masson (Ed.) Marseille France; 1990: n. 3.
19. JM Fain, RE Sheperd, Hormonal regulation or lipolysis. Adv Exper Med Biol 111:43–79, 1979.
20. D Adcock, S Paulsen, RB Shack et al. Analysis of the cutaneous and systemic effects of Endermologie in the porcine model, Aesthetic Surgery Journal. USA 18(6):414–22, 1998.
21. PB Fodor, J Watson, W Shaw et al. Physiological effects of Endermologie: a preliminary report, Aesthetic Surgery Journal. USA 19(1):1–7, 1999.
22. PA Bacci. La fascia superficiale in "Bacci PA" –"Le celluliti", Alberti & C Editori, Arezzo; 2000: parte 4.
23. E Moretti, A Schapira, G Kaplan et al. La fascia superficiale, Rivista panamericana de flebologia y linfologia. Junio; 1993: n.9.
24. M Foeldi. Symposium ueber die sogenannte Zellulitis. Feldberg 1–2 Juni 1983.
25. A Leduc. Le drainage lymphatique, Theorie et pratique, Masson; 1980.
26. PA Bacci. Price en charge de l'oedeme de l'insuffisance veineuse cronique – Angiology Today – n.34:2,3,4, 1998.
27. PA Bacci. Il cosiddetto Lipolinfedema, Flebologia Oggi, Torino – Atti Congresso Nazionale Collegio Italiano Flebologia. Vol.2 N.1:27–32, 1998.
28. PA Bacci, D Klein, M Izzo et al. La patologia linfatica nel Thigh Lifting, Atti Congresso Nazionale SICPRE, Vol.10, 323–31, Ribuffo 1996.
29. A Barile, P Petrigi. Nostra esperienza di impiego della tecnica LPG, Atti 48 congresso SICPRE – Gubbio 1999 –pag. 745.
30. C Campisi. Il linfedema, aspetti attuali di diagnosi e terapia, Flebologia Oggi. Minerva Medica Ed 1:27–41, 1997.
31. P Chang, A Erseg. Noninvasive mechanical body contouring: (endermologie) A one year clinical outcome study update. Aesthetic Plastic Surgery 22:145–53,1998.

32. PB Fodor. Endermologie LPG, does it work?, Aesthetic Surgery Journal. USA 21:68, 1997.
33. PA Bacci. Il ruolo dell'endermologia in medicina e chirurgia plastica, Atti 10 Congresso Nazionale Medicina Estetica SMIEM, Milano. 1999: 20.
34. F Albergati, PA Bacci, P Lattarulo et al. Valutazione sull'attività microcircolatoria della tecnica Endermologie LPG in paziente con PEFS (1997) in "Le celluliti nel 2004", Minelli Editore, Arezzo; 2004.
35. M Comel. Histangeiologie et phlebologie, Folia Angiologica 7:3, 1960.
36. C Allegra, G Pollari, V Ribuffo et al. Pannicolopatia edemato-fibrosclerotica. Minerva Mesoterapica vol.1, 1986.
37. PA Bacci. Il lipolinfedema: riflessioni e osservazioni cliniche, Flebologia Oggi. Torino Minerva Medica 2:10–21, 1997.
38. C Pierard. Cellulite, A.J.D. 22(1):34–37, 2000.
39. M Foeldi. Symposium ueber die sogenannte zellulitis, Feldberg (Au); Ju.,1–2st 1983.
40. M Ceccarelli. Cellulite: approccio diagnostico e terapeutico. Atti 10 Congr Multid Chir Plast e Invecch, Roma, Italy; 9/12 Nov 1989.
41. PA Bacci. Le celluliti, Alberti & C Editor, Arezzo; 2000: 40–46.
42. SB Curri. Aspect morphohistochimiques du tissue adipeux dans la dermohypodermose cellulitique. J Med Est 5:183, 1976.
43. M Binazzi, M Papini. Aspetti clinico istomorfologici in "La cellulite" di Ribuffo – Bartoletti. Salus Ed Roma 7–15, 1983.
44. JF Merlen. La part de la cellulite dans la douleurs vasculaires. Angiologie 3:21–24, 1966.
45. SB Curri. Liposclerosi e microcircolo, La dermoestetica 1:6–7, 1990.
46. PA Bacci. The code TCD: a new classification for cellulitis, Atti Congresso Internazionale della UIP, International Union of Phlebology, San Diego; 31 Agosto 2003.
47. PA Bacci, C Allegra, S Mancini et al. Randomized, placebo controlled double blind clinical study on efficacy of a multifunctional plant complex in the treatment of the so called cellulites, Journal of Aesthetic Surgery and Dermatology Surgery Vol. 5, No. 1, 2003.
48. PA Bacci, C Allegra, S Mancini et al. Valutazione clinica controllata in doppio cieco di prodotti fitocomposti nel trattamento della cosiddetta cellulite, in PA Bacci, S Mariani. "La flebologia in pratica", Alberti & C. Ed, Arezzo –Italy; 2003 - ISBN 88.87936.595.
49. S Bilancini, M Lucchi. Proposition de classification des grosses jambes. Plebologie 42(1):151–56, 1989.
50. S Bilancini, M Lucchi. Approccio al lipedema in Linfologia, n.1:24–26, 1989.
51. PA Bacci. Il lipolinfedema: riflessioni e osservazioni cliniche, Flebologia Oggi, Torino Minerva Medica N.2:pag.10.21, 1997.
52. S Bilancini, M Lucchi, S Tucci. El lipedema: criterios clinicos y diagnosticos, in Angiologia 4(90):133–37.
53. M Binazzi, M Papini. Aspetti clinico istomorfologici, in "La cellulite" ituffo– Bartoletti, Salus Ed. Roma; 1983: 7–15.
54. PA Bacci. La fisioterapia estetica e la tecnica LPG, Minelli Editor, Arezzo; 2004.
55. PA Bacci. La tecnica LPG, in "S Mancini. & Coll, Trattato di Flebolinfologia, Minerva Medica, Torino; 2007".
56. PA Bacci. La cellulite da scoprire, Alberti & C Editori, Arezzo; 2003.
57. F Vinas. Drenaggio linfatico manuale, Les nouvelles esthetiques, RED Edizioni, Marzo; 1993.
58. R Seeley, T Stephens, P Tate. Anatomia e fisiologia, edizioni sorbona, Milano; 1993.
59. FH Netter. Atlante di anatomia e fisiopatologia clinica, Collezione CIBA edizioni; 1996.
60. FG Albergati, PA Bacci. La matrice extracellulare, Minelli Editore, Arezzo Italy; 2004.
61. PA Bacci. Chirurgia estetica mini invasiva con fili di sostegno, Minelli editore, Arezzo; 2007.
62. PA Bacci. Cirugia estetica minimamente invasiva con hilos tensores, Amolca Editor, Caracas; 2007.
63. PA Bacci, PL Rossi. Prevenire e guarire smagliature e cellulite, Minelli editore, Arezzo; 2008.

14 The Use of the Tri-Active™ in the Treatment of Cellulite
Mitchel P Goldman

Mechanism of Action

Tri-Active, as the name implies, uses three mechanisms to treat cellulite (Fig. 14.1). These three mechanisms, diode lasers, contact cooling, and massage work together to restore the body's normal homeostatic environment. The Tri-Active device is equipped with six 808 nm diode lasers that work directly on the endothelial cells lining vascular walls stimulating arterial, venous, and lymphatic flow as well as neovascularization (Fig. 14.2). The contact cooling system decreases edema by causing an initial vasoconstriction followed by a compensatory vasodilatation allowing for pooled fluid to remobilize. The rhythmic massage, when performed in accordance with the specific protocol developed, counteracts circulatory stasis again mobilizing fluids by stimulating lymphatic drainage.

In review, cellulite is caused by the swelling of individual adipocytes with increased fat storage, resulting in the obstruction of vascular and lymphatic flow. The resultant edema impairs the metabolic exchange between blood and adipocytes eventually causing the ensuing fibrosis which gives the cellulitic appearance. The Tri-Active mechanism is based upon this hypothesis. The Tri-Active device improves the circulatory system decreasing the edema that may be present thus restoring cell homeostasis. In addition, the massage stretches the connective tissue, smoothing the interface between the dermis and epidermis.

Parameters

The parameters of the Tri-Active system can be manipulated to optimize patient results, and will be detailed below. The depth and intensity of the rhythmic massage can be controlled by the frequency and duty cycle. The frequency (Hertz) measures the number of aspirations per second. At higher frequencies a superficial mechanical action is achieved, while lower repetition rates stimulate deeper tissue. The duty cycle is the percentage of time the aspiration is active between one aspiration and the next. For example, a duty cycle of 70% indicates that the aspiration is active 70% of the time between the two aspirations. The higher the value, the stronger the action. Thus by manipulating the duty cycle and frequency one can increase or decrease the intensity and depth of the message.

Low level light energy

Low energy lasers have been demonstrated to have beneficial effects on wound healing and biochemical effects on endothelial cells, erythrocytes, and collagen [1–5]. (See Chapter 17 for a complete discussion of low level light energy).

Other Uses

The Tri-Active device has also been used before, during, and after other surgical procedures including liposuction and abdominoplasty. We have noted a marked improvement in irregularities when Tri-Active is performed after liposculpture. This improvement may be due to the redistribution of dystrophic adipose cells.

Contra indications

As is true with other laser devices, Tri-Active should be used cautiously in the following situations including pregnancy, active skin infections, asthma, bronchitis, inflammatory/irritable bowel syndrome, heart failure, hyperthyroidism, hypotension, carotid sinus syndrome, and tumors.

Treatment Protocol

Andrea Pelosi, physiotherapist, developed standardized full body protocols to treat patients with either a gynoid or android/male habitus. These protocols reflect his experience in manual lymphatic drainage [6].

Treatment of the body consists of an intensive phase of 12–15 treatment sessions that last 30 minutes each and are carried out two to three times per week. Once this intensive phase of treatment is finished, the maintenance phase follows with treatments of at least one to two sessions a month.

A separate protocol exists for gynoid and android women. However, only the gynoid protocol will be reviewed, as it is the most frequently used. The treatment areas should be cleaned to remove all lotions and sunscreen. Each phase should be repeated three times unless otherwise noted.

In the initial phase, the abdominal and inguinal lymph nodes are treated. This is followed by the visceral phase, used to stimulate the digestive system. The subsequent drainage phase involves the transverse movements from the inner knees and continues over the entire thigh. Complete the supine treatment by treating the inguinal lymph nodes again (Fig. 14.4).

The patient is then placed in a prone position and the initial phase is repeated with the stimulation of the posterior inguinal node. The drain phase is also repeated, A transverse motion should be carried out from the distal thigh to the proximal thigh. This should be followed by a longitudinal motion, first on the thigh (starting distally) and then on the lower leg (starting distally). Carry out transversal and linear movements on the buttocks as indicated in the figure. Stimulate the vascular pump of the foot by passing the handpiece over the sole of the foot in a transversal manner, starting from the heel. Carry out two to four aspirations in each point, taking more time on the heel. Final lymph node drainage includes the posterior inguinal lymph nodes and popliteal lymph nodes.

Buttocks toning is performed in two consecutive steps; first at low frequency for deep tissue mobilization, followed by a superficial smoothening at max frequency (Fig. 14.5).

Finally, the patient is repositioned in the supine position and the abdominal and inguinal lymph nodes are retreated (Fig. 14.6).

Initial Clinical Studies

The experimental studies in Europe regarding the efficacy of Tri-Active was conducted by Nicola Zerbinati, MD, assistant

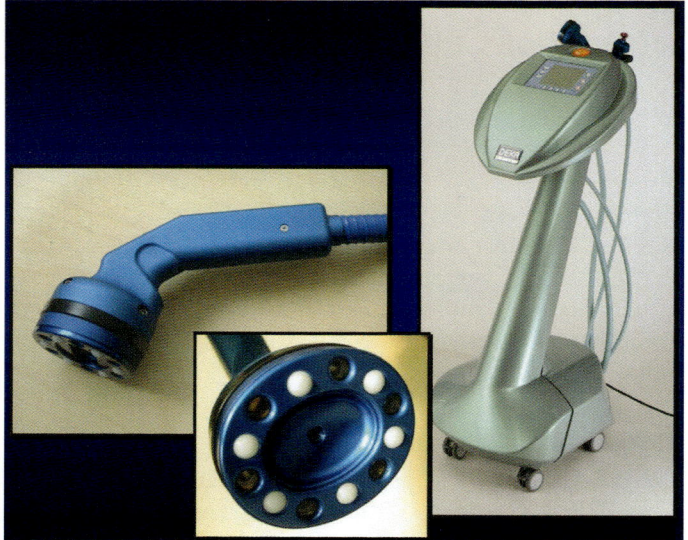

Figure 14.1 The device.

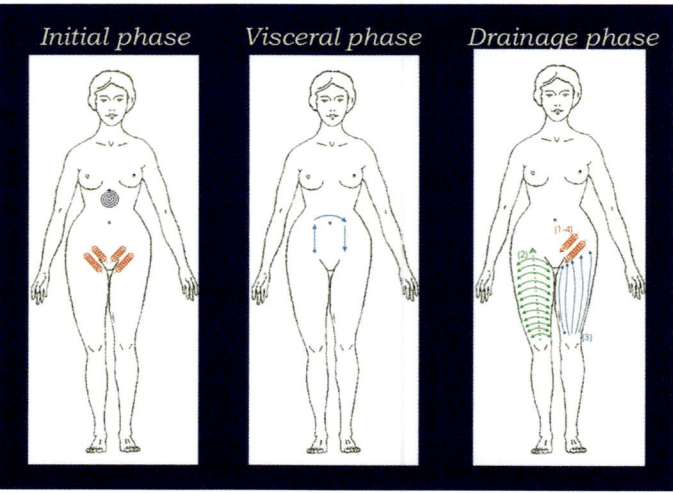

Figure 14.4 Body protocol.

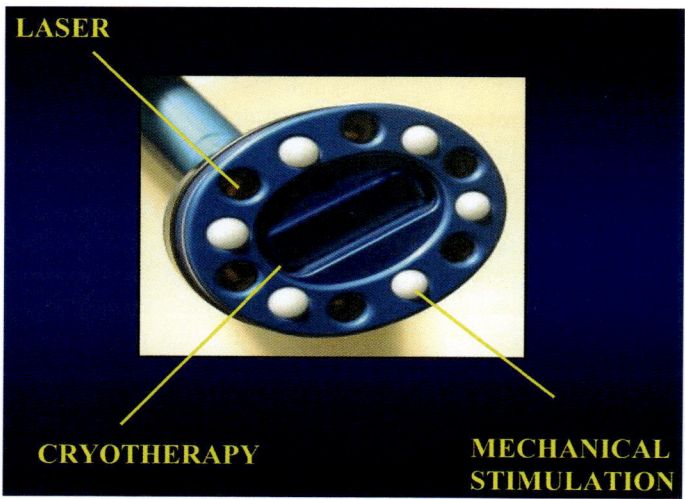

Figure 14.2 Treatment head showing 6 diode lasers, cryotherapy probe and mechanical stimulation.

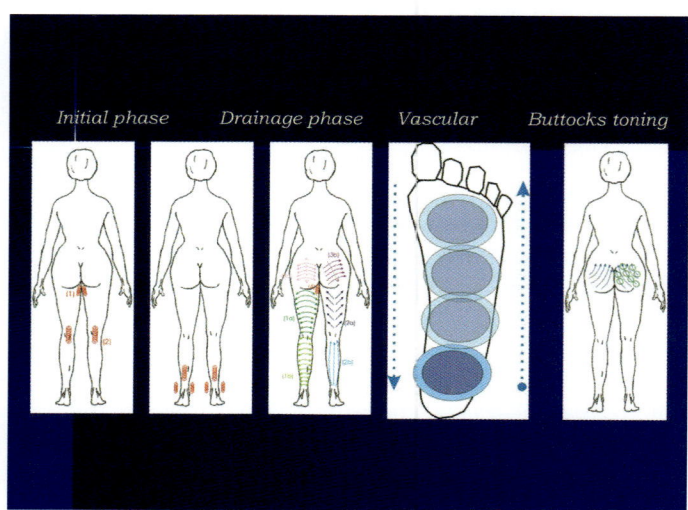

Figure 14.5 Sites for toning.

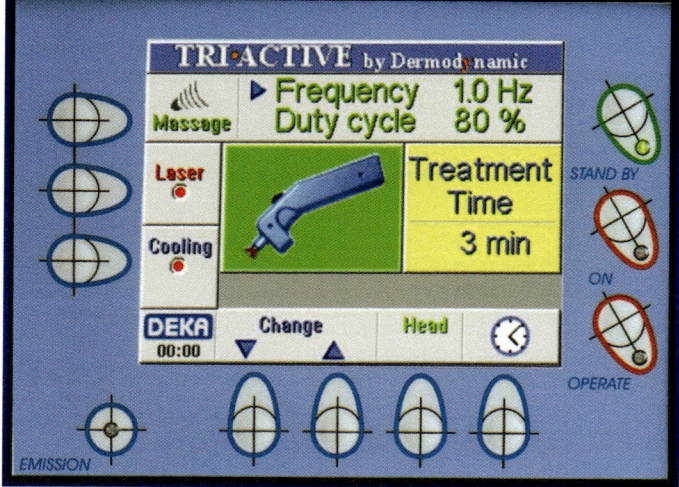

Figure 14.3 Tri-Active screen.

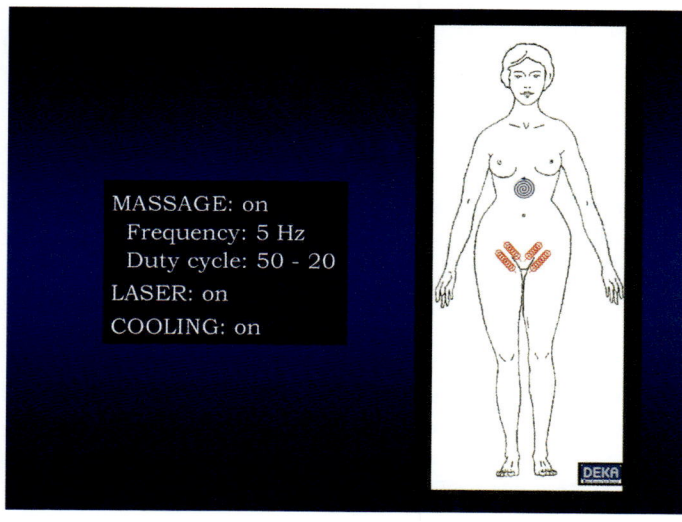

Figure 14.6 Final phase.

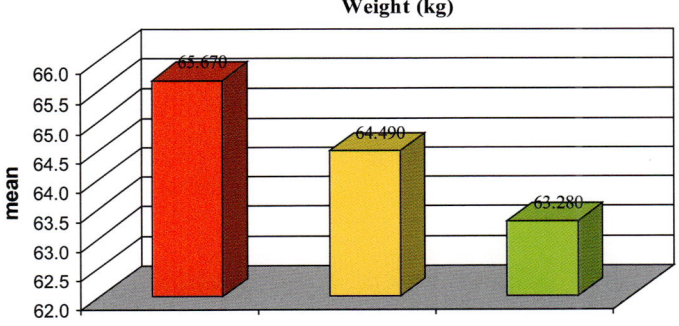

Figure 14.7 From clinical study by Andrea Pelosi and Nicola Zerbinati, MD.

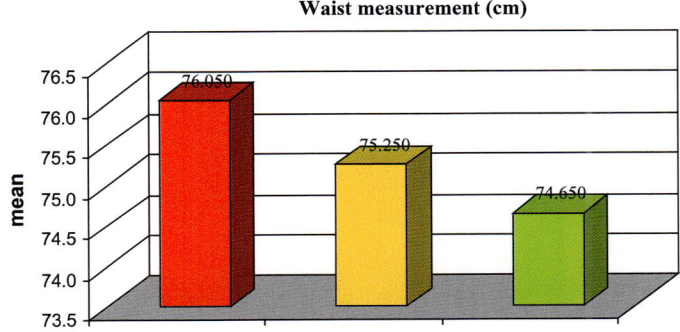

Figure 14.8 From clinical study by Andrea Pelosi and Nicola Zerbinati, MD.

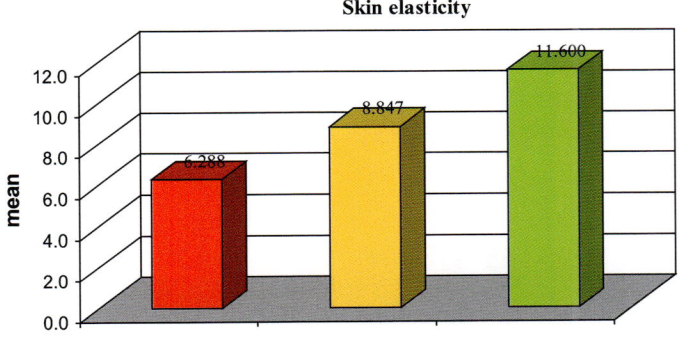

Figure 14.9 From clinical study by Andrea Pelosi and Nicola Zerbinati, MD.

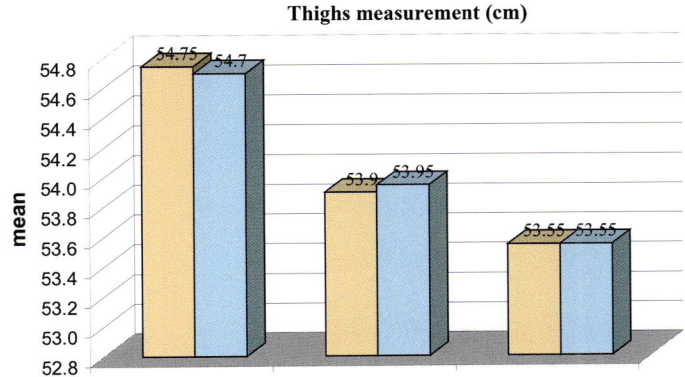

Figure 14.10 From clinical study by Andrea Pelosi and Nicola Zerbinati, MD.

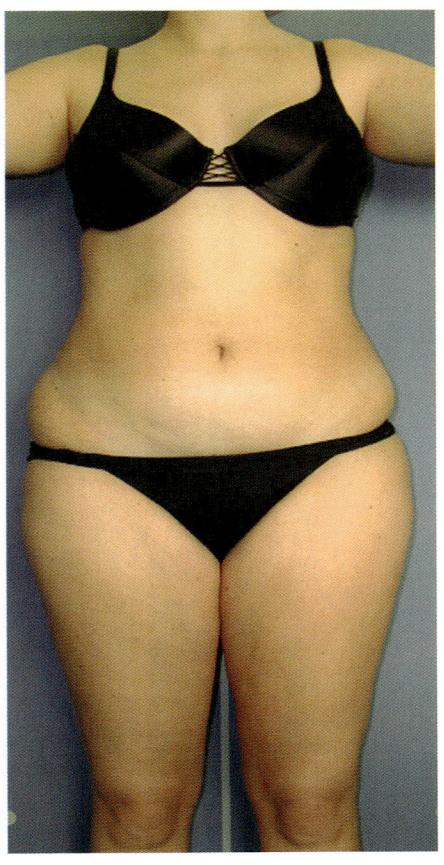

(a)

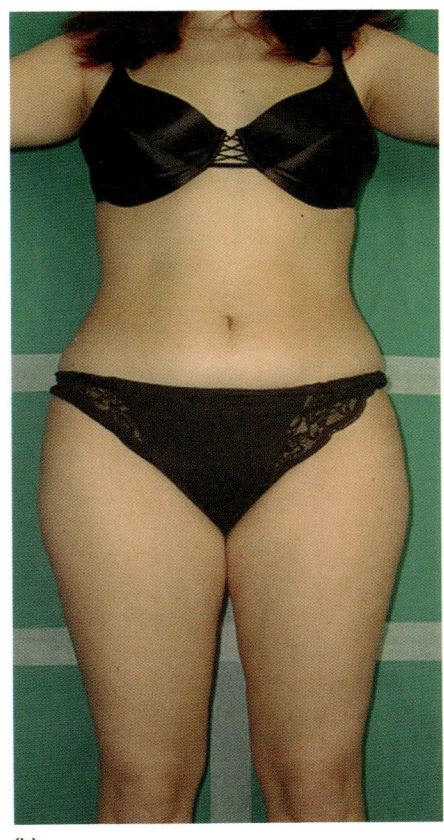

(b)

Figure 14.11 (a) Before treatment, (b) After 20 treatments.

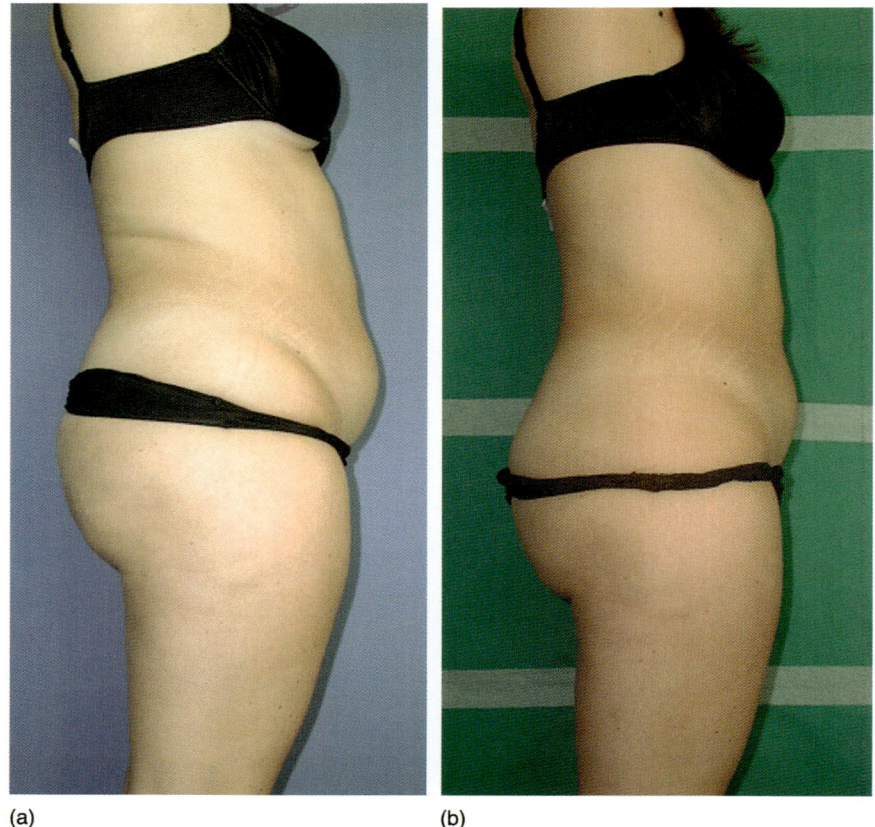

(a)   (b)

Figure 14.12 (a) Before treatment, (b) After 20 treatments.

professor of dermatology, University of Insubria, Milan, Italy [7]. Ten patients were enrolled and each treated with 20-minute sessions three times a week. To evaluate the efficacy of the technique, all patients were requested not to change habits such as diet, physical activity and lifestyle in general. Clinical observation, circumference of the thighs and hips, plicometry, skin elasticity and thermography were recorded. All patients noted an increase in skin tone and a reduction in the circumference of the areas treated. Detailed results of the intensive phase of treatments are presented below.

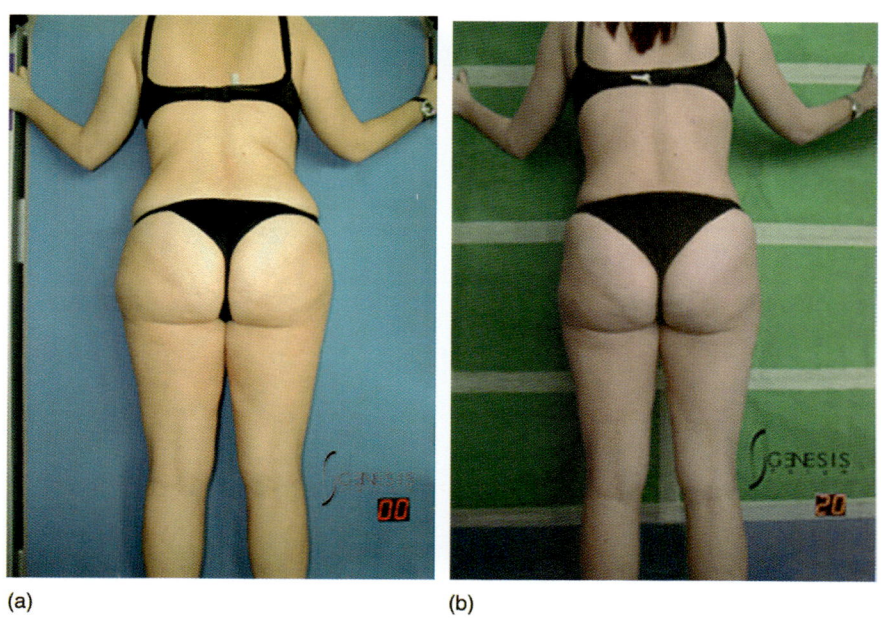

(a)   (b)

Figure 14.13 (a) Before treatment, (b) After 20 treatments.

After 10 sessions:

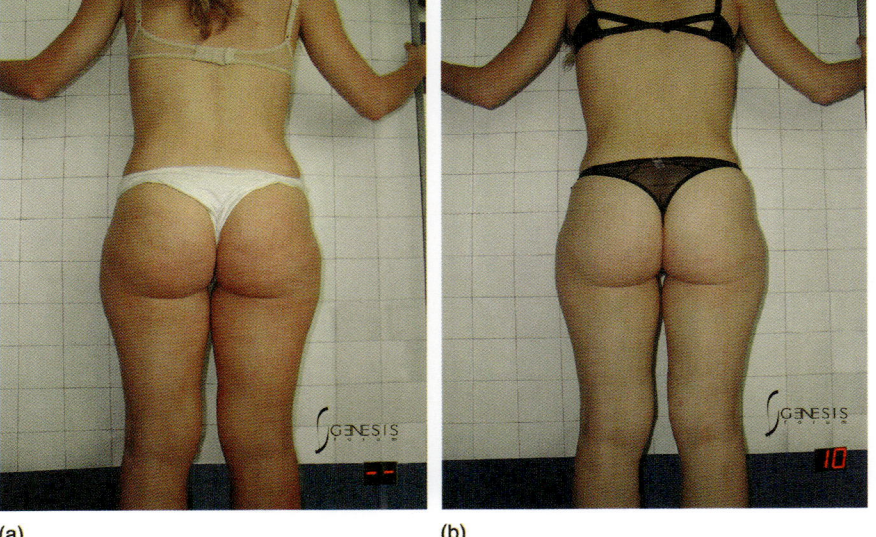

Figure 14.14 (a) Lifting and firming effect of the buttocks, (b) Improves the surfaces and smoothes the skin.

(a)   (b)

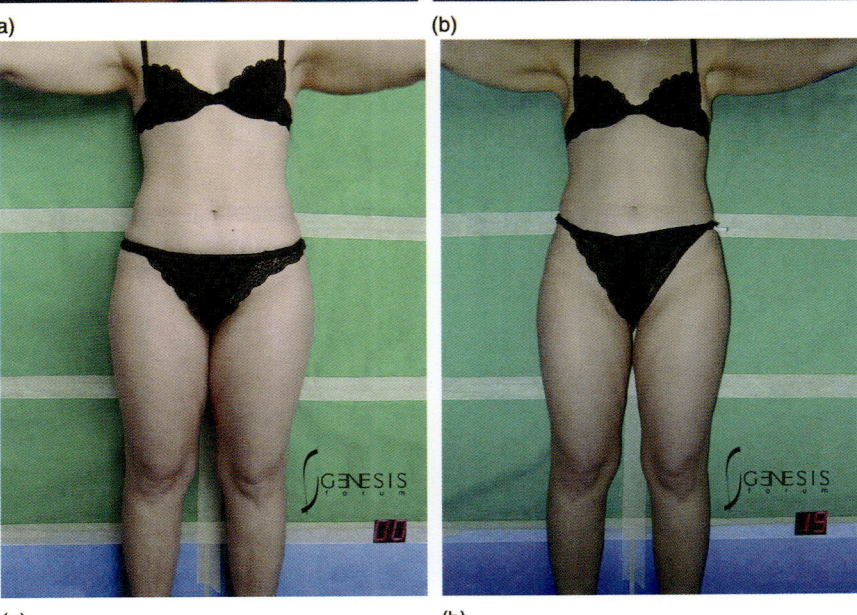

Figure 14.15 (a) Before treatment, (b) After 19 treatments.

(a)   (b)

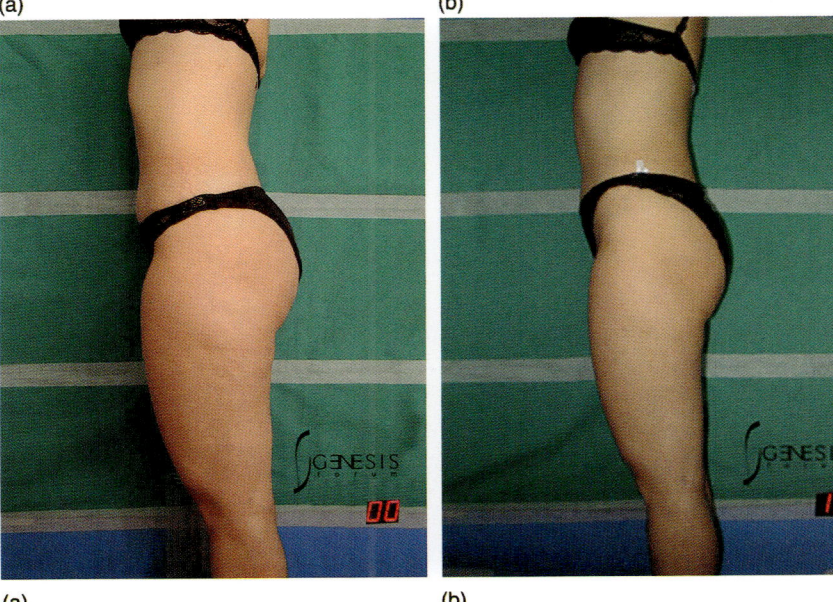

Figure 14.16 (a) Before treatment, (b) After 19 treatments.

(a)   (b)

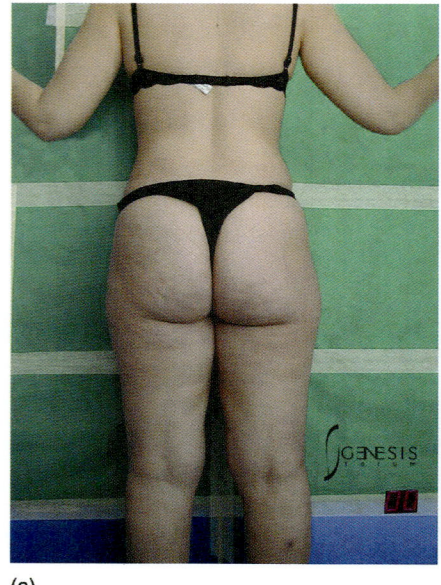 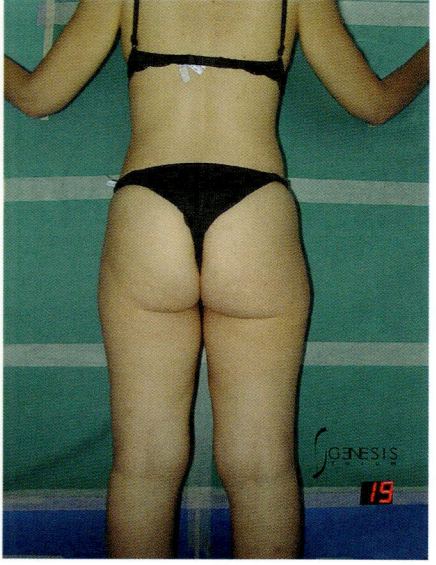

(a)   (b)

Figure 14.17 (a) Before treatment, (b) After 19 treatments.

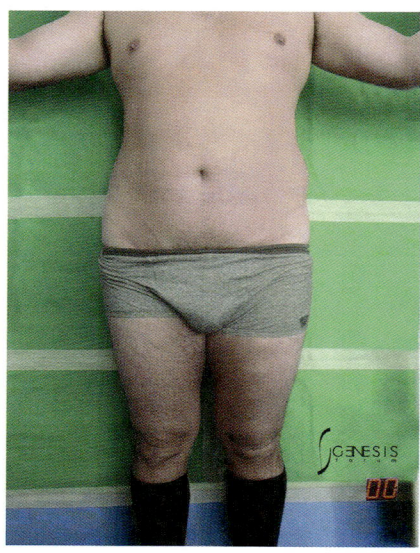 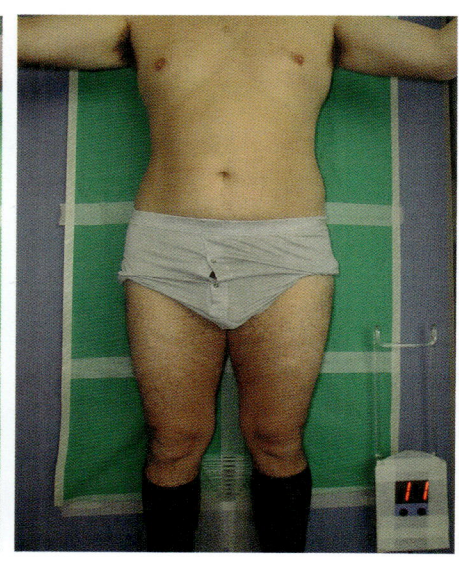

(a)   (b)

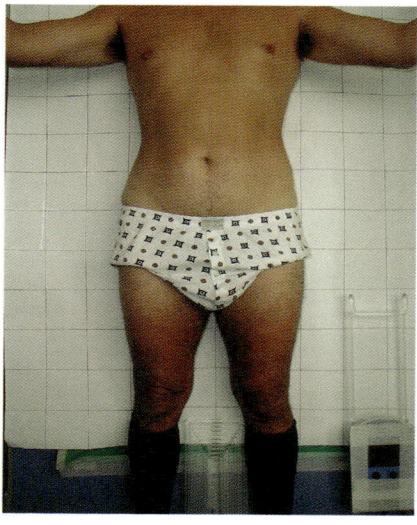

(c)

Figure 14.18 (a) Before treatment, (b) 11 treatments, (c) Follow-up 30 days.

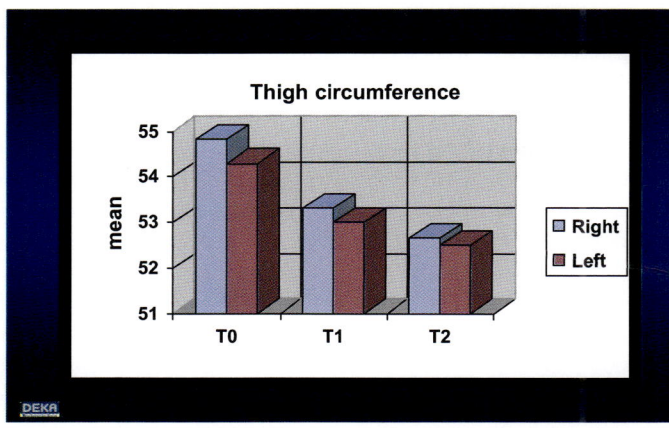

Figure 14.19 From clinical study by Andrea Pelosi and Nicola Zerbinati, MD.

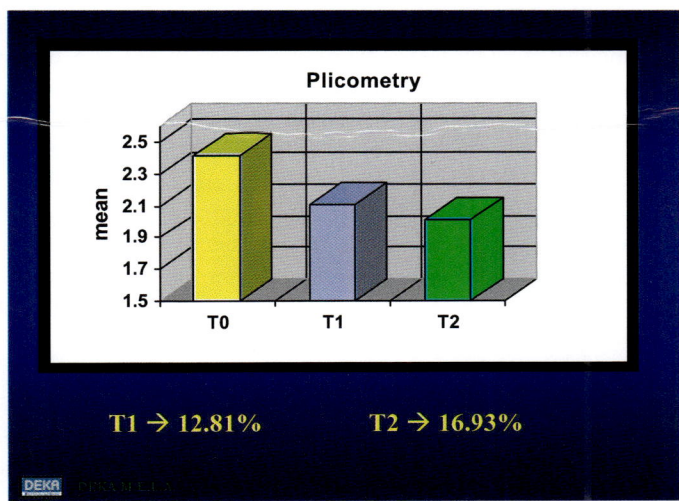

T1 → 12.81%   **T2 → 16.93%**

Figure 14.20 From clinical study by Andrea Pelosi and Nicola Zerbinati, MD.

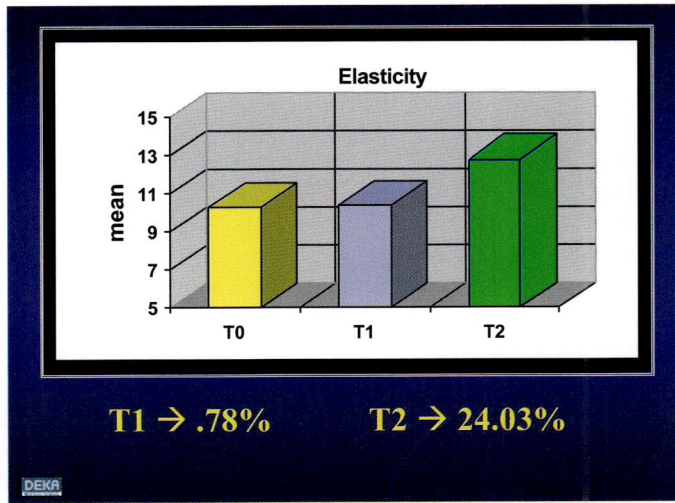

T1 → .78%   **T2 → 24.03%**

Figure 14.21 From clinical study by Andrea Pelosi and Nicola Zerbinati, MD.

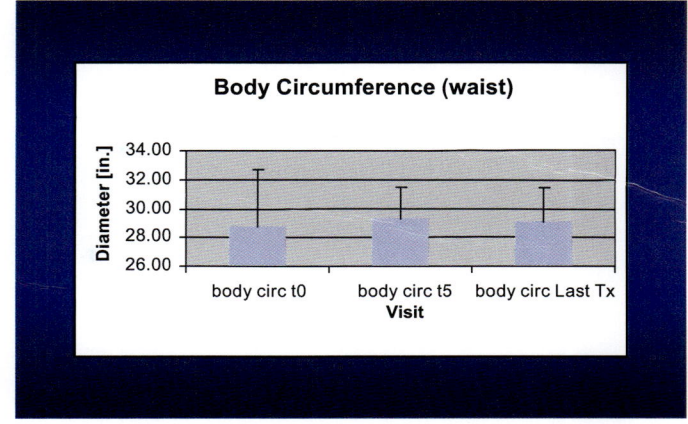

Figure 14.22 Clinical study of Boyce S, Pabby A, Cuchaltkaren P, et al: Clinical evaluation of a device for the treatment of cellulite: TriActive. Am J Cosmetic Surg 2005;22:233–37.

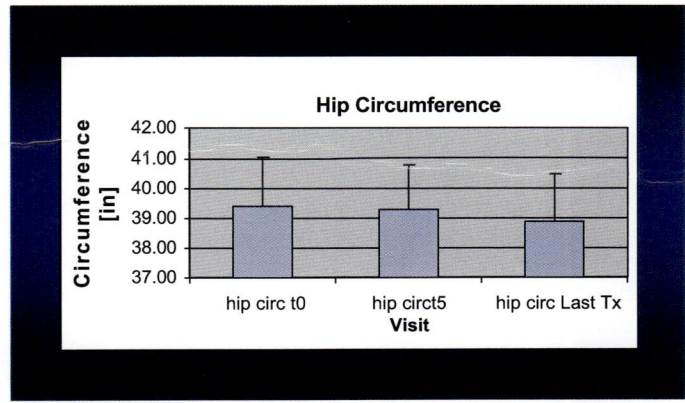

Figure 14.23 Clinical study of Boyce S, Pabby A, Cuchaltkaren P, et al: Clinical evaluation of a device for the treatment of cellulite: TriActive. Am J Cosmetic Surg 2005;22:233–37.

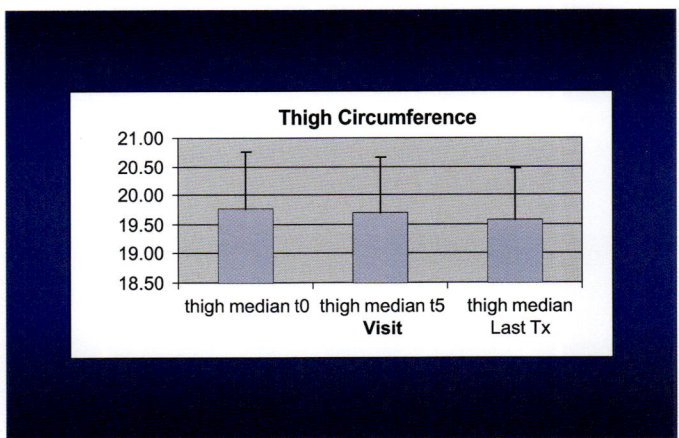

Figure 14.24 Clinical study of Boyce S, Pabby A, Cuchaltkaren P, et al: Clinical evaluation of a device for the treatment of cellulite: TriActive. Am J Cosmetic Surg 2005;22:233–37.

In the initial phase the abdominal and inguinal lymph nodes are treated.

Andrea Pelosi, physiotherapist, conducted a subsequent study to that of Nicola Zerbinati, MD, using the above protocol which he designed and perfected. Pictures obtained during the intensive phase of treatment are presented here (Figs. 14.11–14.21).

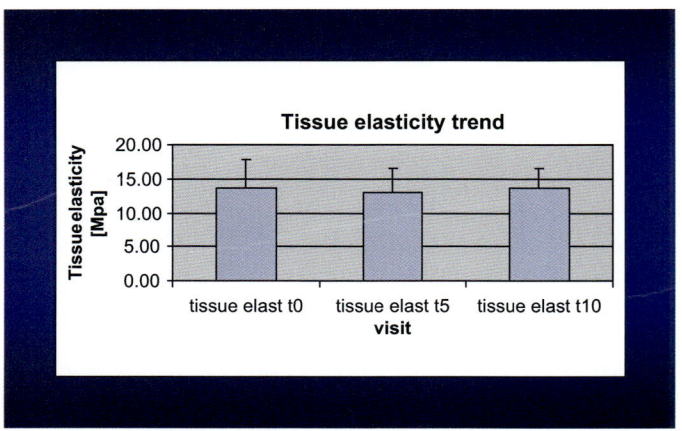

Figure 14.25 Clinical study of Boyce S, Pabby A, Cuchaltkaren P, et al: Clinical evaluation of a device for the treatment of cellulite: TriActive. Am J Cosmetic Surg 2005;22:233–37.

A similar study to those presented above to evaluate the efficacy of the Tri-Active without the lymphatic drainage protocol outlined above confirmed the importance of lymphatic drainage [8]. Thirteen healthy females from 19 years old to 51 years old with a mean age of 36.6 years, with a mean body mass index of 22.26 (19.2 – 29.3) were included in the study. (Normal: 18.5–24.9, Overweight: 25–29.9). Mean starting percentage of body fat of the subjects was 22.18% (16.46–31.02%). (Fit: 21–24% and Acceptable: 25–31%). The subjects underwent biweekly treatments for six weeks for a total of 12 treatments. Treatments were administered locally only on the hips and thighs. Measurement of results included waist, hip, and thigh circumference, elasticity, and thermography.

Analysis of results included a subjective evaluation of pre- and post-treatment photos by five blinded evaluators. An overall improvement of 21% was noted among the treated patients. Most notable improvement was in the appearance of cellulite (23%), skin texture (16%), size (15%), and skin tone (14%). Most notable improvement is shown in Fig. 14.26.

Thermography results evaluated in this study did not show changes of mean temperature, or variations in uniformity of temperature distribution in the treated areas. The results revealed a trend towards modest, but steady improvements in hip and thigh circumferences (Figs. 14.22–14.25)

Comparison to pre-treatment photos also suggests modest improvements in the appearance of cellulite and overall appearance, with those subjects starting with the least symptoms showing the greatest degree of improvement (Fig. 14.26) Comparing these results to those of the previous studies suggest the importance of considering the entire system and method as a whole concept to be diligently performed for maximizing results.

Dr. Michael Gold evaluated the Tri-Active on 10 females with cellulite treated with 15 biweekly sessions [9]. Nine of the 10 subjects completed the study and the one month follow-up period. There were no significant changes in the subject's weight. An approximate 50% improvement in the visual grading scale was noted in 80% of subjects.

Nootheti and Goldman performed the first comparative study to determine the relative efficacy of treatment of cellulite using two novel modalities, Tri-Active versus VelaSmooth [10]. Vela-Smooth is based on a combination of two different ranges of electromagnetic energy which produce heat: infrared light and radio frequency (RF) combined with mechanical manipulation of the skin and also has been demonstrated to improve the appearance of cellulite. (See chapter 15) Patients were treated twice a week for 6 weeks with the randomization of Tri-Active on one side and VelaSmooth on the other side. There were a total of 12 treatments per leg. Cellulite grading was determined utilizing the 4 stage Nurnberger-Muller scale, measurements of thigh circumference were taken before treatment and after the final treatment. Visual inspection and photographic grading was quantified and statistically examined.

In comparing efficacy between VelaSmooth treatment vs Tri-Active treatment, we calculated a 28% vs. a 30% improvement respectively in the upper thigh circumference measurements, while a 56% vs. a 37% improvement was observed, respectively, in lower thigh circumference measurements. These differences in treatment efficacy, using the thigh circumference measurements were found to be non-significant. ($p > 0.05$).

Based on before and after photographs that were blindly evaluated, we found that 25% (5 out of 19) of the subjects showed improvement in cellulite appearance for both Tri-Active and VelaSmooth. The average percent improvement based on random photography grading from a scale of 1–5 (1 representing no improvement and 5 representing most improvement) for the VelaSmooth vs. Tri-Active are 7% and 25%, respectively. This difference is also found to be non-significant ($p = 0.091$). (Fig. 14.26).

Perceived change grade was also calculated based on random side by side comparisons of before and after photographs. Seventy-five precent (15 out of 19) subjects showed improvement in the VelaSmooth leg while 55% (11 out of 19) subjects showed improvement in the Tri-Active leg. The average mean percent improvement was roughly the same for both treatments (22% and 20%, respectively) and showed no statistically significant difference ($p > 0.05$).

Incidence of bruising was reported in 60% of the subjects. Bruising incidence and intensity was 30% higher in the VelaSmooth leg than in the Tri-Active leg. 7 out of 20 subjects reported bruising with VelaSmooth, 1 subject reported bruising with Tri-Active, 3 reported bruising with both VelaSmooth and Tri-Active. Extent of

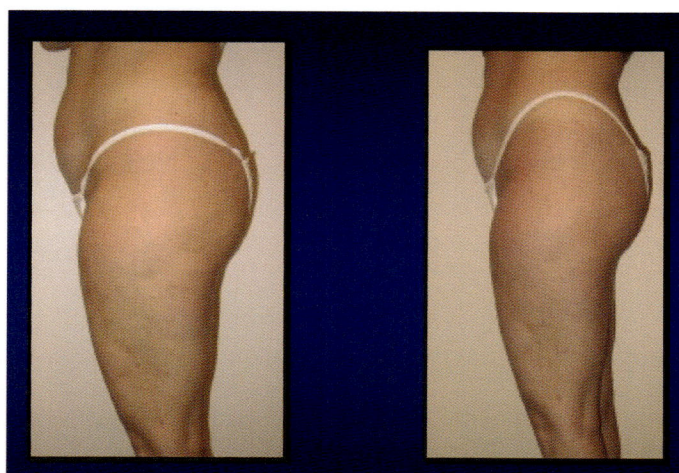

Figure 14.26 After 10 treatments.

bruising ranged from minor purpura to larger and diffused bruises that lasted for an average of a week with no intervention.

Our study revealed that both machines effectively reduced the appearance of cellulite, however when using a p-value of 0.05 there was no statistically significant difference between using Tri-Active versus the VelaSmooth in the reduction of cellulite. Tri-Active provides low-energy diode laser, contact cooling, suction and massage while the VelaSmooth provides a combination of two different ranges of electromagnetic energy: infrared light and radio frequency (RF) combined with mechanical manipulation of the skin. After twice weekly treatment for 6 weeks, there was no statistical significance between the two units in upper or lower thigh circumference measurements, randomized photographic evaluations, or perceived change in before and after photographic evaluations. Incidence and extent of bruising was higher for VelaSmooth than Tri-Active.

REFERENCES

1. AD Agaiby, LR Ghali, R Wilson, M Dyson. Laser modulation of angiogenic factor production by T-lymphocytes. Lasers Surg Med 26(4):357–63, 2000.
2. A Schindl, M Schindl, M Schindl, et al. Increased dermal angiogenesis after low-intensity laser therapy for a chronic radiation ulcer determined by a video measuring system. J Am Acad Dermatol 40:481–4, 1999.
3. GE Romanos, S Pelekanos, JR Strub. Effects of Nd:YAG laser on wound healing processes: clinical and immuno-histochemical findings in rat skin. Lasers Surg Med 16(4):368–79, 1995.
4. I Stadler, R Evans, B Kolb et al. In vitro effects of low-level laser irradiation at 660 nm on peripheral blood lymphocytes. Lasers Surg Med 27(3):255–6, 2000.
5. T Maeda et al. Histological, thermographic and thermometric study in vivo and excised 830 nm diode laser irradiated rat skin. Laser Therapy 2(1):32, 1990.
6. A Pelosi. TRIACTIVE: a three-fold action against cellulite. (Internal study conducted by Deka), 2002.
7. N Zerbinati et al. The Triactive system; a simple and effective way of combating cellulite. (Internal study conducted by Deka, 2002).
8. S Boyce, A Pabby, P Chuchaltkaren et al. Clinical evaluation of a device for the treatment of cellulite: Triactive. Am J Cosmetic Surg 22:233–37, 2005.
9. M Gold. The use of rhythmic suction massage, low level laser irradiation, and superficial cooling to effect changes in adipose tissue/cellulite. Laser Surg Med (Sup) 18:65, 2006.
10. PK Nootheti, A Magpantay, G Yosowitz et al. A single center, randomized, comparative, prospective clinical study to determine the efficacy of the Velasmooth system versus the Triactive system for the treatment of cellulite. Lasers Surg Med 38:908–12, 2006.

15 VelaSmooth and VelaShape
Neil S Sadick

Introduction

Cellulite is a major cosmetic problem, especially for women. The condition is characterized by skin that resembles orange peels or cottage cheese and the presence of dimples in the buttocks and thighs. Cellulite may also occur on the upper arms, breasts, lower abdomen, and other locations where adipose tissue is deposited below the dermis and retained in chambers by subcutaneous fibrous septae. As fat cells become larger, the fat chambers become swollen and compress the surrounding tissue, trapping fluids and making blood circulation more difficult [1]. Slim as well as obese individuals may be affected and excess body weight may accentuate the condition [2–4].

Cellulite has been treated by a variety of procedures described in other chapters of this book. This chapter discusses the use of the VelaSmooth (Syneron Medical Ltd., Israel) and VelaShape (Syneron), both of which utilize Electro-Optical Synergy (ELOS) technology and mechanical manipulation of the skin and fat layer to non-invasively improve the appearance of cellulite. ELOS is a combination of bipolar radiofrequency (RF) and optical energies. The rationale of combining the two types of energy is that the RF energy reduces the amount of optical energy needed to achieve a therapeutic effect. Since RF energy does not heat the epidermis, the likelihood of adverse effects such as scarring and skin pigmentation is reduced [5].

The design of the VelaSmooth (Fig. 15.1) is based on the following principles. RF electrical current is known to heat biological tissue. The amount of heat produced is a function of the tissue impedance, the square of the current intensity, and length of time the skin is exposed to RF energy [6,7]. RF current is not altered by skin type or the presence of chromophores. RF devices may be monopolar, bipolar, or both. In monopolar devices, an active electrode is placed in contact with the area to be treated and a grounding electrode is positioned far from the active electrode. When the device is activated, current flows through the body from the active electrode to the grounding pad, heating the tissue just beneath the active electrode. Since the energy dissipates with distance from the active electrode, only a small amount of heat is generated at the grounding pad. Monopolar RF current penetrates to deep layers of the skin, but the pain during treatment requires the use of anesthesia [7].

In contrast, electrodes of bipolar RF devices are positioned close to each other and both are in contact with the area to be treated. Rather than passing through the entire body, current from the active electrode passes only through the tissue between the two electrodes, following the route of least impedance [4]. Penetration depth is approximately half the distance between the electrodes [7]. The temperature thus increases only in a well-defined volume of tissue [4,8]. If a greater thermal effect on the target tissue is needed, intense infrared light with chromophore-specific wavelengths may be used in addition to RF energy [9]. For example, a combination of RF and IR energy has successfully heated deep layers of tissue [1] and the addition of massage and suction to such a system has been reported to improve the appearance of cellulite [10,11].

Mechanism of Action

The VelaSmooth provides 10 to 100 watts of infrared power, 10 to 100 watts of RF power, 1 MHz RF frequency, and 150 mbar of vacuum suction in 100 to 300-ms pulses, all delivered directly to the skin through a handheld applicator. The IR light spectrum is 680 to 1500 nm and the treated area is 40 × 40 mm. The vacuum suction prepares the skin to receive RF energy that penetrates 10 mm [1,5]. The vacuum suction improves circulation and reduces dimpling by loosening connective tissue around the fat deposits, whereas the IR and RF energies, by heating the skin, enhance the rolling action of the massage unit. Both tissue bulk and dimpling are thus lessened by the massage-induced increase in lymphatic drainage [11].

Sadick and Mulholland have also proposed a mechanism by which the VelaSmooth achieves its therapeutic effect [1]. When the VelaSmooth delivers its infrared (IR) and RF energies to cutaneous tissue, the heat causes the tissue temperature to rise and the local blood supply to the adipose layers to increase. The result is an increase in oxygen availability and in dissociation of oxygen from oxyhemoglobin, which are theorized to promote an increase in fat metabolism. At the same time, the VelaSmooth's mechanical action breaks up the clusters of fat cells, stretches the fibrous bands, and may also facilitate lymphatic drainage by stimulating the removal of fat breakdown products.

Wanitphakdeedecha and Manuskiatti [12] suggested a mechanism by which VelaSmooth treatment improves the bumpiness and dimpling in cellulitic skin. The bumpiness is reduced when the RF current heats adipose tissue at 5 to 10 mm depths, causing lipolysis and fat chamber shrinkage. Penetration of RF energy is enhanced as the rollers knead the skin. The heat also improves peripheral circulation and diffusion of molecules in the treated tissue, thus increasing fat metabolism. Dimpling improves as a result of the repeated kneading of the skin between the rollers, which ruptures fat cell clusters and temporarily stretches the vertical septa and connective tissue.

Patients

Patients seeking treatment of cellulite are first evaluated by history and physical examination. The best candidates have moderate cellulite on the thigh and buttocks and skin contour irregularities that can be monitored regularly by photography as treatment progresses. Treatment can be started when patients have been on a regular diet and exercise program and maintained their weight within 10 pounds for one month [10].

The location and severity of cellulite, previous treatments and response to each, and medical history (diabetes, thrombosis, arterial disease, pregnancy, lactation, patient expectations) should

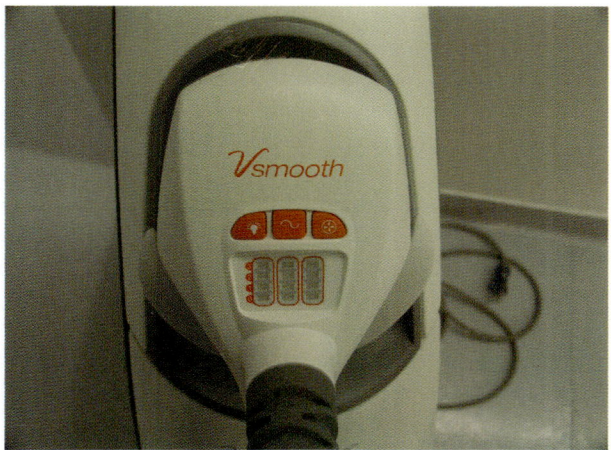

Figure 15.1 The treatment handpiece of the VelaSmooth device (Syneron Medical Ltd., Israel).

be determined. Previous treatments include liposuction, meso-therapy, deep tissue massage, or topical medications. Diabetic patients may be eligible for treatment, but patients with a history of deep venous thrombosis, arterial disease of the legs, or congestive heart failure should not be treated. Pregnant and lactating women are not optimal candidates due to their hormonal variations and the lack of clinical data on the treatment of these women. Patients who expect their cellulite to improve immediately after treatment (by any modality) or who are not willing to undergo a series of treatments for the best results are not good candidates. Finally, patients with diseased, inflamed, or sunburned skin in areas with cellulite are at risk for the development of postinflammatory

hyperpigmentation or other adverse effects after treatment with optical energy, and should therefore not undergo treatment [10].

Patients treated with the VelaSmooth device are shown in Figs. 15.2 and 15.3.

Treatment Protocol

The following is the protocol for a typical 30- to 45-minute session in the author's office. It is used for both the VelaSmooth and VelaShape and is similar to those reported by Alster Tehrani [10], Sadick and Mulholland [1], and Sadick and Magro [5].

1. Hydrate skin with >8 ounces of water up to 1 hour before treatment.
2. If patient bruises easily, give arnica orally or sublingually before treatment.
3. Photograph areas to be treated and record body weight and circumference of thigh or buttocks.
4. Wash skin to be treated with mild soap and water to remove powder, creams, or other material that may interfere with treatment.
5. Dry skin thoroughly.
6. Hydrate skin with a conductive lotion provided by the manufacturer; reapply during treatment if necessary.
7. Using the handheld applicator, treat with four to six passes. Move the handpiece backward and forward several times over the treatment area. Adjust energy levels according to the patient's comfort and tolerance. Use gentle but firm pressure to ensure adequate contact.
8. Treat to erythema and a warm feeling in treated areas (5 to 10 minutes of treatment). These endpoints should disappear in two hours.

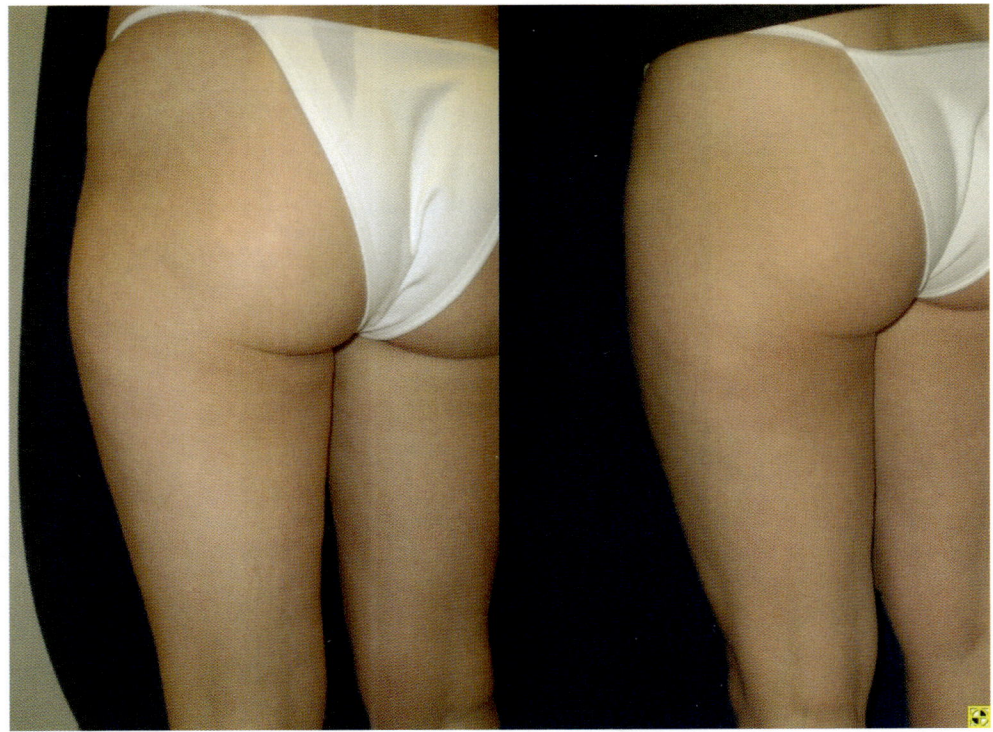

Figure 15.2 A 37-year-old woman before (left) and after three treatments (right) with the VelaSmooth device. Photographs courtesy of Neil S. Sadick, MD.

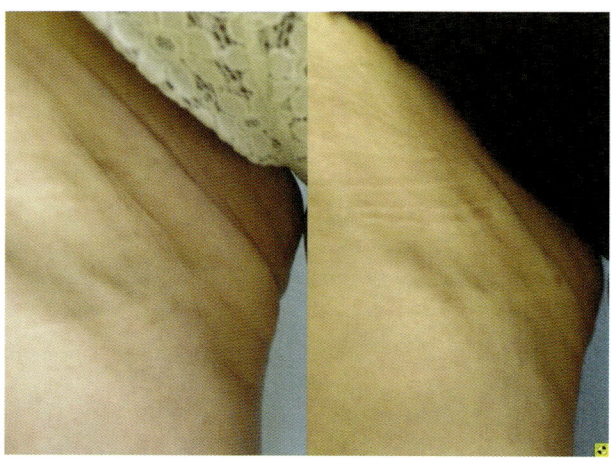

Figure 15.3 A 59-year-old woman before (left) and after eight treatments (right) with the VelaSmooth device. Photographs courtesy of Neil S. Sadick, MD.

9. Hydrate treated area with plenty of water after treatment.
10. If patient was given arnica before treatment, instruct him or her to continue taking arnica orally after treatment and to apply gel containing arnica or vitamin K to treated areas.
11. Instruct patient to avoid hot baths and showers for 24 hours.

Treat twice weekly for four weeks and monthly (or less frequently) thereafter for maintenance. Temporary bruising may occur after the first several treatments.

Clinical Studies

The results of studies of the efficacy and safety of the VelaSmooth for improving the appearance of cellulite are tabulated in Table 15.1.

Sadick and Mulholland [1] evaluated the efficacy by observing changes in the circumference of the thighs and estimating improvement (%) from photographs taken before and after treatment. Energy levels depended on patient tolerance and comfort and were increased with continued treatments. Patients were treated until the appearance of erythema (5–10 min.).

All patients achieved some level of improvement in cellulite appearance and skin smoothing as judged by comparing pre- and post-treatment photographs. Physician-rated improvement was very good to excellent in 23% of patients, good in 35%, and mild in the remaining 42%. Average improvement in cellulite appearance was 40% as judged by a blinded dermatologist. Histological analyses of skin biopsy specimens of the lateral thighs taken from three patients before treatment, after two treatments, and after eight treatments showed no evidence of structural damage, either epithelial or mesenchymal [1].

Alster and Tanzi [11] treated 20 adult women with moderate bilateral thigh and buttocks cellulite. Treatments were given to a randomly selected side (thigh and buttocks) while the other side served as an untreated control. Efficacy was evaluated by (1) thigh circumference measurements before each treatment and at one, three, and six months after the final treatment session and (2) clinical improvement scoring (0 = <25%, 3 = >75%) by two independent, blinded medical assessors who compared pre- and post-treatment photographs.

Eighteen of the 20 patients noticed overall improvement in the appearance of cellulite and 17 would undergo treatment of the untreated thigh. Bruising was limited to the initial sessions and occurred only in two patients. Discomfort during treatment was minimal or absent. Clinical benefit declined slightly at the three and six month evaluations, suggesting that monthly maintenance treatments may be necessary.

Wanitphakdeedecha and Manuskiatti [12] were the first to report cellulite improvement one year after a series of treatments with the VelaSmooth, and for both the thigh and abdomen (Table 15.1).

Table 15.1 Studies evaluating the efficacy and safety of the VelaSmooth device in improving the appearance of cellulite

Reference	No. of women (Skin types)	Location of cellulite	No. of Tx (interval)	Treatment parameters	Efficacy	Adverse effects	Significance of Study
Sadick et al (1)*	35 (II–VI)	Thighs, buttocks	8 to 16, twice weekly	RF = 7, 14, or 20 J/cm^3; IR = 5, 10, or 15 J/cm^2; vacuum = 200 mbar (100, 200, 300 ms)	0.8 inch mean reduction (3.4%) in thigh circumference; maximum reduction 2 inches	Transient swelling, local crusting in a few patients	First study to show the beneficial effect of the VelaSmooth on the appearance of cellulite; included histological studies
Alster et al (11)	20 (I–V)	Thighs, buttocks	8, twice weekly	RF = 20 W; IR = 20 W; vacuum = 200 mbar	Thigh circumference reduced by 0.8 cm (1.4%) on treatment side, no reduction in untreated sides; overall improvement in 90% of patients; mean improvement score ~50%	Transient erythema, bruising	First controlled study to show the efficacy and safety of VelaSmooth

(Continued)

Table 15.1 (Continued)

Reference	No. of women (Skin types)	Location of cellulite	No. of Tx (interval)	Treatment parameters	Efficacy	Adverse effects	Significance of Study
Wanitphakdeedecha et al (12)	12 (III-V)	Abdomen, thighs	8–9, twice weekly	RF = 20 W; IR = 20 W; vacuum = 200 mbar	Abdomen and thigh circumferences reduced 4.04% and 3.50%, respectively, at week 4; mean improvement score ~ 25% for abdomen and ~50% for thighs.	Blister on thigh of 1 patient	First study to evaluate long-term efficacy of VelaSmooth
Nootheti et al (13)	20 (not reported)	Thighs (lower and upper)	12, twice weekly	RF = 1 Mhz IR, vacuum not reported	Lower thigh: 28% of subjects reduced circumference; upper thigh: 56% of subjects reduced circumference; 25% of subjects improved appearance of cellulite; 7% of subjects improved smoothness of skin;	Bruising in 7 patients	First study to compare the VelaSmooth and Tri-Active
Sadick et al (5)	20 (I-VI)	Thighs (lower and upper)	12, twice weekly	Highest energy levels patients could tolerate; vacuum optimized for each patient; circumferences of thighs measured at two locations before and after treatment	0.44 cm overall decrease in lower thigh circumference (0.85%), 0.53 cm decrease for upper thigh circumference (0.90%); >51% visual improvement seen in 50% of subjects at final (8-week) follow-up visit	Mild discomfort, swelling, bruising	Controlled study showing safety and efficacy
Romero et al (4)	10 (II-IV)	Buttocks	12, twice weekly	Highest energy levels patients could tolerate; one buttock treated and the other served as control; treated skin surface evaluated optically at baseline, before final treatment, and 2 months after final treatment; biopsy samples taken	Improvement evident in all patients after 1st session and continued throughout study period; all patients satisfied; histological analyses suggest clinical improvement due to dermal firmness, fiber compaction, and tightened layers of skin	Pain bearable and erythema lasted a few hours	First controlled study to provide objective (optical) data on skin surface at various stages of treatment

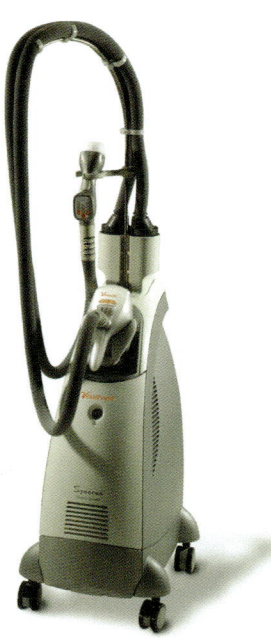

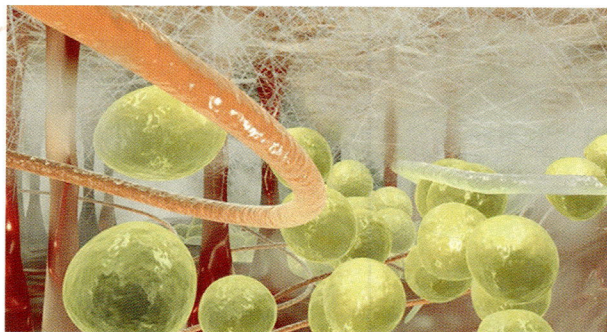

Figure 15.7 After treatment, the fat cells have diminished in size, but did not rupture due to heat-stimulated metabolism of fat cells, mainly IR and RF-induced lipolysis. The heat has also shrunk the connective tissue fibers, resulting in skin tightening. Excess intercellular water and metabolic products have been removed by lymphatic drainage facilitated by the mechanical massage of the rollers. The overall response to treatment leads to circumference reduction and cellulite improvement.

For the thighs, mean circumference reductions were 6.23% immediately after the final treatment, 6.26% four weeks later, and 5.50% one year later. Mean reductions for the abdomens were 6.32%, 4.04%, and 4.64%, respectively. These results suggest that most of the circumferential reductions are maintained for at least one year after the final of eight to nine treatments at two per week.

Nootheti and colleagues [13] compared the efficacies of the VelaSmooth and Tri-Active (Cynosure, Westford, MA) for the treatment of cellulite. The Tri-Active device uses a combination of low-energy diode laser, cooling, suction, and massage. Efficacies were judged by numbers of patients that showed improvement, so actual values of circumferences were not reported. As in earlier studies, improvements were evaluated by comparing

Figure 15.4 The VelaShape device (Syneron Medical Ltd., Israel).

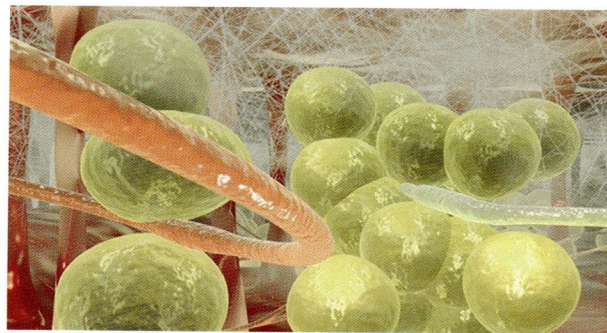

Figure 15.5 The pretreatment subcutaneous layer of large fat cells (adipocytes) below the numerous white strands of connective tissue. Note the white connective tissue fibers that form the fat chamber's septae and the red blood vessels.

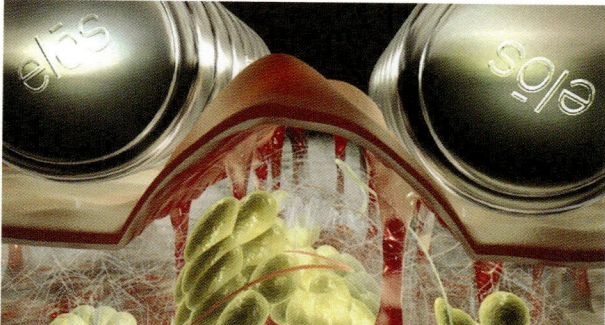

Figure 15.6 Diagram showing the skin layers raised by the vacuum between the rollers. The dermis and hypodermis are now closer to the sources of infrared (IR) and radiofrequency (RF) energies, permitting deeper access and faster heating of both the dermis and hypodermis. Thus, the IR energy heats the dermal layer up to 5 mm deep, and the RF energy heats the hypodermal layer up to 15 mm deep. The outcome of the treatment is described in Fig. 15.7.

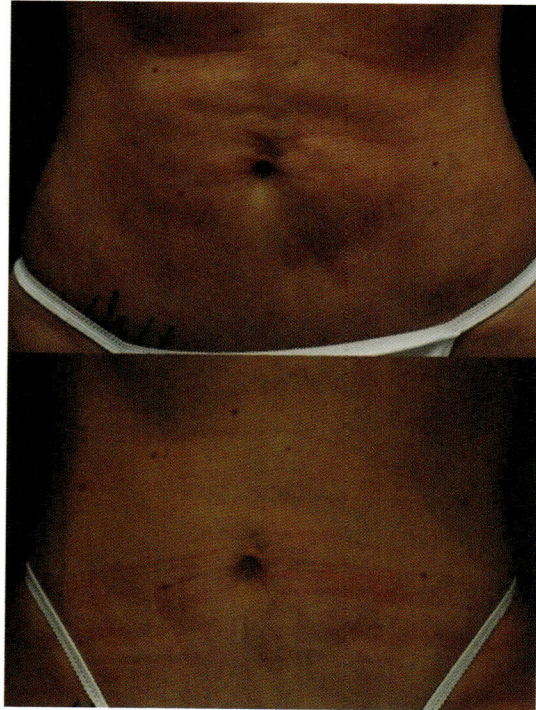

Figure 15.8. A 39-year-old woman before (top) and after 7 treatments (bottom) with the VelaShape device. Photographs courtesy of Neil S. Sadick, MD.

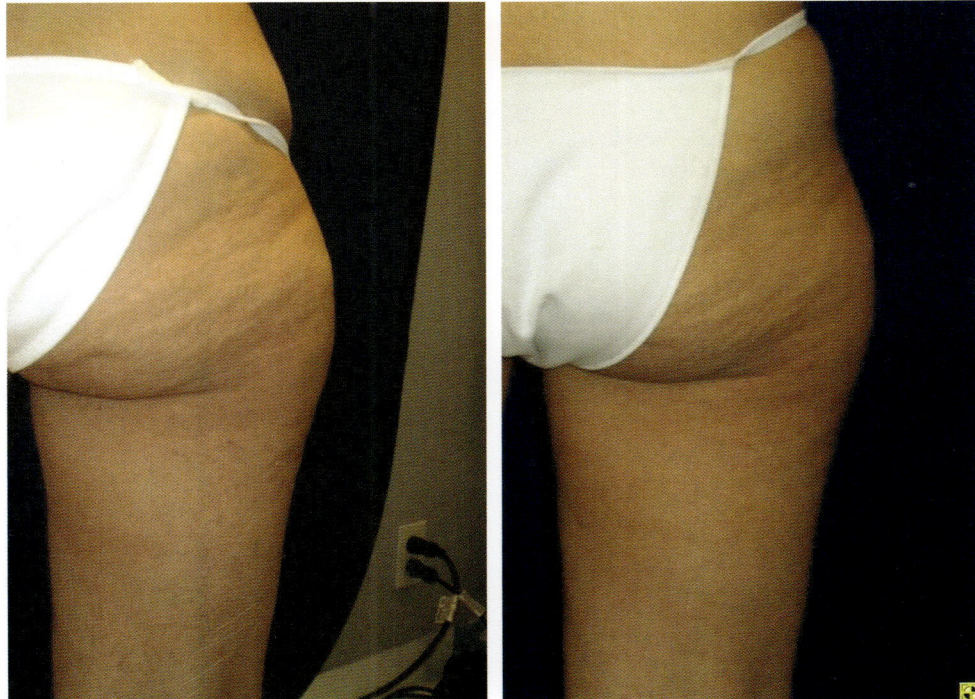

Figure 15.9 A 47-year-old woman before (left) and after 6 treatments (right) with the VelaShape device. Photographs courtesy of Neil S. Sadick, MD.

photographs. The authors concluded that both systems improved the appearance of cellulite to roughly the same degree.

Sadick and Magro [5] showed that the thighs of half of 16 subjects improved more than 25% after 12 treatments. One thigh was treated and the other thigh served as a control. Each thigh was measured at two locations. Significant visual improvement in skin texture and in the appearance of cellulite were noted at the four and eight week follow-up visits by the investigator and an independent evaluator. Thigh circumferences showed a statistically significant decrease only at the four-week follow-up visit, suggesting that maintenance treatments would be necessary to preserve positive results. The authors attributed the transient bruising in five patients to the mechanical manipulation of the skin during treatment. Histological analyses of biopsy specimens from two patients did not reveal morphological changes that correlated with clinical improvement in the appearance of cellulite.

Romero and colleagues [4] evaluated improvement before and after treatment at several time points by two methods: (1) optical analysis of the skin surface to assess changes in tissue depression depth and roughness using three-dimensional profilometry software and (2) patient and blinded clinician evaluation of photographs. The profilometric data showed improvement in skin characteristics at all assessment points. The blinded clinician assessments were generally more positive than the subjective patient assessments, except at the final, two-month follow-up assessment. At the end of the study all participants wanted their untreated buttock to be treated with the VelaSmooth.

Skin biopsy specimens were taken from the buttocks of six of 10 patients before treatment, 2 hours after the first treatment, and two months after the final of 12 treatments. Specimens taken after the final treatment showed improved epidermal and dermal morphology due to tightened dermal collagen and improved organization of epidermal cells compared to the baseline samples. Specimens taken 2 hours after the initial treatment showed dermal fibers aligned with the dermal-epidermal junction, contraction of the papillary dermis, and adipocytes moved close to one another compared with baseline samples. The authors suggested that these histological changes may be due to microinflammatory stimuli produced in the treated tissue and subsequent standard tissue repair.

Velashape

Like the VelaSmooth, the VelaShape (Fig. 15.4) delivers bipolar RF energy, IR light energy, and vacuum suction pulses to the skin surface with a handheld applicator. RF energy penetrates 2 to 20 mm whereas IR energy penetrates up to 3 mm beneath the skin. The vacuum system is the same on both devices. RF power is available at 50 rather than 20 watts (as in the VelaSmooth). The increase in power allows the user to heat the tissue faster, leading to improved efficacy without additional pain or adverse effects. Treatment duration is also shortened by approximately 30% and fewer treatments (4–6) are required to achieve clinical benefit. For example, patients requiring a 16-treatment protocol with the VelaSmooth can achieve a similar result with only four to six treatments with the VelaShape. Additionally the VelaShape platform is available with the VContour applicator. This applicator is smaller and designed for harder to reach areas such as the arms and neck. Recently VelaShape II has been released, which has made further improvements to the ELOS technology. The new platform reduces treatment time by 20% by allowing a higher energy output of 75 W. Additionally it features an advanced ergonomically designed handpiece as well as a new and improved massage system that is completely noiseless and increases patient comfort.

The principles of operation of the VelaShape are shown in Figs. 15.5–15.7.

Patients treated with the VelaShape device are shown in Figs.15.8 and 15.9.

Conclusion

The efficacy and safety of the VelaSmooth device has been shown repeatedly in various studies. The VelaShape promises to reduce treatment duration and number of treatments to achieve clinical benefit comparable to that of the VelaSmooth.

REFERENCES

1. NS Sadick, RS Mulholland. A prospective clinical study to evaluate the efficacy and safety of cellulite treatment using the combination of optical and RF energies for subcutaneous tissue heating. J Cosmet Laser Ther 6:187–90, 2004.
2. Z Draelos, KD Marenus. Cellulite. Etiology and purported treatment. Dermatol Surg 23(12):1177–81, 1997.
3. MM Avram. Cellulite: a review of its physiology and treatment. J Cosmet Laser Ther 6:181–85, 2004.
4. C Romero, N Caballero, M Herrero et al. Effects of cellulite treatment with RF, IR light, mechanical massage and suction treating one buttock with the contralateral as a control. J Cosmet Laser Ther 10:193–201, 2008.
5. N Sadick, C Magro. A study evaluating the safety and efficacy of the VelaSmooth system in the treatment of cellulite. J Cosmet Laser Ther 9:15–20, 2007.
6. G Montesi, S Calvieri, A Balzani, et al. Bipolar radiofrequency in the treatment of dermatologic imperfections: clinicopathological and immunohistochemical aspects. J Drugs Dermatol 6:890–96, 2007.
7. N Sadick. Tissue tightening technologies: fact or fiction. Aesthet Surg J 28:180–88, 2008.
8. N Sadick, L Sorhaindo. The radiofrequency frontier: a review of radiofrequency and combined radiofrequency pulsed-light technology in aesthetic medicine. Facial Plast Surg 21:131–38, 2005.
9. EV Ross, M Smirnov, M Pankratov et al. Intense pulsed light and laser treatment of facial telangiectasias and dyspigmentation: some theoretical and practical comparisons. Dermatol Surg 31(9 Pt 2):1188–98, 2005.
10. TS Alster, M Tehrani. Treatment of cellulite with optical devices: an overview with practical considerations. Lasers Surg Med 38:727–30, 2006.
11. TS Alster, EL Tanzi. Cellulite treatment using a novel combination radiofrequency, infrared light, and mechanical tissue manipulation device. J Cosmet Laser Ther 7:81–85, 2005.
12. R Wanitphakdeedecha, W Manuskiatti. Treatment of cellulite with a bipolar radiofrequency, infrared heat, and pulsatile suction device: a pilot study. J Cosmet Dermatol 5:284–88, 2006.
13. PK Nootheti, A Magpantay, G Yosowitz et al. A single center, randomized, comparative, prospective clinical study to determine the efficacy of the VelaSmooth system versus the Triactive system for the treatment of cellulite. Lasers Surg Med 38:908–12, 2006.

16 Accent® Unipolar Radiofrequency
Jane Unaeze and David J Goldberg

Radiofrequency technology dates back to the 1920's with the introduction of electrocautery. Over the decades, it has been used in multiple specialties for cauterization and ablation. Recently, the use of radiofrequency emerged a non-invasive, non-ablative technology that uses volumetric thermotherapy modify the connective tissue septa and fat in the treatment of cellulite [1]. Although there is no consensus on the etiology of cellulite, growing evidence suggests that a decrease in the microcirculation and weakening of connective tissue with subsequent herniation of subcutaneous adipose tissue into the dermis play a role in its pathogenesis [2,3]. Existing treatment modalities for cellulite range from exercise, weight loss, vibrating machines, suction devices, topical creams, mesotherapy, injectables, surgical subcision, lasers and recently in the last decade radiofrequency devices. The proposed mechanisms for efficacy of radiofrequency in cellulite treatment include thermal injury leading to tightening of dermal fibrous septae, formation of new collagen and collagen remodeling; improved local blood circulation; dissolution of fatty acid and thermal-induced fat cell apoptosis [4,11].

Radiofrequency devices deliver energy in the high frequency electromagnetic spectrum in the 0.3 to 100 MHz range [6] capable of producing temperatures of 65 to 75°C in biologic tissues. The use of radiofrequency in aesthetic dermatology has historically been used in one of two ways: monopolar and bipolar. A monopolar handpiece delivers energy as current between a single electrode tip and grounding plate while a bipolar handpiece applies energy between two points on the tip of a probe [3]. Unipolar radiofrequency is different in that electromagnetic radiation is delivered rather than current and no grounding plate is necessary [3].

The Accent® system (Alma Lasers Inc, Ceasaria, Israel; Fort Lauderdale, FL) is a novel device with a base radiofrequency generator (40.68 MHz) that delivers electromagnetic energy to the patient's skin through unipolar and bipolar handpiece applicators making functional delivery of energy to different depths possible (Figs. 16.1–16.3). It gained US Food and Drug Administration (FDA) cleared approval in 2007 for the treatment of rhytids. It is currently the only unipolar radiofrequency device that has been evaluated for cellulite treatment. Both handpieces are equipped with treatment tips with a built-in continuous cooling system that lessens the risk of epidermal burn [4]. The depth of penetration of heat into the tissue can be modified by varying the level of penetration of the treatment tip and the energy applied [5]. The ability to control the depth of heat that penetrates into the treated tissue using either a unipolar or bipolar applicator makes the Accent® device an attractive therapy for the treatment of cellulite. This chapter focuses on the Unipolar Accent® radiofrequency system for cellulite therapy.

Unipolar radiofrequency energy waves oscillate at a high speed with rapidly alternating electromagnetic fields that displace charged molecules resulting in the rotational movement of water molecules. Such high frequency oscillations produce heat (electrothermolysis) that is dissipated to surrounding tissue depending on the electrical properties of the tissue in contrast to optic energy that depends on the concentration of the chromophore on the skin to achieve the desired effect [3,6]. Controlled thermal injury may result in tissue shrinkage and an inflammatory response with influx of fibroblasts into the treated area leading to neocollagenesis and tightening of the fibrous septa in the dermis, all of which contribute to improving the appearance of cellulite [4,6].

There are some differences between the unipolar and bipolar handpiece applicators of the Accent® device. The radiofrequency power for the Unipolar and Bipolar Accent® handpieces are 100 to 200 watts and 60 to 100 watts respectively. As a result of the higher power, the Unipolar Accent® handpiece heats a greater tissue volume than the Bipolar Accent® handpiece. Bipolar radiofrequency system delivers heat through tissue impedance (Ohm's law) while the Unipolar Accent® system induces rotation of water molecules to produce heat and delivers radiofrequency energy to subcutaneous adipose tissue up to a depth of 20 mm. In contrast the bipolar system, which delivers energy to a depth between 2 to 6 mm, handpiece is useful in treating superficial areas with thin dermis such as the forehead and neck.

The area to be treated is generally marked in grids of 5 × 6 cm (with 15 seconds exposure time) or 10 × 6 cm (30 seconds exposure time) and lubricated with treatment oil to lessen friction. The handpiece is applied to the skin in a continuous fashion with two phases of treatment. In phase I, a therapeutic threshold of ~41°C is reached; in phase II multiple passes are applied to the treatment area leading to homogeneous erythema. Treatments can be repeated up to six to eight times spaced two weeks apart [4].

One of the leading theories on the etiology of cellulite is that a weakened connective tissue lattice in the deep dermis causes herniation of subcuticular fat into the dermis [3]. In cellulite, the microcirculation deposits more fat and retains more interstitial fluids. Fat cells are stored in large groups found between the skin and muscle and separated by fibrous septae. With weight gain, fat cells expand, causing the gap between the muscle and skin to expand. This leads to increased tension on the fibrous septa which might not be able to support the skin. Subsequently, fat cells in the subcutis are pulled into the connective tissue fibers leading to the dimpling of the skin seen in cellulite.

Heating of collagen breaks heat-sensitive bonds and causes denaturalization, a transition process in which the collagen protein transforms from a highly organized crystalline structure to a disorganized gel, which occurs at 65 to 75°C [6]. This temperature range correlates to a surface temperature of 40 to 43°C. The denaturation of collagen caused by the thermal injury is hypothesized to stimulate a wound-healing response where heated fibroblasts are stimulated to produce collagen [5]. Various heat-induced factors affect the behavior of the connective tissue and the amount of tissue contraction. These factors include the peak

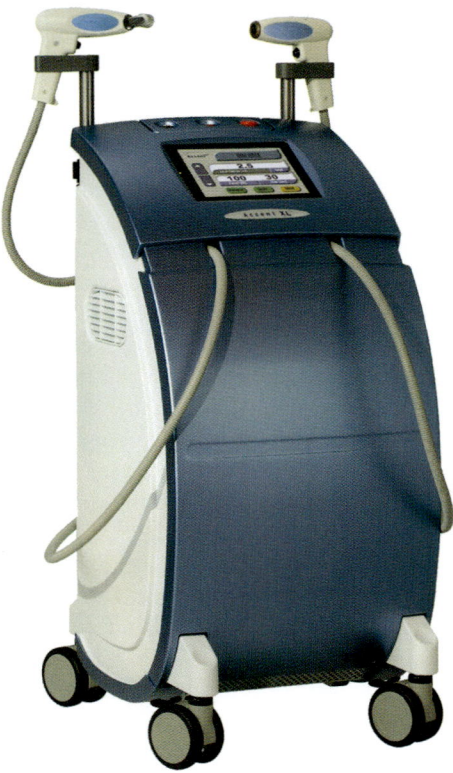

Figure 16.1 The Accent® System. www.almalasers.com

temperature, delivery time of the radiofrequency and the applied mechanical stress during the heating process [6]. Thermal properties of tissue can also be influenced by age, pH, electrolyte milieu, the concentration and orientation of collagen fibers, and the hydration levels of the tissue [2].

After the heat-induced wound healing begins, collagen contraction occurs through an unfolding of the triple helix when

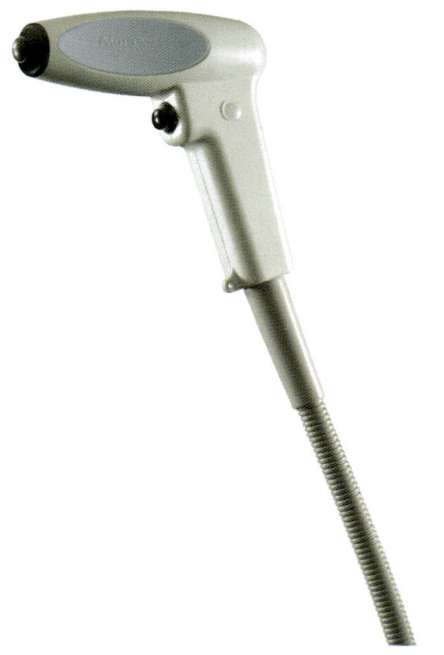

Figure 16.2 Accent® unipolar handpiece.

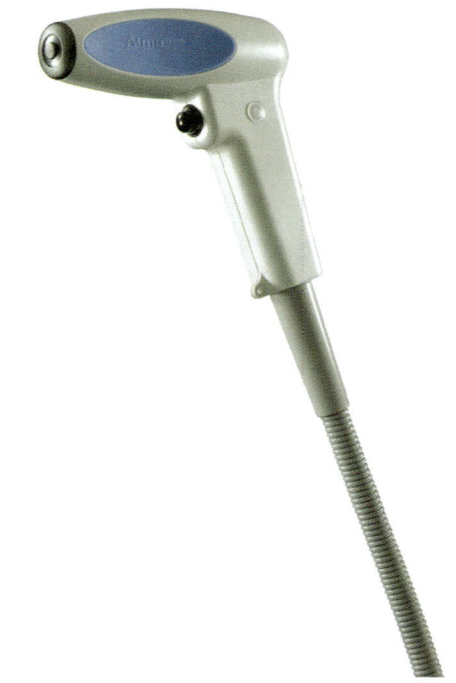

Figure 16.3 Accent® bipolar handpiece.

crossed intermolecular bonds, which are sensitive to heat, are destroyed. In addition, it has been suggested that radiofrequency-induced injury causes collagen contracture due to the breakdown of extramolecular hydrogen bonds with subsequent tightening of the skin [6,7].

There are no conclusive studies showing a direct correlation between temperature and connective tissue contraction. Dermal fibrous band thickening as well as contraction between Camper's fascia and the dermis are possible mechanisms that may contribute to the clinical tightening seen in patients treated with the Accent® device as demonstrated by MRI and ultrasound [6,8]. It has also been proposed that lymphatic drainage of the dissolved fat occurs but this remains to be proven. Radio frequency-induced heating of deep tissue may also improve local blood circulation thereby promoting drainage and replenishment of retained fluids and catabolic products [6]. Induction of rapid oscillations of water molecules by the Unipolar Accent® system would appear to facilitate formation of a uniform and sustained volumetric dermal heating for cellulite treatment [5].

Studies showing improvement of cellulite after radiofrequency therapy are limited by a lack of large randomized control trials, short-term follow-up, and lack of universal standards for assessing the efficacy of treatments studied. In a study by Del Pino and colleagues, 26 females with grade 1 to 3 bilateral cellulite on thighs and/or buttocks received two treatments of unipolar radiofrequency spaced 15 days apart using the unipolar Accent® radiofrequency system. About 70% of the patients showed up to 20% improvement in cellulite appearance as measured by contraction of the distance from dermis to muscle and dermis to Camper's fascia in thigh and buttocks using ultrasound measurements [6]. We also demonstrated the efficacy of the Accent® unipolar device for the treatment of cellulite [8]. In our study, 27 of 30 patients with grade 3 to 4 cellulite of the upper thighs were treated every other week for six sessions with the Accent® unipolar device and showed a

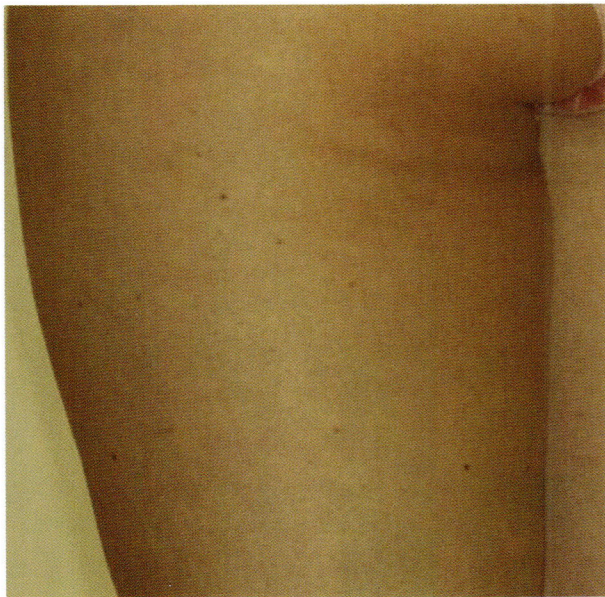

Figure 16.4 Pre-treatment left posterior thigh (Goldberg et al 2008).

mean decrease of approximately 1 inch in leg circumference. There was post-treatment dermal fibrosis without any gross changes in the subcutis noted by MRI. Treatment results lasted at least six months (Figs. 16.4–16.5). In addition a randomized, blinded, split design study compared treated versus untreated control thighs in ten patients with grade 2 to 4 cellulite using the Accent® unipolar device. Three months after the three to six treatments up to 10% improvement was noted in dimple density and distribution. Only a 2% improvement in depth of dimple was observed [3].

Patients are usually able to continue their daily activities uninterrupted af0ter Unipolar Accent® radiofrequency therapy which offers a short treatment session with minimal side effects. Risks of pigment alteration, infection, bleeding, and scarring associated with other modalities such as surgery and laser resurfacing are significantly reduced because radiofrequency is not influenced by competing chromophores on the skin surface [9]. Limitations of the Accent® system include a requirement for multiple treatments to produce a mild to moderate improvement. Given the potential role of fat in the etiology of cellulite, a reasonable concern has been

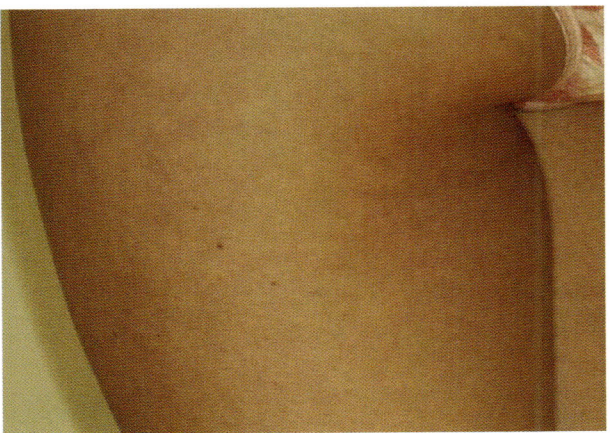

Figure 16.5 Post-treatment with tightening of skin 6 months after treatment (Goldberg et al 2008).

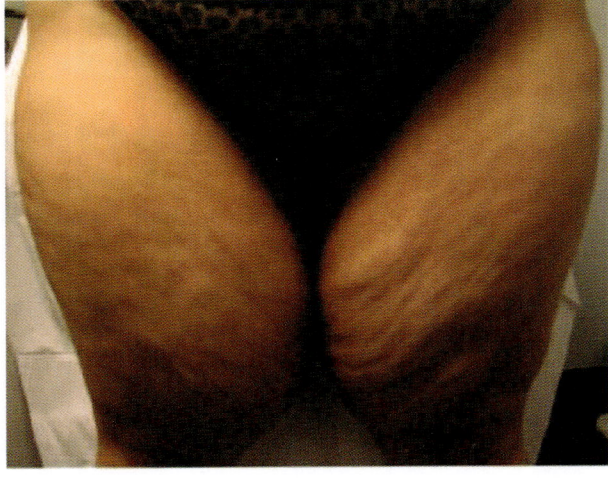

(a)

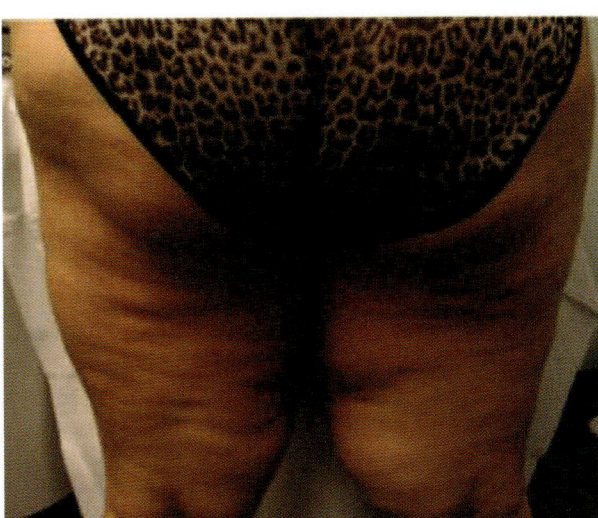

(b)

Figure 16.6a and 6b Right thigh after four treatments at 3 months follow-up with left thigh as control (Alexiades-Armenakas et al 2008).

the possible effect of the cellulite therapy on fat metabolism in the body. However, there are currently no reports of changes in patients' weights, blood lipid profiles or MRI analysis of the fatty layer [8].

Other recent monopolar radiofrequency devices used in cellulite therapy include ThermaCool® (Thermage, Inc, Hayward, CA) which like the Accent® radiofrequency device is also FDA cleared for rhytids. This device, with a new large treatment tip, is now also being used for cellulite treatment. Eventually there will be large studies comparing these two modalities for cellulite treatment. Mayoral reported the case of a patient with upper extremity laxity who received only one treatment with ThermaCool® on one arm while the Accent® treated the other multiple times. Both treatments resulted in improvement of skin laxity but statistical significance was not evaluated [10]. Electron microscopy of post-treatment biopsies of two patients treated with ThermaCool® showed an increase in collagen fibril diameter with blurring between collagen fibril borders up to 5 mm at the 8-week follow-up. The larger diameter of the collagen fibril seemed indicative of shortening of the fibrils [7,9]. Thermal injury is also thought to play a role in stimulating a wound-healing response with the ThermaCool® radiofrequency device [7].

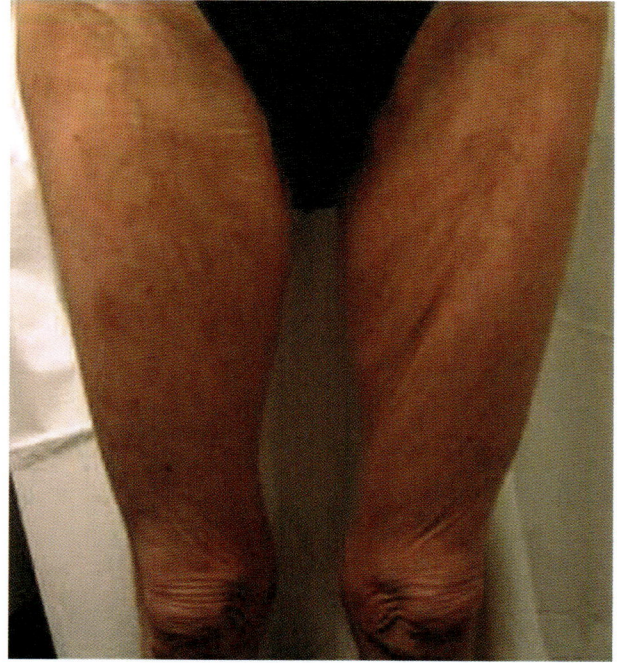

(a)

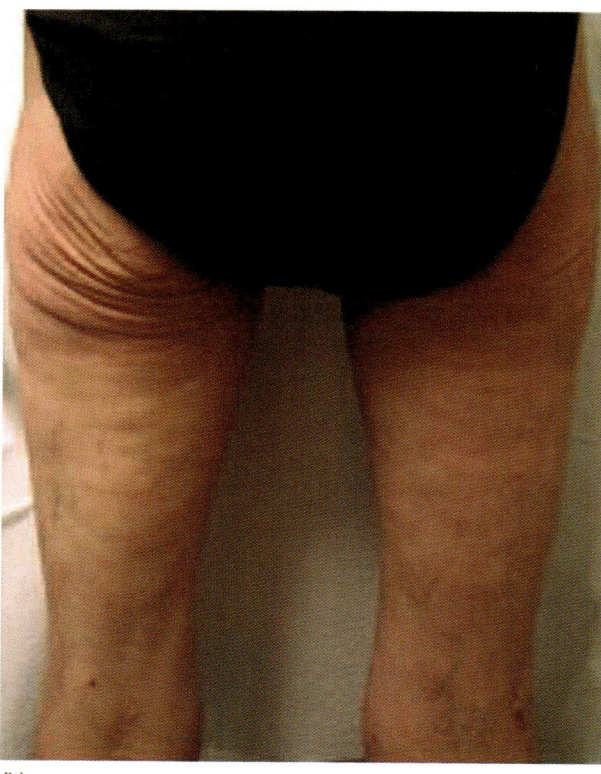

(b)

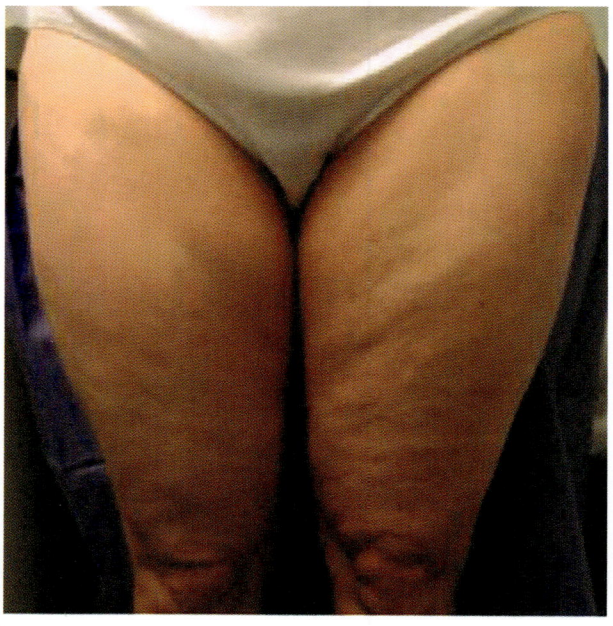

(a)

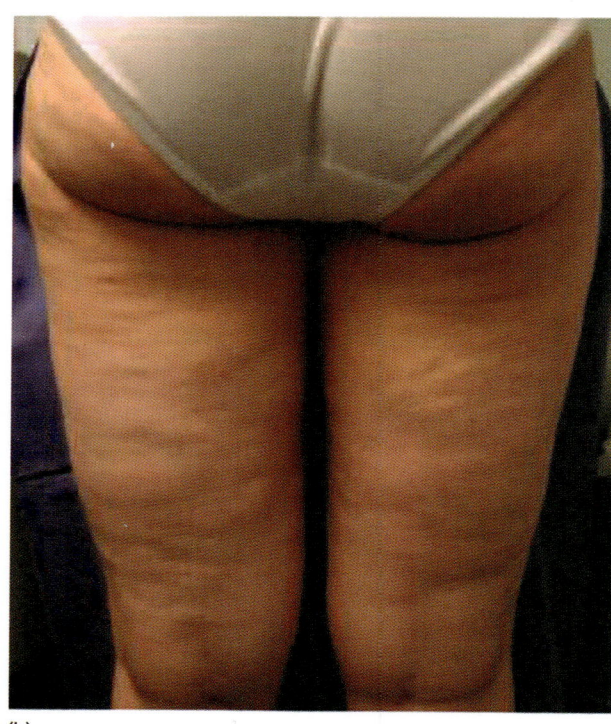

(b)

Figure 16.8a and b Right thigh after three treatments at 3 months follow-up with left thigh as control. (Alexiades-Armenakas et al 2008).

Figure 16.7a and b Right thigh after three treatments at 3 months follow-up with left thigh as control. (Alexiades-Armenakas et al 2008).

The VelaSmooth® device is FDA cleared for the treatment of cellulite. This technology combines bipolar radiofrequency, infrared light and vacuum suction. Studies have shown that up to 12 treatment sessions twice weekly may be required [12,14,15]. Tri-Active® is a diode laser combined with massage therapy also used in cellulite treatment. A study comparing the efficacy of the VelaSmooth®

and Tri-Active® failed to show any statistical difference in treated patients. No studies have compared the Accent ® device to these.

Most patients seem to tolerate radiofrequency therapy well and no major serious adverse events have been reported. Some of the reported side effects with the Accent® unipolar radiofrequency device include small blisters and ecchymosis which usually resolve within a few days without complications. Mild heating sensation and persistent erythema following treatment have also been reported but these generally resolve within 24 hours [3].

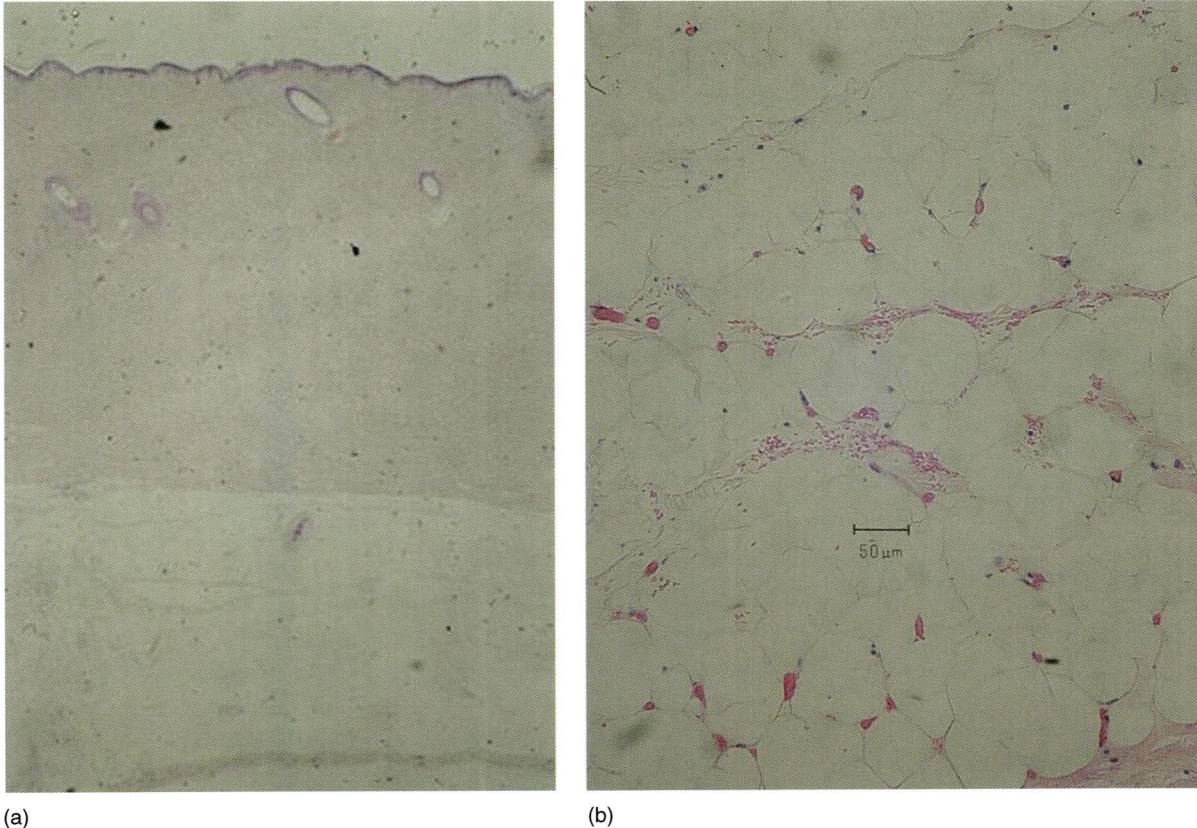

(a)   (b)

Figure 16.9 a and b H & E of Subcutaneous fat: Severe thermal damage after unipolar exposure at 150 watts www.almalasers.com

Accent® radiofrequency treatment offers a promising option for patients who are poor surgical candidates for body contouring or are hesitant about surgical cellulite treatments. Further studies are needed to evaluate the effect of treatment on different tissue depths, impact on factors such mRNA and the extracellular components of cellulite [7].

REFERENCES

1. M Wanner, M Avram. An evidence-based assessment of treatments for cellulite. J Drugs Dermatol 7:341–5, 2008.
2. SP Arcnoczky, A Aksan. Thermal modification of connective tissues: basic science considerations and clinical implications. J Amer Acad Ortho Surg 8:305–13, 2000.
3. M Alexiades Armenakas, JS Dover, KA Arndt. Unipolar radiofrequency treatment to improve the appearance of cellulite. J Cosmet Laser Ther 10:148–53, 2008.
4. A Brown, G de Almedia. Novel Radiofrequency (RF) Device for Cellulite & Body Reshaping Therapy, 2005. www.almalasers.com
5. J Ruiz-Ezparza, J Barba Gomez. The medical face lift: a non-invasive, nonsurgical approach to tissue tightening in facial skin using nonablative radiofrequency. Derm Surg 29:325–32, 2003.
6. E Del Pino, RH Rosado, A Azuela et al. Effect of controlled volumetric tissue heating with radiofrequency on cellulite and the subcutaneous tissue of the buttocks and thighs. J Drugs Dermatol 5:714–22, 2006.
7. BD Zelickson, D Kist, E Bernstein et al. Histological and ultrastructural evaluation of the effects of a radiofrequency-based non-ablative dermal remodelling device: a pilot study. Arch Derm 140:204–9, 2004.
8. DJ Goldberg, A Fazeli, AL Berlin. Clinical, laboratory, and MRI analysis of cellulite treatment with a unipolar radiofrequency device. Dermatol Surg 34:204–9, 2008.
9. GH Fisher, LG Jacobson, LJ Bernstein et al. Nonablative radiofrequency treatment of facial laxity. Dermatol Surg 31(9 Pt 2):1237–41, 2005.
10. FA Mayoral. Skin tightening with a combined unipolar and bipolar radiofrequency device. J Drugs Dermatol 6:212–4, 2007.
11. EV Ross, JR McKinlay, RR Anderson. Why does carbon dioxide resurfacing work? A review. Arch Dermatol 135:444–54, 1999.
12. TS Alster, EL Tanzi. Cellulite treatment using a novel combination radiofrequency, infrared light, and mechanical tissue manipulation device. J Cosmet Laser Ther 7:81–5, 2005.
13. NS Sadick, RS Mulholland. A prospective clinical study to evaluate the efficacy and safety of cellulite treatment using the combination of optical and RF energies for subcutaneous tissue heating. J Cosmet Laser Ther 6:187–90, 2004.
14. N Sadick, C Magro. A study evaluating the safety and efficacy of the VelaSmooth system in the treatment of cellulite. J Cosmet Laser Ther 9:15–20, 2007.
15. PK Nootheti, A Mogpantay, G Yosowitz et al. A single center, randomized, comparative, prospective clinical study to determine the efficacy of the VelaSmooth system versus the Tri-active system for the treatment of cellulite. Lasers Surg Med 38:908–12, 2006.

17 Scientific Bases for the Use of Low-Level Light Energy on the Treatment of Cellulite

Gordon H Sasaki

Cellulite, referred to as skin dimpling, dells and nodularities, is most commonly located in the upper lateral and posterior thighs and lower buttocks. This condition represents a frequent physiologic and unsightly appearance, whose classification [1–2], etiology [3–7], anatomy [8] and management [9–11] are subjects of continued deliberation. Despite its prevalence and intensive interest in the lay and medical press [12], no agreement exists on the causes of its presentation, thereby confusing efforts to manage it.

Cellulite expresses itself most commonly in postpartum women [26] who demonstrate an increased number or volume of adipocytes in certain predictable locations. During pregnancy, females may begin to exhibit the early stages of cellulite on their lower abdomen, thighs and buttocks. It is of interest that a woman's body possesses about 21 to 22 billion adipocytes, while men have only about 17 to 18 billion cells. Infrequently, cellulite may be seen in women with normal body fat distribution and body weight ratios. Cellulite is rarely detected in men, even though they may accumulate increased fatty girths around their lower abdomen, hips and lumbar regions. Furthermore, this gender-specific predisposition is corroborated at the histological level, not only by the presence of thinner, arched and almost perpendicular and parallel supporting septae [3], but also by a more irregular dermo-hypodermal boundary produced by increased normal protrusions of adipocytes that accompany the numerous adnexal structures (hair follicles, sebaceous glands) into the reticular and papillary dermis. These normal micro-anatomical structural findings in women, confirmed by sonography, MRI and spectroscopy [13,14] favor the clinical expression of cellulite, whenever there exists a gender-linked regional accumulation of localized fat [15,16] and/or the presence of compressive forces [9] upon the adiposal layers. If one pinches the skin between the thumb and index finger (the so-called pinch test), the fat bulges upward within the fat chambers, producing the typical orange peel appearance [7]. These factors facilitate the migration and "herniation" of fatty tissue into the dermal layer in both slender and obese women.

Cellulite is also more commonly displayed in lax rather than firm skin. Since skin is sensitive to hormonal changes, skin aging is accelerated in women owing to hormonal fluctuations during pregnancy and menopause and from distention over regional accumulations of fatty deposits. Therefore, it is not surprising that cellulite-affected skin has been shown to exhibit biomechanical properties of increased skin laxity in contrast to skin without cellulite in cellulite-prone and non-prone areas in women [17,19]. Although microvascular ischemia [4], microlymphatic obstruction [18] and inflammatory etiologies [9] cannot be excluded for the development of cellulite, current evidence supports that gender-related differences in the skin, subcutaneous fat and septal architecture, and localized tissue pressure contribute more to the presence of cellulite than do these aforementioned factors.

Since cellulite is more likely to occur within lax skin in obese women, its unsightly appearance may be improved, first, by rejuvenating the overlying skin and subdermal septal network and, secondly, by reducing the presence of fat bulges that intrude through the dermo-subcutaneous barrier. Preliminary studies employing low-level light therapy, in the form of energy generated by light emitting diodes (LED), have demonstrated modest and temporary results in the management of cellulite. This chapter will discuss LED therapy and its role in the treatment of this common and annoying condition.

Introduction

The 40-year development of low-level light energy therapy from laser light sources for reasonable therapeutic results rather than dramatic surgical outcomes began with the work of Endre Mester [1–4] in 1968. Ever since one FDA-approved device was cleared in 2002 for "providing temporary relief of minor chronic neck and shoulder pain of musculoskeletal origin", low-level light laser energy has been used in physical therapy to relieve pain, reduce edema and improve wound healing of leg ulcers [5–9]. Light emitting diodes (LEDs), as a source for quasi-monochromatic or narrow bandwidths of light, were also introduced as an alternative low-level light energy device to provide skin and other wound benefits in aesthetic and reconstructive cases. Despite the reported advantages for either low-level laser or LED energy technology, the purported beneficial effects have remained controversial and uncertain [10–13]. The *in vitro, ex vivo* or *in vivo* effects have been anecdotal, contradictory, or non-transferable from animal to clinical studies, in part due to flawed methodology or minimally detectable end-points [14–16]. In addition, there has been a lack of convincing data that demonstrates its actions at the subcellular level to account for the perceived beneficial clinical outcomes. In spite of these misgivings, this chapter will review the LED physics, LED-induced histological, ultrastructural and biochemical changes, patient indications, pre-treatment preparation, techniques and clinical efficacy and side effects of LED phototherapy in its role in the management of cellulite.

LED Theory for Cellulite Skin Treatment

Low-level LED energy therapy may be defined as light treatment that produces no immediate detectable temperature elevation in the treated tissue and no visible morphological alteration in the tissue structure [17]. Low-level light devices typically emit 2–200 mW (0.2 to > 0.02 W), with power density ranging from 0.05 W/cm² to greater than 5 W/cm². At this energy level, specific cells can simultaneously regulate up or down their intracellular activities in a nonthermal manner. Photomodulation of living cellular activities by LED wavelengths has been shown to increase collagen and elastin production in fibroblasts, increase

ATP production in healing cells, reduce the production of inflammatory interleukins, inhibit the production of matrix metalloprotease (collagenase), increase lymphatic drainage, and stimulate new vessel growth. Such cellular responses result in improved skin rejuvenation without the anticipated side effects of other thermally based skin care treatments. The clinical benefits of LED treatments can be observed in aesthetic skin rejuvenation and in reducing dermatitis even after radiation therapy. There have been a number of studies demonstrating the most efficient and effective way to apply this energy, the results of which depend on 1) the LED light source, 2) type of non-coherent light, 3) optimal wavelength and physics, and 4) power for photobiomodulation.

LED Source

The most common LED light source consists of diode heads for producing electromagnetic radiation at specific preset wavelengths (Table 17.1) that are non-coherent, non-polarized, and for all intensive purposes, non-thermal or low-thermal in origin. Most therapeutic devices precisely mount a number of LED diodes either in an articulated, multipanal array or in handpieces that differ in their design to account for the divergence of individual beams to maximized interference patterns, the exposed surface treatment area, and internal dosimetry.

Non-coherent LED Light

The successful use of non-coherent light-emitting diodes in low-level light energy therapy suggests that a coherent radiation field of a laser is not an essential light property to evoke a cellular response [17,18]. Based on quantum physics, Frohlich anticipated that any living matrix of protein dipoles within cells would oscillate from applied energy and then signal integrated intracellular processes for growth, repair, defense and other functions [19–21]. The excitations within cytoskeletal microtubules have been proposed as the mechanism to mediate these intracellular processes [22,23].

Optimal Wavelength and Physics

The dosimetry of any LED treatment must be considered in two parts, the **external dosimetry** which involves quantum energies directly controlled by the provider (within the limits of the device) and the **internal dosimetry**, which is difficult to determine *in vivo* because the optical properties and heterogeneity of the tissue at each wavelength are not known. Mathematical diffusion models [27], however, project that the light energy fluence rate (the rate at which photochemical reactions occur at the cellular level) falls to 0.07% of its effective initial value at the skin surface (external dose) at a distance of 5 mm of penetration depth into the tissue. Interpolation of data [28] from mathematical models in fair Caucasian skin suggest that red light (630 nm), for example, penetrates on the average of 1–2 mm, while near-infrared light

Table 17.2 Clinical Assessment of Improvement of Periorbital Rhytids

	Digital photography analysis	Profilometry	Skin elasticity
Group 1 (830 nm)	95.2%	33.0%	19.0%
Group 2 (633 nm)	72.3%	26.0%	14.0%
Group 3 (633/830 nm)	95.5%	36.0%	16.0%
Group 4 (sham)	13.3%	No change	No change

(800–900 nm) penetrates about twice as much. The often claimed red light penetration of 5–10 mm by commercial systems does not take into account tissue attenuation that results in only 1% of the incident light playing a phototherapeutic role within the deeper tissues. Since thigh skin thickness varies from 1 mm to as much as 3 mm (average 1.5 mm), the majority of photobiomodulation effects are expected to occur within the skin level. Red light (630 to 640 nm) provides the optimum wavelength for photobiomodulation. At this range, the most favorable amount of fibroblasts and keratinocyte proliferation and microcirculation in skin is observed.

Power for Photobiomodulation

Internal dosimetry is a measure of the rate that a quantity of LED-induced photons penetrate and interact with mitochondrial non-specialized photoacceptor antennae molecules (flavoprotein NADH-dehydrogenase and cytochrome *c* oxidase) within targeted cells in the epidermal and dermal layers. At this low energy level, an activated molecule can cause measurable biochemical reactions. The induced cascades of differing redox reactions produce an immediate response in seconds, such as the conversion of adenosine diphosphate (ADP) that can up-regulate or down-regulate by gene expression a wide range of pathway actions [29]. On the other hand, LED energy can also produce many other secondary biochemical reactions in cells that occur hours or days later after the LED irradiation is switched off. Of particular interest is the consistent finding that biological reactions occur in cells that are not directly irradiated by non-thermal LED energy, commonly referred to as the "bystander effect". It is believed that the irradiated cells may release intercellular signaling molecules that propagate the photobiomodulation effects between cells even

Table 17.1 Common LED Wavelengths for Possible Cellulite Treatment

Blue	415 nm
Yellow	590
Red	660
Near-infrared	830–950

Table 17.3 Treatment gels

Active gel	Placebo gel
Bupleurum falcatum extract 7%	
Caffeine 1%	
Coenzyme A: 100 ppm	
Phosphatidylcholine 15%	
Ethoxydiglycol	Ethoxydiglycol
Denatured alcohol	Denatured alcohol
Hydroxypropyl cellulose	Hydroxypropyl cellulose
Centrimonium bromide	Centrimonium bromide
Edetate tetrasodium	Edetate tetrasodium
Butylated hydroxytoluene	Butylated hydroxytoluene
Tromethamine/tromethamine HCl	Tromethamine/tromethamine HCl
Water	Water

Controlled Biochemical, Histological-Ultrastructural and *in vitro*/Clinical Studies

Two recent peer-review publications [24,25] have reported encouraging results after LED exposures in clinical trials that utilize randomized, double blinded, placebo-controlled methodologies. In the first clinical study of 76 patients, hemifaces received either 830 nm near-infrared alone (Group 1), 633 nm red alone (Group 2), a combination of 633 nm and 830 nm (Group 3), or a sham treatment light (Group 4), twice a week for four weeks. The cumulative data, as listed in Table 17.2, indicated not only that LED energy results in objective improvements in skin over sham controls, but also that a greater clinical efficacy was observed with longer (more penetration) wavelengths and with combined 800 nm and 633 nm wavelength exposures.

In this study, isolated human cultured cells, exposed to each wavelength in the LED spectra, also demonstrated further corroboration to the beneficial results that were observed clinically in non-thermal photorejuvenation of skin.

The second randomized, double-blinded clinical study examined the effectiveness and safety of a topical anti-cellulite gel and LED (red and near-infrared) light on Grade III thigh cellulite [25]. Each patient lightly massaged in the same manner 5 cc of the active anti-cellulite gel to one thigh and 5 cc of the placebo gel to the opposite thigh twice daily in a home program for three months. The active and placebo gels, listed in Table 17.3, were identical in appearance and shielded throughout the entire study from both the patients and evaluators. Twice weekly, each thigh was treated for 15 minutes with LED red (660 nm) and near-infrared (950 nm) for a total of 24 treatment sessions over 12 weeks (Fig. 17.1). After the study was completed, all participants were informed of their treatments and offered the active gel and LED light to their placebo-treated thighs.

At the end of three months, eight of nine patients treated with the phosphatidylcholine-based, anti-cellulite gel and LED treatments were downgraded to a lower cellulite grade by clinical examination, digital photography, and pinch test assessment (Figs. 17.2–17.6). Although the exact beneficial mechanisms of action of this unique combined treatment are not completely understood, a synergism of treatment modalities may be occurring. With a randomized double-blinded assignment of active gel

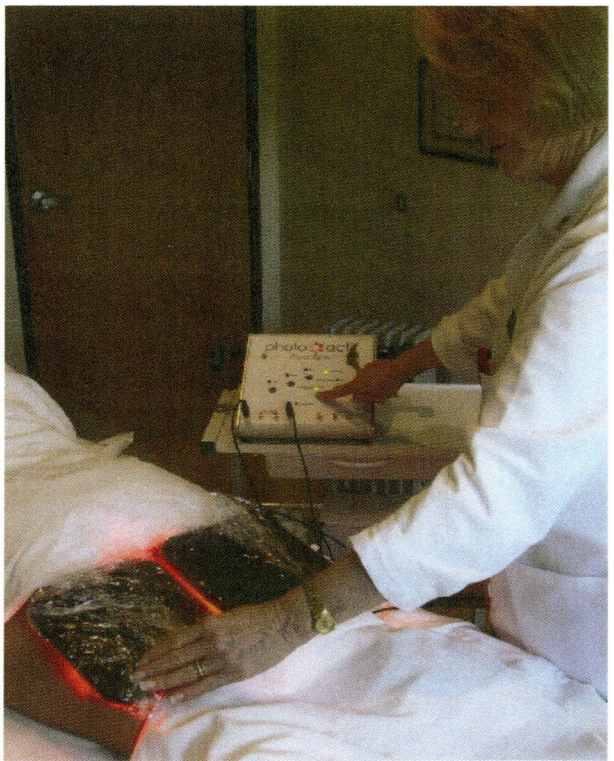

Figure 17.1 LED red and infrared treatment for 15 minutes twice weekly after application of anti-cellulite active gel or placebo.

with the deeper dermis, resulting in modulations in cell functions, cell proliferations and repair of compromised cells. LED-induced photobiomodulations are specifically coded by the preset wavelengths, fluencies, pulsing on-times and off-times, and dedicated duty cycles that result in at least 24 immediate diverse cellular actions. More than one of the cellular actions (e.g., synthesis of ATP, mRNA and reverse transcriptase-polymerase change reactions, collagen and elastin production, increased levels of tissue inhibitor of matrix metalloprotease, decreased levels of matrix metalloprotease, and induced mitosis or apoptosis can be initiated, inhibited, or modulated by LED energy from one or more wavelengths by unknown regulatory mechanisms.

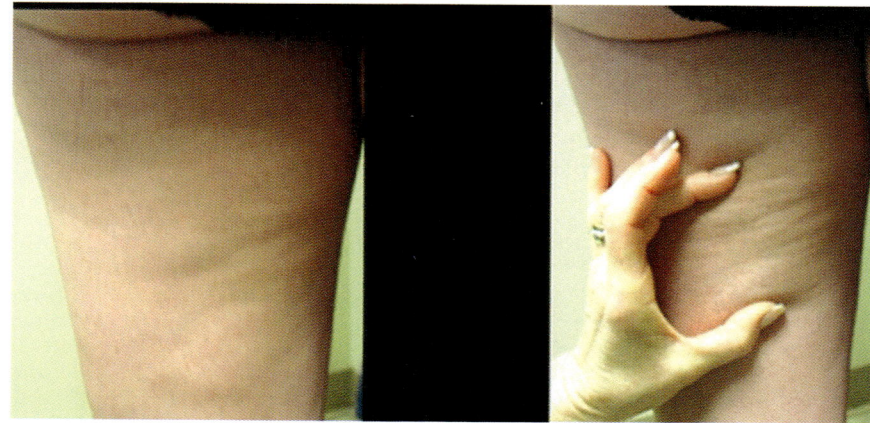

Figure 17.2 Pinch test of patient #1 demonstrating Class III grading of cellulite.

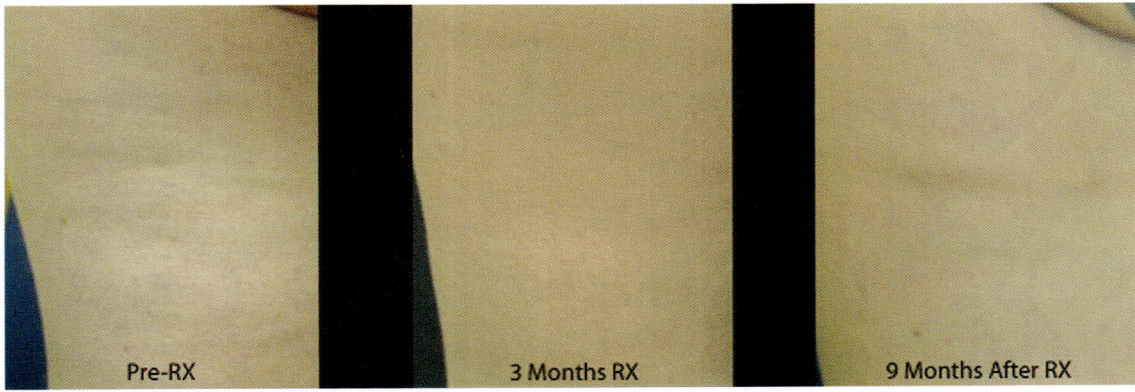

Figure 17.3 Patient #1 had no weight change throughout the study period. Cellulite returned after nine months of no treatment.

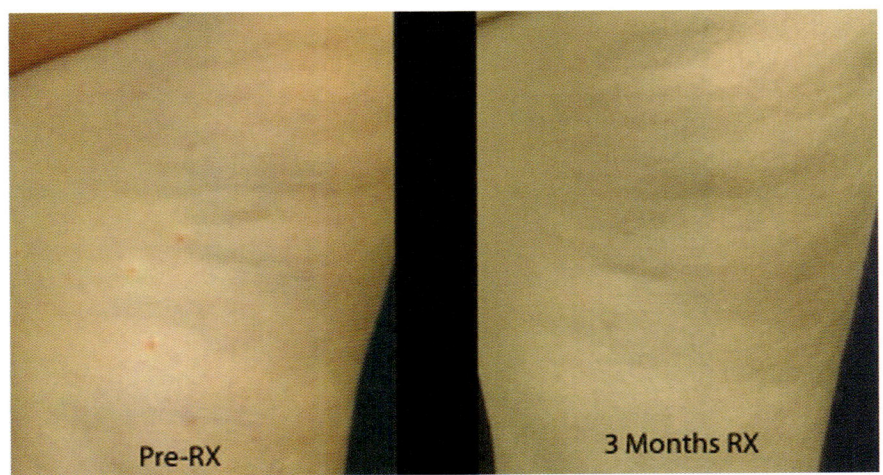

Figure 17.4 Patient #1 demonstrated no changes in cellulite from placebo treatment.

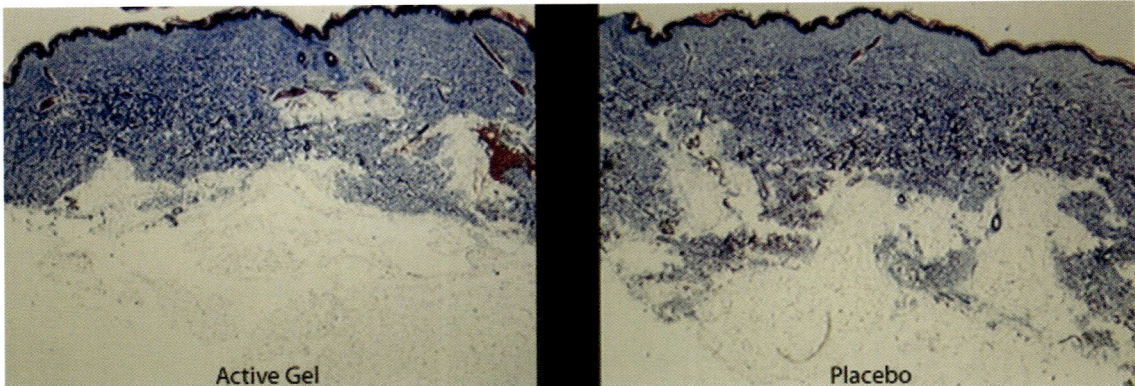

Figure 17.5 Biopsy from patient #1 after three months of active gel and placebo treatments.

versus placebo in combination with LED treatment, it is assumed that other variables such as weight, BMI, percentage of body fat, degree of physical activity, diet, skin hydration and error in measurements will have been evenly spread out to minimize their effects on final outcomes.

Conclusions

While the exact mechanisms of LED for skin rejuvenation are still unclear, recent studies suggest that low levels of specific LED light energy can target particular receptors within cells and subcellular mitochondrial components to induce pro-collagen synthesis, down

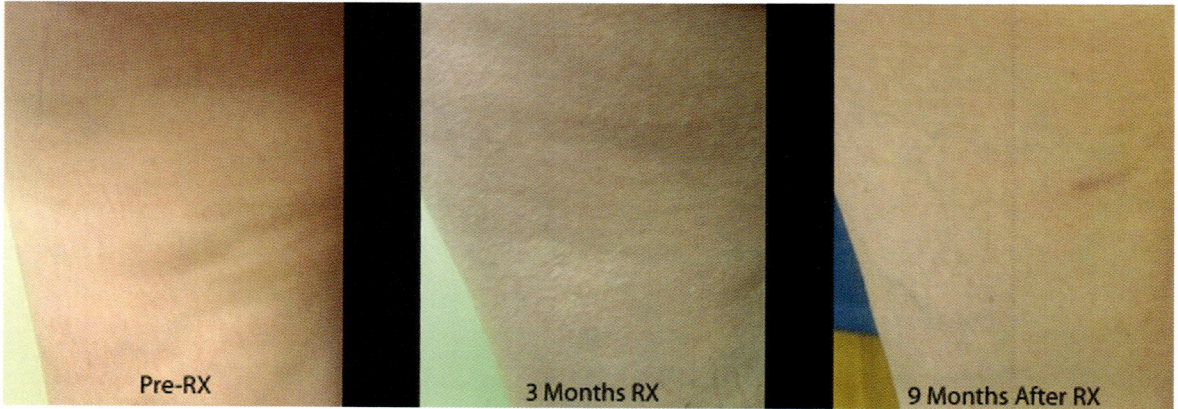

Figure 17.6 Patient #8 gained 2.5 lbs during the study but demonstrated improvement in cellulite at three month of active gel treatment and four month. Later off treatment.

regulate matrix metalloprotease-1 (MMP-1 or collagenase) activity, as well as increase local blood flow and reduce pathways for tissue inflammation. The effects of LED light on skin and septal collagen have been reported in the cited studies and possibly contribute to the clinical improvements in cellulite. The benefit of LED light by itself on the reduction of adipocytes in areas of cellulite has yet to be determined in future studies.

REFERENCES

1. E Mester. The stimulating effect of low power laser rays on biological systems. Laser Rev 1:3–9, 1968.
2. E Mester, T Spiry, B Szende. Effect of laser rays on wound healing. Am J Surg 122:532–25, 1971.
3. E Mester, AF Mester. A Mester. The biomedical effects of laser application. Lasers Surg Med 5:31–39, 1988.
4. AF Mester, A Mester. Wound healing. Laser Therapy 1:7–15, 1989.
5. K Flemming, N Cullum. Laser therapy for venous leg ulcers. Cochrane Database Syst Rev 2000:CD001182, 2000.
6. DA Hendrick, A Meyers. Wound healing after laser surgery. Otolaryngol Clin North Am 28:969, 1995.
7. L Brousseau, V Welch, G Wells et al. Low level laser therapy (classes I, II, and III) for the treatment of osteoarthritis. Cochrane Database Syst Rev 2000:CD002046, 2000.
8. C Lucas. LJ Criens-Poublon, CT Cockrell et al. Wound healing in cell studies and animal model experiments by low level laser therapy: Were clinical studies justified? A systematic review. Lasers Med Sci 17:110, 2002.
9. T Oshiro, RG Calderhead. Development of low reactive-level laser therapy and its present status. J Clin Laser Med Surg 9:267, 1991.
10. EL Nussbaum, I Biemann, B Mustard. Comparison of ultrasound/ultraviolet-c and laser for treatment of pressure ulcers in patients with spinal cord injury. Phys Ther 74:812–23, 1994.
11. M Malm, T Lundeberg. Effect of low power gallium arsenide laser on healing of venous ulcers. Scand J Plast Reconstr Hand Surg 25:249–51, 1991.
12. M Iusum, J Kimchy, T Pilar et al. Evaluation of the degree of effectiveness of biobeam low level narrow band light on the treatment of skin ulcers and delayed postoperative wound healing. Orthopedics 15:1023–26, 1992.
13. I Bihari, Mester Ar. The biostimulative effect of low level laser therapy of longstanding crural ulcers using helium neon laser, helium neon plus infrared lasers and noncoherent light: preliminary report of a randomized double blind comparative study. Laser Ther 1:75–78, 1989.
14. H Beckerman, RA de Bie, LM Bouter. The efficacy of laser therapy for musculoskeletal and skin disorders: a criteria-based meta-analysis of randomized clinical trials. Phys Ther 72:483–91, 1992.
15. C Lucas, RW Stanborough, CL Freeman et al. Efficacy of low laser therapy on wound healing in human subjects: a systematic review. Lasers Med Sci 15:84–93, 2000.
16. A Schindl, M Schindl, H Pernerstorfer Schon et al. Low-intensity laser therapy: a review. J Invest Med 48:312–26, 2000.
17. PR King. Low level laser therapy: A review. Laser Med Sci 4:141–48, 1989.
18. GD Baxter, A Bell, JM Allen et al. Low level laser therapy: Current clinical practice in Northern Ireland. Physiotherapy 77:171–82, 1991.
19. H Frohlich. Long-range coherence and energy storage in biological systems. Int Quantum Chem 2:641, 1968.
20. H Frohlich. Long range coherence and the actions of enzymes. Nature 228:1093, 1970.
21. H Frohlich. The extraordinary dielectric properties of biological materials and the actions of enzymes. Proc Natl Acad Sci U.S.A. 72:4211, 1975.
22. SR Hameroff, RC Watt. Information processing in microtubules J Theor Biol 98:549, 1982.
23. S Rasmussen, H Karampurwala, R Vaidyanath et al. Computational connectionism within neurons: A model of cytoskeletal automata subserving neural networks. D Physica 42:428, 1990.
24. SY Lee, CE You, K Park, J Choi et al. A prospective randomized, placebo-controlled, double-blinded, and split-face clinical study on LED phototherapy for skin rejuvenation: Clinical, profilometric, histologic, ultrastructural and biochemical evaluations and comparison of three different treatment

settings. J Photochem and Photobiol B: Biology 88:5167, 2007.

25. GH Sasaki, K Oberg, B Tucker, M Gaston. The effectiveness and safety topical PhotoActif phosphatidylcholine-based anti-cellulite gel and LED (red and near-infrared) light on Grade II-III thigh cellulite: a randomized, double-blinded study. J of Cosmetic and Laser Therapy 9:87–96, 2007.

26. ZD Draelos, KD Marenus. Cellulite: etiology and purported treatment. Dermatol Surg 23:1177, 1997.

27. AJ Welch, G Yoon, van MJC Gemert. Practical models for light distribution in laser-irradiated tissue. Lasers Surg Med 6:484–93, 1987.

28. RR Anderson, JA Parrish. Optical properties of human skin. In: JD Regan, JA Parrish (eds) The science of photomedicine. New York: Plenum Press; 1982: 147–94.

29. DH McDaniel, J Newman, R Geronemus, et. al. Non-ablative non-thermal LED photomodulation-a multicenter clinical photoaging trial. Lasers Surg Med 15:22, 2003.

18 SmoothShapes® Treatment of Cellulite and Thigh Circumference Reduction: When Less Is More

Michail M Pankratov and Serge Mordon

Introduction

Cellulite is a skin condition characterized by a dimpling, uneven, or "cottage cheese" skin texture occurring almost exclusively in post-pubertal females. It is most commonly seen in the thighs and buttocks, but may also be apparent in the breasts, back, hips, abdomen or upper arms. It occurs even in the slim and fit or otherwise healthy women, but the appearance of cellulite is naturally exacerbated by an excess of fat. There is no uniform theory for the origin of cellulite and purported etiologies vary from morphological differences between male and female skin anatomy (the hypodermal connective tissue strands run diagonally in male skin and vertically in female skin), to hormonal involvement (cellulite is frequently present in androgen-deficient males and not seen in pre-pubertal females), to lipodystrophy (gynoid lipodystrophy is one of the synonyms for cellulite) and circulatory disorders, to hereditary factors [4,5,8,15,31,43,48,60,65,66,70,73,77]. It is very likely that all these factors play some role in the origin of cellulite.

The regional fat accumulation is responsible for vertical stretching of the superficial fat lobules protruding into the lower reticular dermis producing irregularities and dimpling of the skin at the surface. Advanced stages of cellulite are associated with deterioration of dermal vasculature, deposition of hydrophilic byproducts [48], and retention of excess fluid within the dermis and adjacent interstitial structures. Ensuing edema leads to vascular compression, cellular changes and tissue hypoxia. In time, continuing tissue congestion leads to thickening and sclerosis of fibrous septae causing a dimpled appearance. Some investigators reported the presence of chronic inflammatory cells, e.g., macrophages and lymphocytes, in fibrous septae of cellulite biopsies [43].

Although our understanding of cellulite has grown exponentially in the last few years, we still rely on highly subjective measures such as digital photography, or other somewhat primitive and outdated methods of classification. For example, the Nürnberger and Müller Severity Scale, proposed more than 30 years ago [60], is used to assign patients to one of four clinical stages (0–III) based on clinical alterations observed at rest and with pinch test or muscular contraction. This severity scale leaves too much room for subjectivity in evaluation and comparison of changes over time, making settled but appreciable changes in cellulite appearance hard to correlate with changes on the severity scale. Several attempts to develop a new classification system or to modify and expand the existing severity scale to incorporate some objective biometric measurements did not gain wide acceptance and remains a domain of individual users [6,25,32,33].

There are a few objective methods for demonstrating and monitoring of cellulite conditions and its changes over time: specialized 3-D photography, high-resolution MRI and high frequency ultrasound [23,25,49,54,64,71,72,76]. Unfortunately, these tests are not readily available, cost-effective, or easily justified when treating a cosmetic, non-life threatening condition.

Advanced stages of cellulite involve multi-level pathologic changes in affected tissue, i.e., cellular, metabolic, circulatory, physiologic, and biomechanical; and therefore treatment modalities require interventions capable of dealing with many if not all of these pathologic changes in order to deliver effective and long-lasting improvement.

Treatments for Cellulite

Currently available treatments for cellulite include surgical techniques (liposuction, subcision, and laser- and ultrasound-assisted liposuction) [29,30,46], mechanical manipulation (endermologie, lymphatic massage, etc.), topical creams, energy-based devices (light, ultrasound, acoustic shock, radio frequency, electrical stimulation, etc.), mesotherapy and injection lipolysis [11,47] as well as combinations of the above-mentioned techniques.

The benefits of the many available treatments for cellulite vary from marginal to somewhat effective, but are not without drawbacks and limitations. For example, liposuction and laser- and/or ultrasound-assisted liposuction are unlikely to "cure" cellulite and in many cases require additional interventions to improve appearance of cellulite [4,81]. Mesotherapy and injection lipolysis are capable of inducing local lipolysis and improve skin condition and cellulite appearance but are invasive and associated with numerous side effects, including pigmentary changes and fibrosis.

There is no shortage of energy sources (laser light, ultrasound, acoustic shock, radiofrequency, electrical stimulation, low temperature (cold), mechanical massage and vacuum, etc.) that are being used or proposed for ablative as well as non-ablative intervention in the treatment of cellulite [2,7,14,21,44,59,63,81,83]. Techniques employing energy sources for ablative fat reduction and cellulite treatment are subject to the same complications and side effects as any surgical intervention. Non-ablative energy-based techniques are safe and nearly free of side effects when administered by a well-trained operator, but the efficacy and longevity of the therapeutic benefits are unpredictable.

The effectiveness of these treatments and longevity of therapeutic benefits is dependent upon many variables, including frequency, duration and total number of treatments, size of the treatment area, power levels of employed energy sources, and intensity of vacuum and mechanical effort as well as operator's technique [44]. A patient's age, severity of cellulite and contributory medical conditions may also affect the outcome of the treatment regimen. Cellulite management with devices employing mechanical massage and suction require monthly maintenance treatments following the original treatment regimen in order to sustain the therapeutic benefits; otherwise, these benefits tend to disappear within three months.

Patients treated with the devices employing light and/or light and radiofrequency as well as other energy sources find that their therapeutic benefits begin to diminish around three months post-therapy with almost all benefits reversed by six months. Accordingly, they are also advised to return for maintenance treatments not later than six months.

The chase for a better non-invasive treatment of cellulite and fat reduction continues with more and more players entering the market utilizing established modes and energy sources and introducing new ones: acoustic shock, low temperatures, microwaves, etc.

Clinical Study Utilizing Low Intensity Light Therapy

Anecdotal observations of successful treatment of cellulite using low intensity light therapy (LILT) combining HeNe (632 nm) and GaAs (904 nm) laser radiation were discussed at various symposia but never published in a refereed journal. However, some *in vitro* studies have demonstrated that exposure of adipose tissue samples collected from lipectomy to 635 nm wavelength light from a 10 mW diode laser for six minutes (3.6 J/cm²) produced near total emptying of fat from these cells through, what the authors postulated were, transitory pores in the membranes of adipocytes [35,55–58]. In addition, they observed that these transitory changes didn't cause destruction of adipocytes or other interstitial structures.

These findings led to an inception of laser-assisted liposuction where LILT is administered transcutaneously for 6–15 minutes (in an hour prior to liposuction). It became an adjunct, intraoperative procedure. Practitioners of this technique mostly agree that there are significant benefits to patients in post-operative recovery: fewer side effects, less swelling, less bruising, less discomfort, decrease in post-operative use of pain medication, etc., but there is no consensus on whether it also simplifies liposuction procedure in terms of ease of performing liposuction, reduced time in surgery, or enhanced emulsification of extracted fat [12,35]. Although some studies have failed to reproduce Dr. Neira's results [12,53] the hypothesis of "transitory pores" was not overturned because there were significant differences between the device, wavelength, and method of application used by Dr. Neira and the other studies.

For the purpose of non-destructive treatment of cellulite and fat reduction, another wavelength that can penetrate relatively deep into the skin and has preferential affinity for lipids, (i.e., absorbed better in fat than surrounding tissue) was added to the mix in order to complement the pore-inducing effect of the 635 nm wavelength and assist in fat evacuation from adipocytes. It has been established for some time [50] and recently reconfirmed by Anderson et al. [3] that four infrared wavelength bands—915 nm, 1205 nm, 1715 nm and 2305 nm—have about 50% more absorption in lipid-rich tissue than in aqueous tissue.

Combining the visible 650 nm wavelength for its adipocyte membrane pore-inducing properties and the infrared 915 nm wavelength for its lipid-liquefying properties creates a dual-band light source capable of positively affecting skin adipose tissue. Augmenting this dynamic distinct light duo with suction (vacuum) and mechanical massage produces an entirely new process that was termed Photomology® and defined as:

> "Exclusive process that treats cellulite and subcutaneous fat by combining dynamic light and laser energy along with vacuum massage to gently stimulate natural cell processes and modify cell activity."

The study under discussion was designed to evaluate the effectiveness of the dual-band (630 and 900 nm) laser light for the improvement of appearance of cellulite and removal of discrete subcutaneous deposits of adipose tissue from the thighs of otherwise healthy volunteer subjects. It was conducted in two phases: first a pilot study of 12 subjects, followed by a second, much larger multi-center study. Pre- and post-treatment MRI scans were used to accurately document changes in fat and photography, physical examination and questionnaires were used to assess and document changes in cellulite. In the pilot study, the bi-dimensional MRI fat images demonstrated remarkable reduction in fat thickness by as much as 35% relative to the control group. According to the investigators:

> "weight loss per se appeared to be random and did not correlate to findings of changes found in a single thigh… However, the use of MRI was found to be a reliable cross indicator of fat change in the treated legs. Furthermore, the use of MRI was found to be a reliable means of monitoring the longevity of the results, which was confirmed to have persisted as far as 13 months post treatment" [94].

Encouraged by the success of the pilot study, the investigators set to replicate these findings in a large group of volunteer subjects in the multi-center, IRB-approved, clinical investigation [45].

Subjects

One hundred two healthy female volunteers between the ages of 18 and 50 with mild to moderate cellulite (≤15% overweight from a standard actuarial table) on the thighs were enrolled in the IRB-approved study with 74 subjects meeting eligibility requirements completing the treatments and follow-up. Prior to treatment, cross-sectional MRI scans of both thighs were taken. Subjects were randomly assigned to have one thigh treated with the combination of laser and massage, while the contra lateral thigh served as the "control" and was subjected to massage treatment only. Subjects were "blinded" as to which leg received laser plus massage treatment vs. massage alone.

Device

904 nm 1 watt laser diode with the spot size of 3 mm and 0.5 watt of 632 nm HeNe laser were scanned over large treatment area (30.5 × 15 cm) at a frequency of 30 Hz, thus covering the entire area in 2 seconds.

Pixel densitometry of each layer of each MRI image was employed to objectively and consistently calculate changes in the fat pad. The pixel counts of the respective anatomic elements identified in each image were calculated. Selective outlining of the entire thigh, fat, muscle, and bone was performed. The total cross-section of the thigh was calculated in cm² using standard software algorithms. The pixel count of the thigh minus the fat layer was calculated and subtracted from the complete thigh surface area to produce an objective representation of fat thickness.

Treatment

Each subject underwent 12–14 treatment sessions two to three times a week over a four- to six-week period. MRI scans of both thighs were performed pre- and post-treatment. Subcutaneous peri-muscular fat pads were measured on MRI images by a "blinded" independent radiologist who had no knowledge of the laser vs. non-laser treated side. Volumetric determination technique was used to quantify the difference in fat deposits based on pixel densitometry of the respective anatomic constituents identified in the MRI. Changes in skin condition were evaluated using digital photographs by blinded observers and subjects' questionnaires.

Results
Sixty-five subjects with complete pre- and post-treatment data were included in the analyses. As measured by the MRI, there was a statistically significant difference over time between the laser plus massage treated thigh vs. the massage-only treated thigh (p < 0.001), with the average fat thickness in the experimental leg decreasing by an average of 1.19 cm² vs. an increase of an average 3.82 cm² in the control leg (Fig. 18.1). There was a high degree of patient satisfaction with the treatment and therapeutic results:

    Subjects who experienced improvement – 82%
    (the percentage improvement was not noted)
    Pleased with the results – 89%
    Would participate in the treatment again – 73%
    Would recommend this treatment to a friend – 73%
See also Figs. 18.2–18.4.

Five subjects returned for an additional follow-up examination including MRI evaluation 13 months or longer after completion of the study. Four of these subjects maintained some improvements on the laser plus massage treated thigh, while the control thigh continued to demonstrate an increase in the circumference based on the MRI measurements [94].

Discussion
The therapeutic effect of low intensity light therapy is no longer in question [19,26–28,34,51,52,69]. However, the question remains as to how the light works at the cellular, tissue, and organ levels, and what are the optimal parameters for the most effective therapeutic effects for various medical conditions. It is believed that, on the cellular level, light first interacts with mitochondria leading to an increase in ATP production, modulation of reactive oxygen species, and induction of transcription factors [1,16,18,19]. These effects lead to increased cell proliferation and migration, especially, fibroblasts, modulation in levels of cytokines, growth factors and inflammatory mediators, and increased tissue oxygenation. The ability of monochromatic light to modify cellular function of living tissue, enhance healing and restore its normal function is a basis for the treatment of numerous dermatological, musculoskeletal, and neurological conditions [1,13,19,22, 26,28,34,51,52,67–69,74,75,79,80,82,84,85,87].

Light traversing living tissue is subjected to scattering and absorption which are both wavelength-dependent phenomena. Absorption of monochromatic visible and near-infrared light at the cellular level by components of the cellular respiratory chain is at the heart of the beneficial therapeutic effect [20,24,61]. Mitochondria are conceivably the principal unit within the cell controlling the LILT response and by being at the core of a chain reaction within the cell that originates with improving respiratory and ion-transporting activity in the cell and culminating in beneficial therapeutic reaction on cellular, tissue, and systemic levels [9,10,27].

Phototherapy produces primary, secondary and tertiary effects which collectively enhance tissue repair and produce pain relief [17,38,42,62,74,75,78,86]. Primary effects in the cells, often referred to as photoreception, occur through direct interaction of photons with cytochromes. Secondary effects, e.g., cell proliferation,

protein synthesis, growth factors secretion, myofibroblast contraction, neurotransmitter modification, etc., occur in the same cells as primary and can be initiated by light as well as other stimuli. Tertiary effects, e.g., tissue repair and pain relief, are the indirect responses of distant cells to photon-induced changes in other cells. These effects are the least predictable because they are influenced by cellular as well as environmental factors.

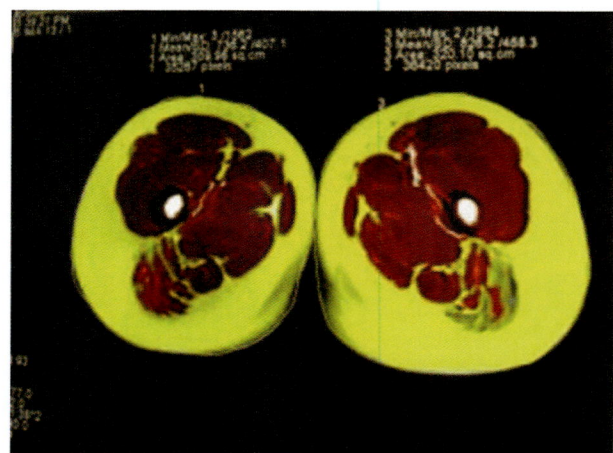
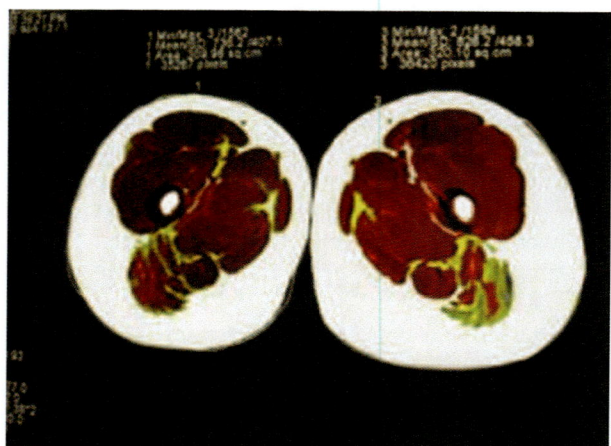
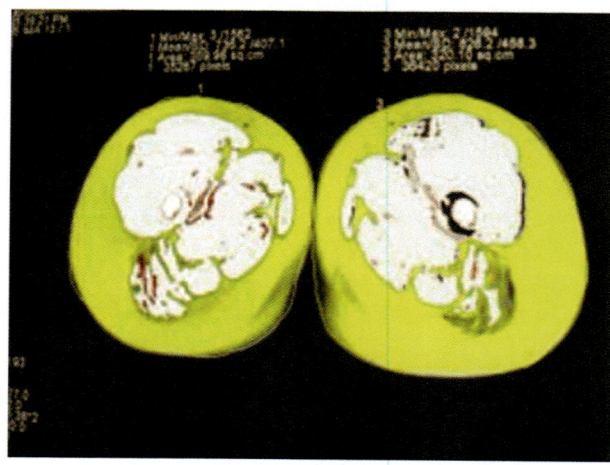

Figure 18.1 Horizontal images of the laser-massage and massage-only thighs of an individual treated in this study. The volume of each leg was measured by pixel densitometry. Pixel counts of the entire thigh exclusive of the fat layer were subtracted from the pixel counts of the entire thigh to obtain pixel counts of the fat layer (from ref. 94, with permission).

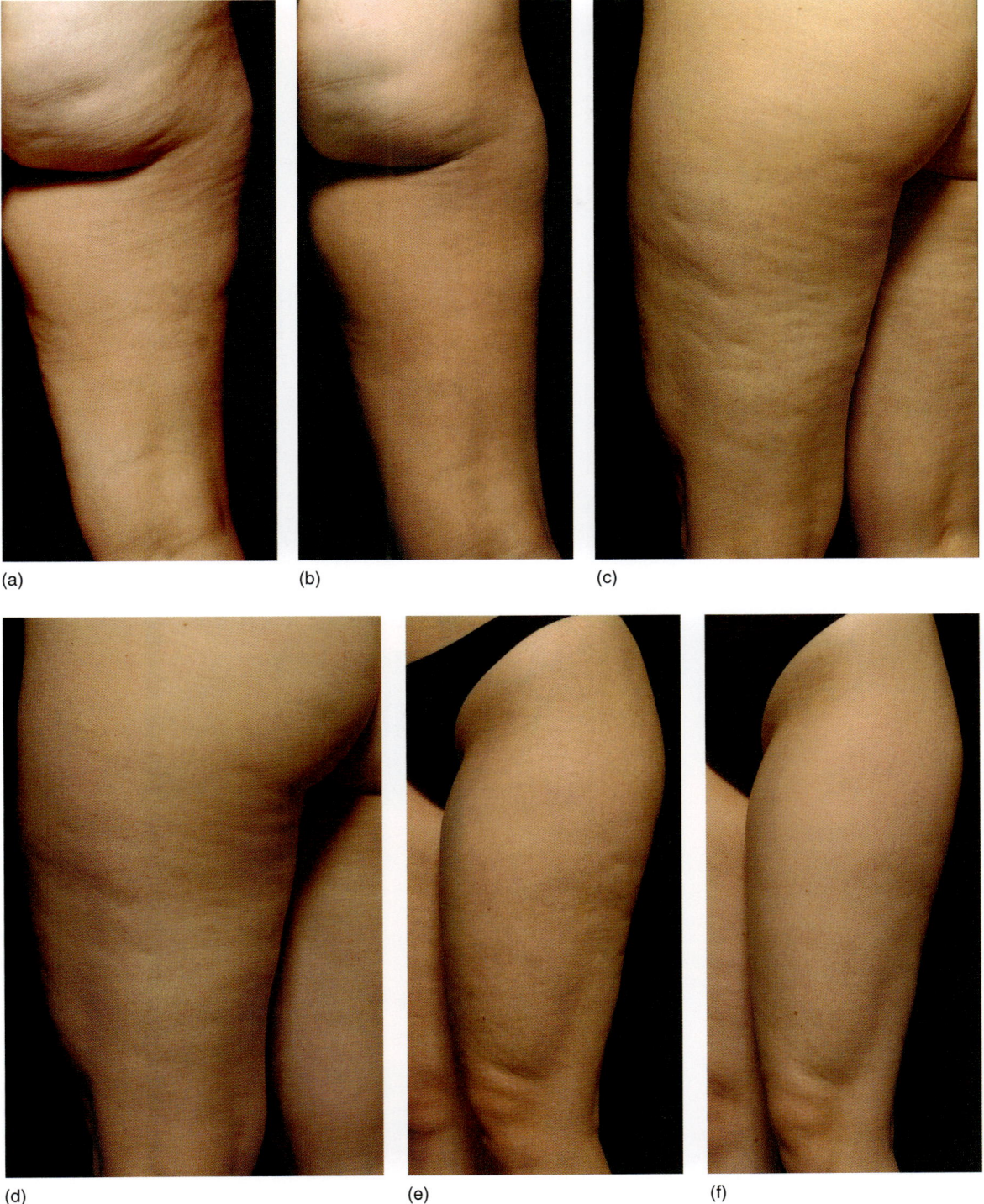

(a)   (b)   (c)

(d)   (e)   (f)

Figure 18.2 (a,b) A patient before and one month after eight treatments (by courtesy of Robert Weiss, MD); (c,d) a patient before and three months after eight treatments (by courtesy of Khalil A Khatri, MD); (e,f) a patient before and three months after eight treatments (by coutesy of Khalil A Khatri, MD).

It is believed that the most beneficial effects are achieved in the 600–950 nm wavelength range with the exception of 700–770 nm wavelength range which is considered ineffective. Hence the choice of a monochromatic wavelength is an important consideration when considering treatment of superficial or deeply located tissues: shorter wavelengths for more superficial applications and longer wavelengths for deeper penetration [9,27,36,37,39].

Given the positive results from the multi-center study for the treatment of cellulite and statistically significant results for the decrease in fat, a new prospective, randomized, controlled multi-center, IRB study was initiated to assess the therapeutic benefit of a higher watt system of for the reduction of thigh circumferences.

Clinical Study Utilizing LILT and a High Power Infrared Wavelength for Thigh Circumferential Reduction

Study Design
The multi-center study was designed to evaluate the effectiveness, reproducibility and longevity using LILT and a high power infrared

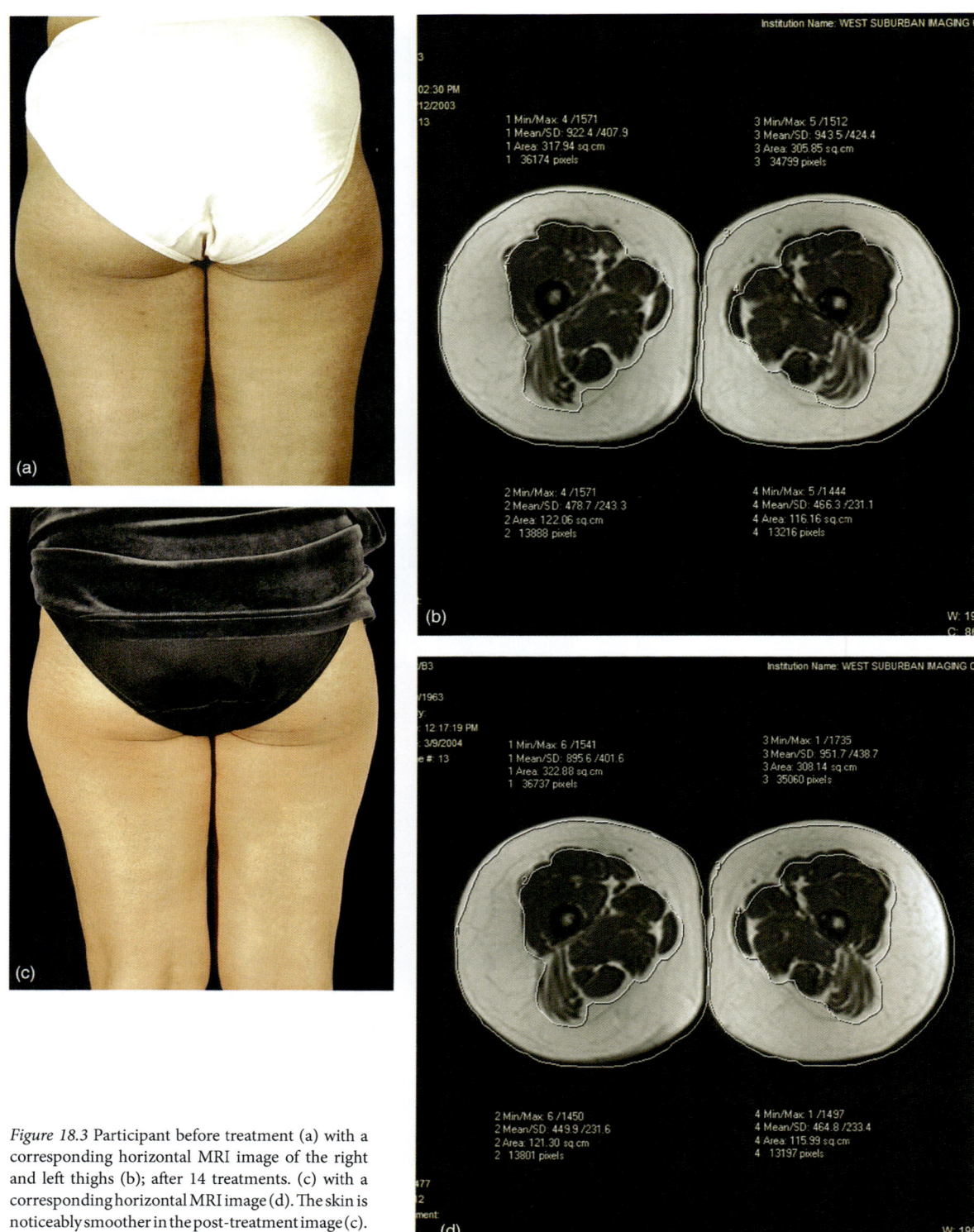

Figure 18.3 Participant before treatment (a) with a corresponding horizontal MRI image of the right and left thighs (b); after 14 treatments. (c) with a corresponding horizontal MRI image (d). The skin is noticeably smoother in the post-treatment image (c). (From ref. 94, with permission.)

wavelength to treat mild to moderate cellulite in female patients, to produce sustainable improvement in cellulite appearance and thigh reduction in subcutaneous fat as validated by standard measurements, imaging and subjective patient evaluations.

Subjects
Six clinical sites participated in the multi-center, IRB-approved, single-blinded clinical study with female subjects between the ages of 18–45, skin type I to VI. The number of subjects per site varied from 10 to 26. The subjects consisted of 83 premenopausal females with mild to moderate visible cellulite on thighs and with various Body Mass Indexes (BMI) ranging from normal to overweight. Subjects were randomly assigned to have one thigh treated with the combination LEDs, laser diodes, vacuum and massage and the other thigh served as the control.

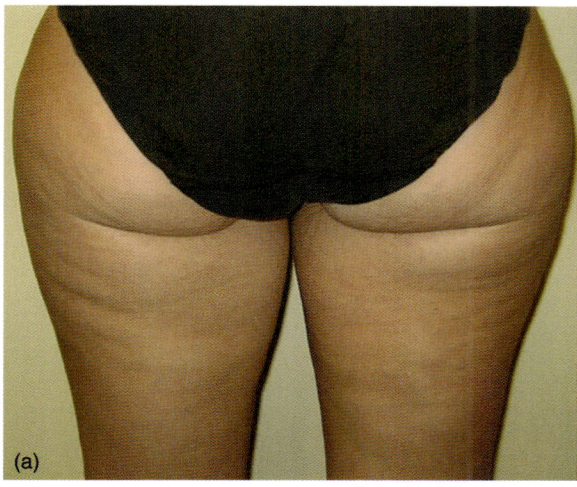 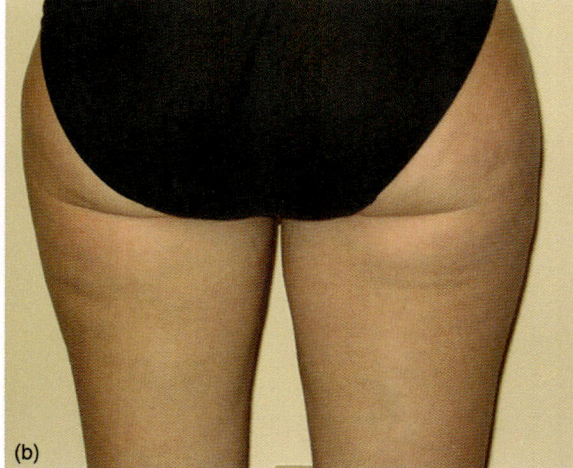

(a) (b)

Figure 18.4 Participant before treatment (left) and 2 weeks after nine treatments with the SmoothShapes device (right). In the post-treatment photograph, the skin of the upper thigh and lower buttocks is smoother and tighter and the circumference of both treated areas is noticeably reduced. (From ref. 94, with permission.)

Device
915 nm 10 watts of laser diodes and 650 nm 1 watt of LED delivered through a 70 mm × 40 mm aperture with integrated vacuum and contoured rollers for massage.

Treatment
Each subject underwent a total of eight treatment sessions, administered twice a week for four weeks. The entire circumference of one thigh was treated for 30 minutes at each treatment session.

Weight, digital photographs and thigh circumference were recorded pre-treatment, during treatments and at one month and three-month follow-up visits. Both the treated and the control thighs had three measurements taken with a spring-loaded tape at each of three locations on the thigh: upper, mid- and lower. Location for measurement was determined with a laser-based level device and recorded in the subjects chart for accuracy and reproducibility during follow-up measurements.

Results
Eighty-three subjects who completed one-month follow-up and had no data points missing throughout the study were included in the final one-month data analysis. At one month post-treatment, when comparing the treated and control thighs, the circumference reduction was statistically significant ($p < 0.001$, Student's t-test) with positive responding subjects recording a combined average loss of 3.5 cm ranging from −0.2 cm to −8.7 cm [93].

Seventy-two subjects who completed three-month follow-up were included in the final three-month data analysis. When comparing the treated and control thighs, the circumference reduction was statistically significant ($p < 0.001$, Student's t-test) with positive-responding subjects recording a combined average loss of 2.9 cm ranging from −0.1 cm to −8.7 cm [93].

SmoothShapes®— Mechanisms of Action
LILT therapy produces no significant temperature elevation and no immediate, visible structural changes in the cells, tissues, or organs. It modulates the level of cellular activity that eventually improves local blood circulation and metabolism, reduces inflammatory response to injury and improves cell survival, modifies

perception of pain (nociception) and improves tissue condition that causes pain. Although photobiostimulating effects of LILT can occur in the absence of temperature elevation there is evidence that moderate temperature elevation to the level of "high-fever" in the treated tissue ($\leq 40°$ C) would facilitate many of the same functions and activities that LILT alone is attempting to improve: local blood circulation, metabolic activity, chemical reaction, etc. [88].

Photomology® process for non-destructive, modulating action of LILT in combination with moderate temperature elevation in the irradiated tissue is at the root of the therapeutic effects of dual-band light application for improvement in the appearance of cellulite and fat reduction by the SmoothShapes® technology. This improvement appears to be the result of the tertiary effects of phototherapy that together with primary and secondary effects to enhance tissue repair [36–41].

The SmoothShapes® system (Elemé Medical, Inc, Merrimack, NH) utilizes the Photomology® process that combines dual-band light therapy 650 nm red light from LEDs with near-infrared 915 nm from laser diodes with mechanical massager and vacuum to reduce discrete subcutaneous adipose tissue and improve the appearance of cellulite and reduce thigh circumferences (Fig. 18.5). The laser diode and LED light sources operate in continuous mode and deliver 11 watts of combined optical power integrated into a delivery system with the message and vacuum components.

The 650 nm wavelength was selected for its action in modifying permeability of the adipocytes' membranes and enhancement of fat emulsification. This wavelength falls into a so-called optical window where there is relatively minimal absorption in hemoglobin, water and other skin components, except for melanin, which allows for adequate penetration to the subcutaneous fat level.

The choice of 915 nm wavelength was based on its preferential absorption in lipids. This wavelength penetrates well into the tissue with even less scattering than 650 nm but gets absorbed by the lipids in fat. This selective absorption by lipids that induces temperature elevation and temperature measurements with thermocouples in a subset of patients demonstrated that temperature could reach 46°C.

Because the lipid bilayer components of the cell membranes are held together only by forces of hydration, the lipid bilayer is

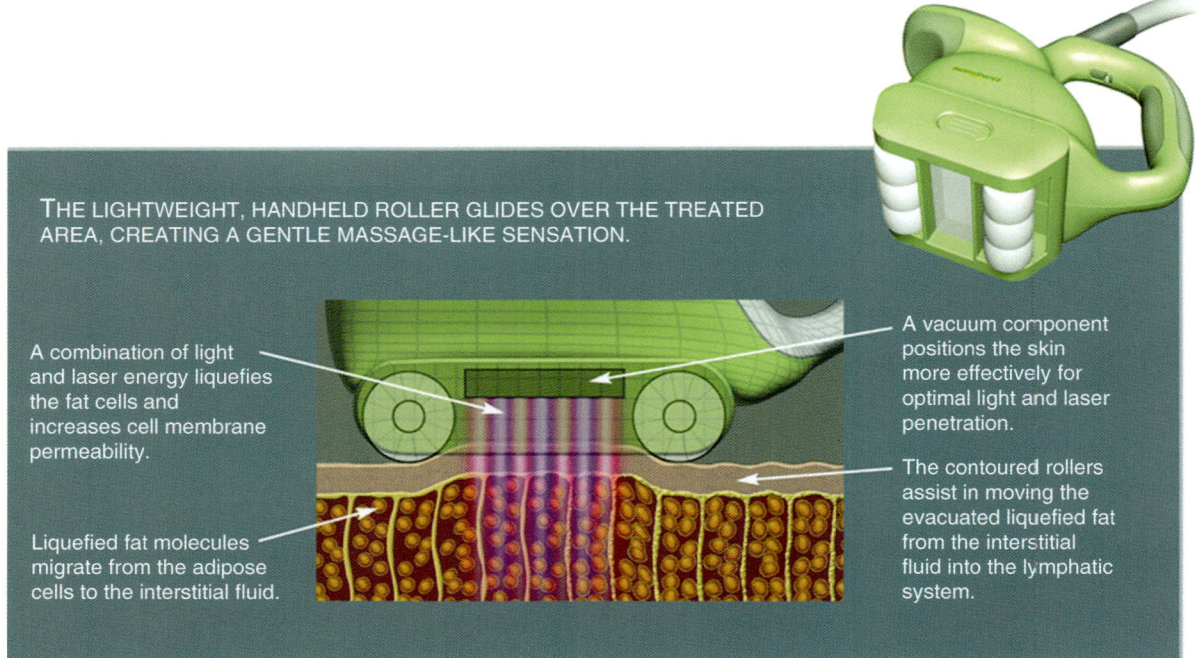

THE LIGHTWEIGHT, HANDHELD ROLLER GLIDES OVER THE TREATED AREA, CREATING A GENTLE MASSAGE-LIKE SENSATION.

A combination of light and laser energy liquefies the fat cells and increases cell membrane permeability.

A vacuum component positions the skin more effectively for optimal light and laser penetration.

Liquefied fat molecules migrate from the adipose cells to the interstitial fluid.

The contoured rollers assist in moving the evacuated liquefied fat from the interstitial fluid into the lymphatic system.

Figure 18.5 SmoothShapes® system mechanism of action.

the most vulnerable to heat damage. Even at temperatures of only 6°C above normal (i.e. 43°C), the structural integrity of the lipid bilayer is lost [92].

Hamilton has demonstrated that 1) fatty acid transport is mainly governed by a diffusion mechanism through the adipocyte membrane and 2) this mechanism is modified by heat-induced membrane permeabilization which begins to appear at temperatures between 43°C and 45°C [91].

Gaylor measured the stability of mammalian skeletal muscle cell membranes in isolated cell cultures to supraphysiologic temperature by determining the kinetics of the onset of altered membrane permeability to intracellular carboxyfluorescein dye and proposed a set of coefficients before cell membrane rupture. He demonstrated that activation energy necessary to thermally induce membrane permeabilization in adipocyte cells is very low 238 KJ/l.mol [90]. This temperature elevation also increases the blood flow. An increase in adipose tissue blood flow is of physiological importance by facilitating the removal of FFA (free fatty acid) from adipose tissue [89].

Finally, mechanical roller massage therapy plays a role in reducing cellulite. Combined with laser heating, the rollers exert pressure on the skin and subcutaneous tissues, and the suction draws a fold of skin and fat into the vacuum space. This deep kneading and stretching of the body tissues also improves the blood flow and reinforces removal of FFA.

To summarize, both wavelengths are implicated in producing other beneficial therapeutic effects discussed earlier:

- Improved local blood and lymphatic circulation
- Improved metabolic activity of treated tissue at the tissue and cellular level
- Induce mild inflammatory reaction thus attracting fibroblasts that lead to new collagen production and deposition manifesting in thicker dermis

Mechanical massager with suction has a proven track of:

- Improved blood and lymphatic circulation
- Modification of underlying connective and muscular tissue leading to tissue tightening
- Modification of subcutaneous fat layer

Conclusion

In both the preliminary LILT and the second study of circumferential reduction of the thighs the SmoothShapes® system with Photomology™ demonstrated that a high degree of effectiveness, ~80%, was reproduced and showed longevity up 13 months. Additionally, there was a high degree of participant satisfaction with the treatment which they found virtually painless, pleasant and relaxing. There is some indication that cellular and tissue changes incited by the dual-band LILT therapy may have produced long-lasting effects.

The search for longer-lasting non-ablative treatment of cellulite and subcutaneous fat will continue, but the authors acknowledge this new approach combining LILT and laser appears promising.

Acknowledgement
Authors are thankful to the following individuals for their knowledge, data, experience and valuable comments and corrections: Elliot Lach, MD, Tracey Corby, RN, Mary Stoll, RN, William McGrail, and Andrea Morrison, RN.

REFERENCES
1. H Abrahamse, D Hawkins, N Houreld. Effect of wavelength and fluence on morphology, cellular and genetic integrity of diabetic wounded human skin fibroblasts. In: MR Hamblin, RW Waynant, J Anders (eds). Mechanisms for low-light therapy, Proceedins of SPIE vol 6140, 6140006:1–13, 2006.

2. TS Alster, M Tehrani. Treatment of cellulite with optical devices: An overview with practical considerations. Lasers Surg Med 38:727–30, 2006.

3. RR Anderson, W Farinelli, H Laubach et al. Selective photothermolysis of lipid-rich tissues: a free electron laser study. Lasers Surg Med 38:913–19, 2006.

4. MA Avram. Cellulite: a review of its physiology and treatment. J Cosmet Laser Ther 6:181–85, 2004.

5. PA Bacci. Anatomy of cellulite and interstitial matrix. In: MP Goldman, PA Bacci, G Leischoff et al. (eds). Cellulite: pathophysiology and treatment. Taylor and Francis, New York; 2006: pp 29–40.

6. PA Bacci. Clinical-therapeutic classification: BIMED-TCD. In: MP Goldman, PA Bacci, G Leischoff et al. (eds). Cellulite: pathophysiology and treatment. Taylor and Francis, New York; 2006: pp 115–41.

7. PA Bacci. The role of endermologie in treatment of cellulite. In: MP Goldman, PA Bacci, G Leischoff et al. (eds). Cellulite: pathophysiology and treatment. Taylor and Francis, New York; 2006: pp 171–87.

8. PA Bacci, G Leisbaschoff. Pathophysiology of cellulite. In: MP Goldman, PA Bacci, G Leischoff et al. (eds). Cellulite: pathophysiology and treatment. Taylor and Francis, New York; 2006: pp 41–74.

9. SK Bisland, BC Wilson. To begin at the beginning: the science of bio-stimulation in cells and tissues. In: MR Hamblin, RW Waynant, J Anders (eds). Mechanisms for low-light therapy, Proceedins of SPIE vol 6140, 6140002:1–10, 2006.

10. R Bortoletto, NS Silva, RA Zangaro et al. Mitochondrial membrane potential after low-power laser irradiation. Laser Med Sci 18:204–206, 2004.

11. M Braun. Lipodissolve for body sculpting. In: MP Goldman, PA Bacci, G Leischoff et al. (eds). Cellulite: pathophysiology and treatment. Taylor and Francis, New York; 2006: pp 301–22.

12. SA Brown, RJ Rohrich, J Kenkel et al. Effect of low-level laser therapy on abdominal adipocytes before lipoplasty procedure. Plast Reconstr Surg 113:1796–804, 2004.

13. A Capon, E Souil, B Gauthier et al. Laser-assisted skin closure (LASC) by using 815-nm diode laser system accelerates and improves wound healing. Lasers Surg Med 28:168–75, 2001.

14. P Chang, J Wiseman, T Jacoby et al. Noninvasive mechanical body contouring: (endermologie) a one year clinical outcome study update. Aesthetic Plast Surg 22:145–53, 1998.

15. ZD Draelos, KD Marenus. Cellulite: Etiology and purported treatment. Dermatol Surg 23:1117–81, 1997.

16. M Dyson. Cellular sub-cellular aspects of low level laser therapy (LLLT). In: T Oshiro, RG Calderhead (eds). Progress in laser therapy: selected papers from the October 1990 ILTA Congress, John Wiley & Sons, New York; 1991: pp 221–22.

17. M Dyson. Primary, secondary and tertiary effects of phototherapy: a review. In: MR Hamblin, RW Waynant, J Anders (eds). Mechanisms for low-light therapy, Proceedins of SPIE vol 6140, 6140005:1–12, 2006.

18. SO El Said, M Dyson. Comparison of the effect of multiwavelength light produced by a cluster of semiconductor diodes and of each individual diode on mast cell number and degranulation in intact and injured skin. Lasers Surg Med 10:559–68, 1990.

19. CS Enwemeka. Laser biostimulation of healing wounds: specific effects and mechanism of action. J Orthop Sports Physiotherapy 9:333–38, 1988.

20. CS Enwemeka. Attenuation and penetration of visible 632 and invisible 904 infra-red light in soft tissue. Laser Ther 13:95–101, 2001.

21. PB Fodor. Endermologie (LPG) does it work? Aesthetic Surg J 21:68, 1997.

22. L Gan, C Tse, RM Pilliar et al. Low-power laser stimulation of tissue engineering cartilage tissue formed on a porous calcium polyphosphate scaffold. Lasers Surg Med 39:286–93, 2007.

23. M Gniadecka. Potential for high-frequency ultrasonography, nuclear magnetic resonance, and Raman spectroscopy for skin studies. Skin Res Tech 3:139–46, 1997.

24. V Grimblatov, A Rubinshtein, M Rubinshtein. Spectral dosimetry in low light therapy. In: MR Hamblin, RW Waynant, J Anders (eds). Mechanisms for low-light therapy, Proceedins of SPIE, vol 6140, 614000S:1–6, 2006.

25. G Guillard, JM Lagarde. Skin lesions segmentation and quantification from 3D body's models. Skin Res Tech 11:123–31, 2005.

26. AK Gupta, N Filonenko, N Salansky et al. The use of low energy photon therapy (LEFT) in venous leg ulcers: a double-blind, placebo-controlled study. Dermatol Surg 24:1383–86, 1998.

27. MR Hamblin, TN Demidova. Mechanisms of low level light therapy. In: MR Hamblin, RW Waynant, J Anders (eds). Mechanisms for low-light therapy, Proceedins of SPIE; vol 6140, 6140001:1–12, 2006.

28. D Hawkins, N Houreld, H Abrahamse. Low level laser therapy (LLLT) as an effective therapeutic modality for delayed wound healing. Ann NY Acad Sci 1056:486–93, 2005.

29. DM Hexsel, R Mazzuco. Subcison: a treatment for cellulite. Int J Dermatol 39:539–44, 2000.

30. D Hexsel, R Mazzuco. Subcision®. In: MP Goldman, PA Bacci, G Leischoff, D Hexsel et al. (eds). Cellulite: pathophysiology and treatment. Taylor and Francis, New York; 2006: pp 251–62.

31. D Hexsel, T Dal'Forno, S Cignachi. Definition, clinical aspects, associated conditions, and differential diagnosis. In: MP Goldman, PA Bacci, G Leischoff et al. (eds). Cellulite: pathophysiology and treatment. Taylor and Francis, New York; 2006: pp 7–28.

32. D Hexsel, T Dal'Forno, C Hexsel et al. Cellulite severity scale. J Am Acad Dermatol 56(Suppl. 2):AB59, 2007.

33. D Hexsel, T Dal'Forno, C Hexsel. Severity scale of cellulite. J Europ Acad Dermatol Venerol 91:FC3.9, 2007.

34. LR Horwitz, TJ Burke, D Carnegie. Augmentation of wound healing using monochromatic infrared energy. Adv Wound Care 12:35–40, 1999.

35. RF Jackson, G Roche, KJ Butterwick et al. Low-level laser-assisted liposuction: A 2004 clinical study of its effectiveness for enhancing ease of liposuction procedures and facilitating the recovery process for patients undergoing thigh, hip, and stomach contouring. Am J Cosmetic Surg 21:191–198, 2004.

36. T Karu. Photobiology of low-power laser effects. Health Phys 56:691–704, 1989.

37. T Karu. Laser biostimulation: a photobiological phenomenon, J Photochem Photobiol B3:638–40, 1989.

38. T Karu. Primary and secondary mechanisms of action of visible to near-IR radiation on cells. J Photochem Photobiol B 49:1–17, 1999.

39. T Karu, NI Afanas'eva. Cytochrome c oxidase as the primary photoacceptor upon laser exposure of cultured cells to visible and near IR-range light. Dokl Akad Nauk 342:693–95, 1995.

40. TI Karu, LV Pyatibrat, GS Kalendo. The effect of He-Ne laser irradiation on the adhesive properties of the cell membranes. J Int Radiat Biol Med 115:622–23, 1993.

41. TI Karu, LV Pyatibrat, GS Kalendo et al. Effects of monochromatic low-intensity light and laser irradiation on adhesion of HeLa cells in vitro. Lasers Surg 18:171–77, 1996.

42. S Kasai, T Kono, Y Yamamoto et al. Effect of low-power laser irradiation on impulse conduction in anesthetized rabbits, J Clin Laser Med Surg 14:107–109, 1996.

43. AM Kligman. Cellulite: facts and fiction. J Geriatr Dermatol 5:136–39, 1997.

44. M Kulick. Evaluation of the combination of radio frequency, infrared energy and mechanical rollers with suction to improve skin surface irregularities (cellulite) in limited treatment area. J Cosmet Laser Ther 8:180–95, 2006.

45. E Lach, S Pap. Laser treatment for cellulite: a non- invasive alternative to liposuction. Lasers Surg Med Suppl 16:32, 2004.

46. G Leibaschoff. Surgical treatment. In: MP Goldman, PA Bacci, G Leischoff et al. (eds). Cellulite: pathophysiology and treatment. Taylor and Francis, New York; 2006: pp 211–50.

47. G Leibaschoff. Mesotherapy in the treatment of cellulite. In: MP Goldman, PA Bacci, G Leischoff et al. (eds). Cellulite: Pathophysiology and Treatment. Taylor and Francis, New York; 2006: pp 263–86.

48. T Lotti, I Ghersetich, C Grappone et al. Proteoglycans in so-called cellulite. Int J Dematol 29:272–74, 1990.

49. GW Lucassen, WLN van der Sluys, JJ van Herk et al. The effectiveness of massage treatment on cellulite as monitored by ultrasound imaging. Skin Res Tech 3:154–60, 1997.

50. D Manstein, AV Erofeev, GB Altshuler et al. Selective photothermolysis of lipid-rich tissue. Lasers Surg Med Suppl 13:6, 2001.

51. T Marovino. Cold lasers in pain management. Practical pain management; Sept/Oct 2004.

52. DH McDaniel, RG Geronemous, RA Weiss et al. LED photomodulation reverses acute UV induced skin damage. Lasers Surg Med (Suppl 16):30, 2004.

53. AP Medrado, E Trindale, SRA Reis et al. Action of low-level laser therapy on living fatty tissue of rats. Lasers Med Sci 21:19–23, 2006.

54. F Mirrashed, JC Sharp, V Krause et al. Pilot study of dermal and subcutaneous fat structures by MRI in individuals who differ in gender, BMI, and cellulite grading. Skin Res Tech 10:161–68, 2004.

55. R Neira, C Ortiz-Niera. Low level laser assisted liposculpture: clinical report of 700 cases. Aesthetic Surg J 22:451–55, 2002.

56. R Niera, R Jackson, D Dedo et al. Low-level laser-assisted lipoplasty appearance of fat demonstrated by MRI on abdominal tissue. Am J Cosmet Surg 18:133–40, 2001.

57. R Neira, J Arroyave, H Ramirez et al. Fat liquefaction: effect of low-level laser energy on adipose tissue. Plast Reconstruct Surg 110:912–22, 2002.

58. R Neira, L Toledo, J Arroyave et al. Low-level laser-assisted liposuction: the Neira 4 L technique. Clin Plast Surg 33:117–27, 2006.

59. PK Nootheti, A Magpantay, G Yosowitz et al. A single center, randomized, comparative, prospective clinical study to determine the efficacy of the Velasmooth system versus the TriActive system for the treatment of cellulite. Lasers Surg Med 38:908–12, 2006.

60. F Nürnberger, G Müller. So-called cellulite: an invented disease. J Dermatol Surg Oncol 4:221–29, 1978.

61. EL Nussbaum, J van Zuylen. Transmission of phototherapy through human skin: dosimetry adjustment for effects of skin color, body composition, wavelength and light coupling. In: MR Hamblin, RW Waynant, J Anders (eds). Mechanisms for low-light therapy, Proceedins of SPIE; vol 6140, 614000H:1–8, 2006.

62. T Ohno. Pain suppressive effect of low power laser irradiation: a quantitative analysis of substance P in the rat spinal dorsal root ganglion. Nippon Ika Daigaku Zasshi 64:395–400, 1997.

63. A Pabby, MP Goldman. The use of TriActive™ in the treatment of cellulite. In: MP Goldman, PA Bacci, G Leischoff et al. (eds). Cellulite: pathophysiology and treatment. Taylor and Francis, New York; 2006: pp 189–95.

64. F Perin, C Perrier, JC Pittet et al. Assessment of skin improvement treatment efficacy using the photograding of mechanically-accentuated macrorelief of thigh skin. Int J Cosmet Sci 22:147–56, 2000.

65. GE Piérard. Commentary on cellulite: skin mechanobiology and the waist-to-hip ratio. J Cosmetic Dermatol 4:151–52, 2005.

66. GE Piérard, JL Nizet, C Pierard-Franchimont. Cellulite: from standing fat herniation to hypodermal stretch marks. J Am Dermatopathol 22:34–37, 2000.

67. MA Porgel, JW Chen, K Zhang. Effects of low-energy gallium-aluminum-arsenide laser irradiation on cultured fibroblasts and keratinocytes. Lasers Surg Med 20:426–32, 1998.

68. W Posten, DA Wrone, JS Dover et al. Low level laser therapy for wound healing: mechanism and efficacy – A review. Lasers Surg Med (Suppl. 16):30, 2004.

69. W Posten, DA Wrone, JS Dover et al. Low-Level laser therapy for wound healing: mechanism and efficacy. Dermatol Surg 31:334–40, 2005.

70. P Quatresooz, E Xhauflaire-Uhoda, C Piérard-Franchimont et al. Cellulite histopathology and related mechanobiology. Int J Cosmet Sci 28:3, 207–10, 2006.

71. B Querleux. Cellulite characterization by high-frequency ultrasound and high-resolution magnetic resonance imaging. In: MP Goldman, PA Bacci, G Leischoff et al. (eds). Cellulite: pathophysiology and treatment. Taylor and Francis, New York; 2006: pp 105–14.

72. B Querleux, C Cornillon, O Jolivet et al. Anatomy and physiology of subcutaneous adipose tissue by in vivo magnetic resonance imaging and spectroscopy: relationships with sex and presence of cellulite. Skin Res Technol 8:118–24, 2002.

73. M Rosenbaum, V Prieto, J Hellmer et al. An exploratory investigation of the morphology and biochemistry of cellulite. Plast Reconstr Surg 101:1934–39, 1998.

74. A Schindl, M Schindl, H Pernerstorfer-Schon et al. Low intensity laser therapy: A review. J Invest Medicine 48:312–26, 2000.

75. A Schindl, M Schindl, H Schon et al. Low-intensity laser irradiation improves skin circulation in patients with diabetic microangiopathy. Diabetes Care 21:580–84, 1998.

76. LK Smalls, CY Lee, J Whitestone et al. Quantitative model of cellulite: three dimensional skin surface topography, biophysical characterization and relationship to human perception. J Cosmet Sci 56:105–20, 2005.

77. LK Smalls, M Hicks, D Passeretti et al. Effect of weight loss on cellulite: gynoid lypodystrophy. Plastic Reconstr Surg 118:510–16, 2006.

78. CWR Steinlechner, M Dyson. The effect of low-level laser therapy on macrophage-modified keratinocyte proliferation. Laser Ther 5:65–73, 1993.

79. G Tam. Low power laser therapy and analgesic action. J Clin Laser Med Surg 17:29–33, 1999.

80. TL Thomasson. Effects of skin-contact monochromatic infrared irradiation on tendonitis, capsilitis, and myofascial pain. J Neurol Orthop Med Surg 16:242–45, 1996.

81. M Van Vliet, A Ortiz, MM Avram et al. An assessment of traditional and novel therapies for cellulite. J Cosmet Laser Ther 7:7–10, 2005.

82. H Wakabayashi, M Hamba, K Matsumoto et al. Effect of irradiation by semiconductor laser on response evoked in trigeminal caudal neurons by tooth pulp stimulation. Lasers Surg Med 13:605–10, 1993.

83. R Wanitphakdeedecha, W Manuskiatti. Treatment of cellulite with a bipolar radiofrequency, infrared heat, and pulsatile suction device: a pilot study. J Cosmetic Dermatol 5:284–88, 2006.

84. C Webb, M Dyson, WHP Lewis. Stimulatory effect of 660 nm low laser energy on hypertrophic scar-derived fibroblasts: possible mechanisms for increase in cell counts. Lasers Surg Med 22: 294–301, 1998.

85. RA Weiss, DH McDaniel, RG Geronemus et al. Non-ablative, non-thermal light emitting diode (LED) phototherapy of photoaged skin. Lasers Surg Med (Suppl. 16):31, 2004.

86. W Yu, JO Naim, H McGowan et al. Photomodulation of oxidative metabolism and electron chain enzymes in rat liver mitochandria. Photochem Photobiol 66:866–71, 1997.

87. K Zitzlsperger, J Counters, S Tasi et al. Photomodulation using Gentlewaves LED with and without rejuvenating masque products. Lasers Surg Med (Suppl. 16):30, 2004.

88. United States Patent Application (2004) Publication No. US 2004/0162596.

89. J Bulow, J Madsen. Influence of blood flow on fatty acid mobilization form lipolytically active adipose tissue. Pflugers Arch 390(2):169–74, 1981.

90. D Gaylor. Physical mechanism of cellular injury in electrical trauma. Cambridge, MA, USA, Massachusetts Institute of Technology; 1989.

91. JA Hamilton, RA Johnson, B Corkey, F Kamp. Fatty acid transport: the diffusion mechanism in model and biological membranes. J Mol Neurosci 16(2-3):99–108, 2001; discussion 151–7.

92. NA Moussa, EN Tell, EG Cravalho et al. Time progression of hemolysis of erythrocyte populations exposed to supraphysiologic temperatures. J Biomech Eng 101:213–17, 1979.

93. M Gold, N Fournier, K Hails et al. Unpublished data.

94. E Lach. Reduction of subcutaneous fat and improvement in cellulite appearance by dual-wavelength, low-level laser energy combined with vacuum and massage, Journal of Cosmetic and Laser Therapy. 10:202–09, 2008.

19 High Frequency Ultrasound Evaluation of Cellulite Treated with the 1064 nm Nd:YAG Laser

Régine Bousquet-Rouaud, Marie Bazan, Jean Chaintreuil, and Agustina Vila Echague

Introduction

Treatments in aesthetic dermatology are evolving towards non-invasive techniques, whose efficacy has yet to be proven. Infrared lasers and radiofrequency devices used for the treatment of cellulite have been the subject of several recent publications [1–6]. Numerous therapies have been advertised for the treatment of cellulite, but little scientific evidence demonstrates that any of these treatments is beneficial. In fact, much of this evidence is subjective or based upon patient self-assessment.

Therefore, the use of ultrasound imaging, which is widespread in other specialties, is of potential interest here, for reasons of simplicity and objectivity.

According to various studies, cellulite concerns 85 to 98% of post-pubertal females. The term "cellulite" originated in France more than 150 years ago [7–8]; it describes the "orange peel" syndrome or quilted appearance in areas with subcutaneous fat and has received no definitive explanation so far [9–15]. This condition is most commonly observed on the thighs, the abdomen and the arms; it occurs at an early age, even in thin young girls. Despite the lack of morbidity or mortality associated with this syndrome, the female population expresses a high demand for treatment. Numerous therapies have been suggested [16–20], among which Endermologie–LPG and mesotherapy are the best known [21,22]. None of them has been proven as a permanent cure for cellulite.

At present, three devices have received FDA approval for "temporary improvement in the appearance of cellulite": a mechanical massage machine (Endermologie, LPG, Fort Lauderdale, FL); a combination of laser, radiofrequency and vacuum (VelaSmooth/VelaShape, Syneron Medical Ltd., Yokneam, Israel); and a combination of laser and mechanical vacuum (SmoothShapes, Eleme Medical Ltd., Merrimack, NH).

Laser and radiofrequency treatment have been chosen according to the physiopathology of cellulite or, at least, to the most commonly accepted hypotheses [23–25]. The anatomical description of cellulite is a combination of superficial adipose tissue enlargement, fibrosis of the conjunctive fibers in the septae, skin laxity and water retention. The degree of combination of these factors varies, depending mainly on age and hormonal events. Two leading hypotheses have been formulated to explain the physiopathology of cellulite: (i) a gender-related dimorphism in the skin architecture, resulting in a perpendicular orientation of the connective tissue septae [13] and possibly responsible for fat indentation or herniations; (ii) vascular changes and abnormal deposits of glycosaminoglycans in the extracellular matrix of the dermis, leading to fluid retention, hypoxia and chronic inflammation [10,26,27].

A distinctive structural feature of cellulite is the presence of subcutaneous fat herniations into the reticular and papillary dermis [11–15]. The micro-anatomical basis of this condition is still being debated.

According to the hypothesis that altered connective tissue creates herniations of fat at the dermalhypodermal interface [28,29], the 1064 nm Nd:YAG laser was used to induce a thermal injury into the deep dermis and the hypodermis. Lasers radiating from 1064 nm to 1450 nm have been used to produce non-specific dermal heating and to trigger a wound-healing response resulting in the formation of new collagen [30,31]. The actual chromophore of the 1064 nm Nd:YAG laser is not precisely identified; the absorption by water and by lipids at this particular wavelength appears weak as described by Anderson et al. in 2006 [32]. Nevertheless, the 1064 nm Nd:YAG laser has proven safe and somewhat successful in non-ablative facial treatments [33–36]. The same properties that ensure a deep penetration into the skin and result in bulk heating of the dermis may appear valuable in the treatment of cellulite.

The purpose of the present study was twofold: (i) to investigate the 1064 nm laser radiation as a long-term treatment of cellulite, (ii) to evaluate the results using high frequency ultrasound imaging, a technique considered, alike magnetic resonance imaging (MRI), to be an adequate tool to assess the efficacy of any cellulite treatment [11,13,14,29,37,38].

The study was designed using a combination of high fluence (30J/cm^2), 18 mm spot size and a long pulse duration (30 ms) in order to enhance the penetration in the skin. Protection of the epidermis was achieved by using cryogen (tetrafluoroethane).

The expected results were a deep remodelling action in the conjunctive septae between the adipocyte lobules of the hypodermis.

Materials and Methods

The study was conducted between February and July of 2006 and was approved by Institutional Review Boards and Ethics Committees for the protection of human subjects.

Twelve female patients were enrolled in the study. All subjects signed an informed consent before being enrolled in the study. This randomized study was designed to assess the efficacy and safety of the Candela Nd:YAG 1064 nm laser for the treatment of cellulite. The efficacy was judged from the improvement in the appearance of cellulite and from the evaluation of dermal thickness changes. Treatments were done at three- to four-week intervals. Patients were eligible to participate in the study if they were female, 20 to 56 years old (mean age: 47.4 ±12 years), skin phototypes I–IV presenting with spontaneous or induced cellulite and with a body mass index less than 28 (Table 19.1). They were treated on their left or right thigh; the contralateral side was not treated and served as control for visual comparison.

Table 19.1 Demographics of Patients, Therapeutic Outline and Results

Patient no.	Age	Weight (kg)	Height (m)	BMI	Cellulite stage	Cellulite type	Side treated	Satisfaction index
1	57	57	1.69	19.96	2	Hard	left	2
2	50	67	1.73	22.39	2	Hard	right	4
3	48	56	1.07	19.38	2	Hard	left	4
4	58	51	1.58	20.43	2	Hard	right	3
5	49	58	1.07	20.07	2	Hard	left	4
6	48	62	1.61	23.92	2	Hard	left	2
7	59	69	1.07	23.88	3	Soft	right	3
8	20	64	1.07	22.15	2	Hard	right	1
9	55	64	1.68	22.68	3	Soft	left	3
10	45	48	1.63	18.07	2	Hard	right	4
11	24	50	1.06	19.53	2	Hard	left	2
12	56	64,5	1.62	24.58	3	Soft	right	3

Other inclusion criteria were stable weight, regular and unchanged physical activity, unchanged caloric intake and identical hormonal status. Exclusion criteria included: pregnancy, severe cellulite involving pain and/or tenderness in the thighs; patients who had had surgical procedures including liposuction and mesotherapy, or recent medical treatment (endermology or massage); patients with venous and/or lymphatic insufficiency, with photosensitivity or ingesting sun-sensitizing or anti-coagulant medications; patients with a history of keloids, neuropathy, coagulopathy or diabetes and patients who were unable or unwilling to comply with the study requirements. Subjects with pacemakers or metallic implants or Fitzpatrick V or VI were not enrolled either.

Screening and Measurements
The severity of cellulite was scored according to the Nürnberger-Muller scale:

Stage 0: no orange-peel skin
Stage 1: orange-peel not visible but appearing when skin is pinched
Stage 2: visible orange-peel skin in standing position
Stage 3: visible orange-peel skin in decubitus position

The texture of cellulite was also evaluated as hard, adherent to deep planes, or soft with no adherence to deep planes, not painful and flaccid. Each participant was weighed before each treatment. A photograph was taken before each treatment, including front, side and back views of the thighs, using the Canfield Monostand device (Canfield Scientific, Fairfield, NJ) with a dedicated camera set at fixed focal length and under constant lighting.

Ultrasound Image Acquisition and Image Processing
Ultrasound assessment was performed using the Dermascan, Ver 3 (Cortex technology, Denmark), equipped with a 20 MHz transducer, providing a 60 x 200 micron resolution and a penetration depth of 10 to 15 mm. The resulting images were 12 mm in width and 13 mm in height. The transducer was held on the skin at a constant pressure. Contact between the skin and the transducer was established by using a thin layer of gel.

The dermal thickness was measured as the distance between the epidermis and the hyperechogenic layer that characterizes the hypodermis. As the determination of the hypodermic boundary is sometimes uncertain and therefore subjective, an automatic image-processing method was developed to determine this limit, strictly based on echogenicity and requiring no human interpretation.

The image processing was performed using different tools provided by Visiquest 4.5 (Accusoft Corp, Northborough, MA) [39–43].

The automatic analysis process is described in full in Appendix 1.

Laser Treatment
The Nd:YAG laser (GentleYag, Candela Corp, Wayland, MA), with a wavelength of 1064 nm was used on the 12 patients, with the following parameters: spot size of 18 mm, pulse duration set at 30 ms, fluence of 30 J/cm^2, cryogen (Dynamic Cooling Device) of 20 to 30 ms and no post-laser cryogen. These parameters were the same for all patients.

Each target area—posterior side of the thigh—received one single set of separated pulses at 1.5 Hz applied in linear fashion, without pulse overlap, which led to a slight transient erythema in most patients. Each area was treated three times: at the time of entry into the study, one month and two months later. No anesthetic cream was used.

Immediately after treatment, the subjects were asked to rate the pain from 0 to10 (none to very bad) and the clinical side effects, purpura, edema, erythema and blistering were also assessed.

Follow-up Procedure
The follow-up evaluation was conducted one month and three months after the third treatment.

The following parameters were evaluated: photo before and after, ultrasound assessment as described above and patient satisfaction index rated on a scale from 1 to 5 (1 not satisfied, 2 slightly satisfied, 3 somewhat satisfied, 4 satisfied, 5 very satisfied).

Statistical Analysis
A statistical analysis was performed to assess the significance of the ultrasound measurements of dermal thickness and dermal echogenic density. A non-parametric Wilcoxon test was used to test the differences between baseline and follow-up assessments. A value of $p < 0.05$ was considered statistically significant.

Results
The age of the group was 47.4 ± 12.7 (extremes 20–59) years. The Body Mass Index was 24.4 ± 2.1 (extremes 18.07–24.58). Nine patients presented with a cellulite stage of two and three patients presented with a cellulite stage of three.

The twelve patients underwent 36 laser sessions and 35 ultrasound examinations. Eleven patients from the group were satisfied with the procedure, the frequency and the comfort of the treatment.

One patient (aged 20) did not return for the second follow-up visit after the third treatment because no improvement had occurred either clinically or through ultrasound assessment.

The patient satisfaction index gave the following results for the eleven subjects three months after the third treatment: three patients were little satisfied (satisfaction grade two), four patients were somewhat satisfied (satisfaction grade three), four patients were satisfied (satisfaction grade four).

The average satisfaction index among the eleven patients who completed the protocol was 3.09 ± 0.83. Counting the patient who dropped out as dissatisfied (grade 1), the average satisfaction index became 2.92 ± 1.00.

A significant correlation between the satisfaction grade and the improvement in the ultrasound parameters was tested. The significance was not reached, due to one patient who ranked second for the improvement in ultrasound parameters and scored a satisfaction grade 2.

Satisfaction responses of individual patients were similar concerning the procedure, the comfort and the observed improvement. The most frequently reported improvements were tissue firmness, tactile perception of tighter skin and reduction of surface irregularities.

The photographs taken in the standing position showed a slight improvement of the dimpling aspect and a reduction of the gluteal fold, in some patients. Examples are shown in Fig. 19.1 and 19.2.

Immediately after each session, some erythema was observed, at different times and of varying intensity, depending on the patient. This erythema disappeared within 2–48 hours; no hyperpigmentation or edema occurred. No other side effect was reported.

Ultrasound Examination
Qualitative aspects
The epidermis appears on the screen as a more or less straight white line of varying thickness, depending on the area. The dermis, like the hypodermis, is shown as dense areas interspersed with hypoechogenic areas (Fig. 19.1 and 19.2). After treatment, the hypoechogenic areas often appeared to be reduced in number and size and the dermal thickness was reduced, resulting in a more compact aspect of the skin. These subjective results were confirmed by quantitative measurements as follows.

Quantitative aspects
The precision of the method used to provide an automatic evaluation of the dermis thickness and a semi-automatic evaluation of the dermal echogenic density was assessed by repeating the measurements ten times on two healthy subjects at the forearm level, repositioning the probe each time.

Subject one, male, aged 52, presented a dermal thickness of 3.50 ± 0.26 mm. The resulting coefficient of variation was 7.31%. The corresponding dermal echogenic density, expressed as a percentage ratio of the segmented area to the total area, was 25.51% ± 2.42%. The resulting coefficient of variation was 9.50%.

Subject two, female, aged 23, presented a dermal thickness of 3.82 ± 0.25 mm. The resulting coefficient of variation was 6.55%. The corresponding dermal echogenic density, expressed as a percentage ratio of the segmented area to the total area, was 20.61% ± 1.78%. The resulting coefficient of variation was 8.64%.

Individual precision measurements are shown in Fig. 19.3 (dermal thickness) and Fig. 19.4 (dermal echogenic density).

In the study, patient dermal thickness and echogenic density were assessed at the treatment site before treatment (T0), one month after the third treatment (T1) and three months after the third treatment (T2).

At T1, 10 patients out of the 12-patient group had a reduced dermal thickness and 10 patients presented with an increase in dermal echogenic density. One patient did not show any reduction in dermal thickness but an increased echogenic density and one patient with a reduction in dermal thickness also presented a slight reduction in echogenic density.

For the group, dermal thickness improved from 3.21 ± 0.49 mm at time T0 to 2.75 ± 0.62 mm at T1 ($p < 0.05$). Echogenic density improved from 32.41% ± 5.12% at time T0 to 40.30% ± 11.96% at T1 ($p < 0.05$).

At T2, 10 patients out of the 12-patient group had a reduced dermal thickness. Ten patients presented with an increase in dermal echogenic density. One patient did not show any reduction in dermal thickness but presented with an increased echogenic density and one patient with a reduction in dermal thickness presented with a slight reduction in echogenic density.

For the group, dermal thickness improved from 3.21 ± 0.49 mm at time T0 to 2.54 ± 0.44 mm at T2 ($p < 0.01$). Echogenic density improved from 32.41% ± 5.12% at time T0 to 45.15% ± 11.80% at T2 ($p < 0.01$).

Individual patient measurements at time T0, T1 and T2 are shown in Fig. 19.5 (dermal thickness) and in Fig. 19.6 (dermal echogenic density).

Therefore, reduction in dermal thickness appears to be the objective translation of the clinical skin improvement, i.e tightening.

Discussion
In recent years, various physical and mechanical techniques have been proposed to improve cellulite on prevalent anatomical sites, mainly on the thighs but also on the arms and abdomen [16–22]. Endermologie aims at draining water from adipose lobules into the lymphatic system. This technique developed in France in the 1970s utilizes a patented, electrically powered handheld device to aspirate and massage the affected areas between the two revolving rollers in order to improve lymphatic drainage. Collis and co-workers [21], in a controlled trial of 52 patients, found no statistical difference between thigh measurements while 11 of the 35 subjects described some (self-assessed) improvement. Moreover, the slight ecchymosis which occurs on the treated areas due to the massage and suction, may increase alteration of the dermal vasculature, creating hypoxia, increasing proteoglycan deposition and actually worsening cellulite [26]. Mesotherapy aims at inducing a more or less specific action on inflammation and vascular abnormalities and/or adipolysis [22] in the case of phosphatidylcholine. But current scientific studies are yet to be published.

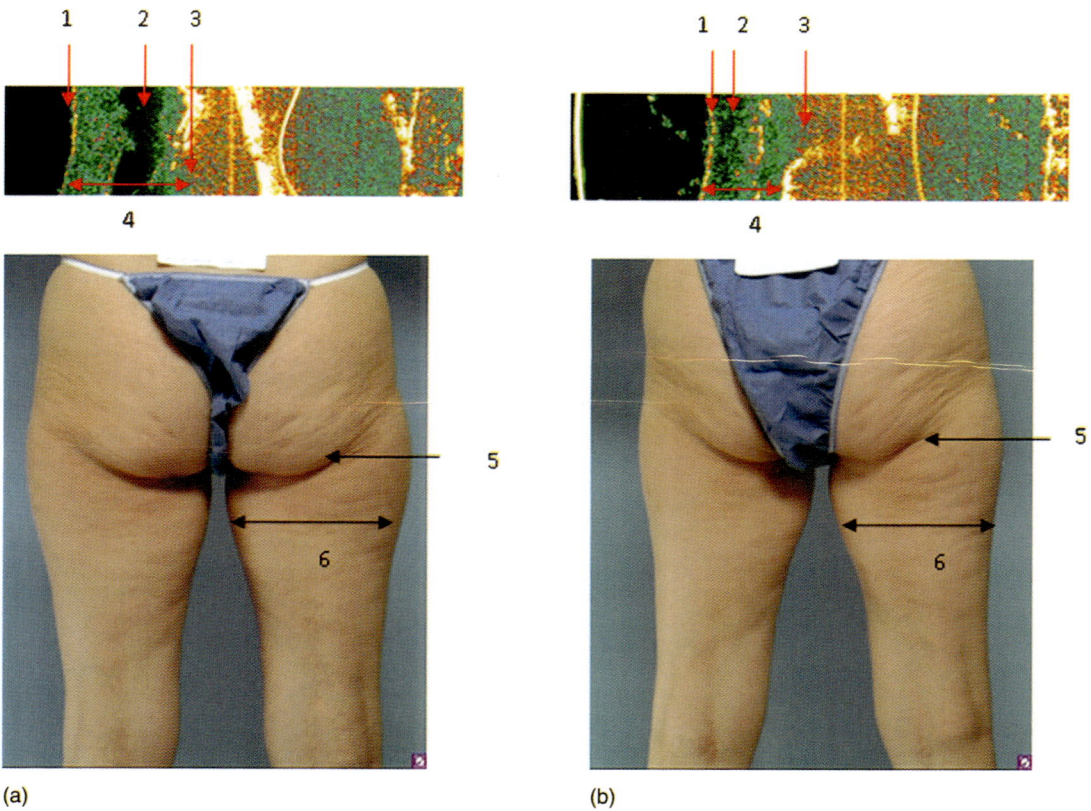

Figure 19.1 (a) Pre-treatment, posterior side of the right thigh of a 58-year-old woman and ultrasound image. (b) Three months after treatment. 1:Epidermis; 2: Hypoechogenic area with herniations; 3: Hyperechogenic area: hypodermis boundary ; 4: Dermis thickness; 5: Reduction in gluteal fold; 6: Reduction in thigh circumference.

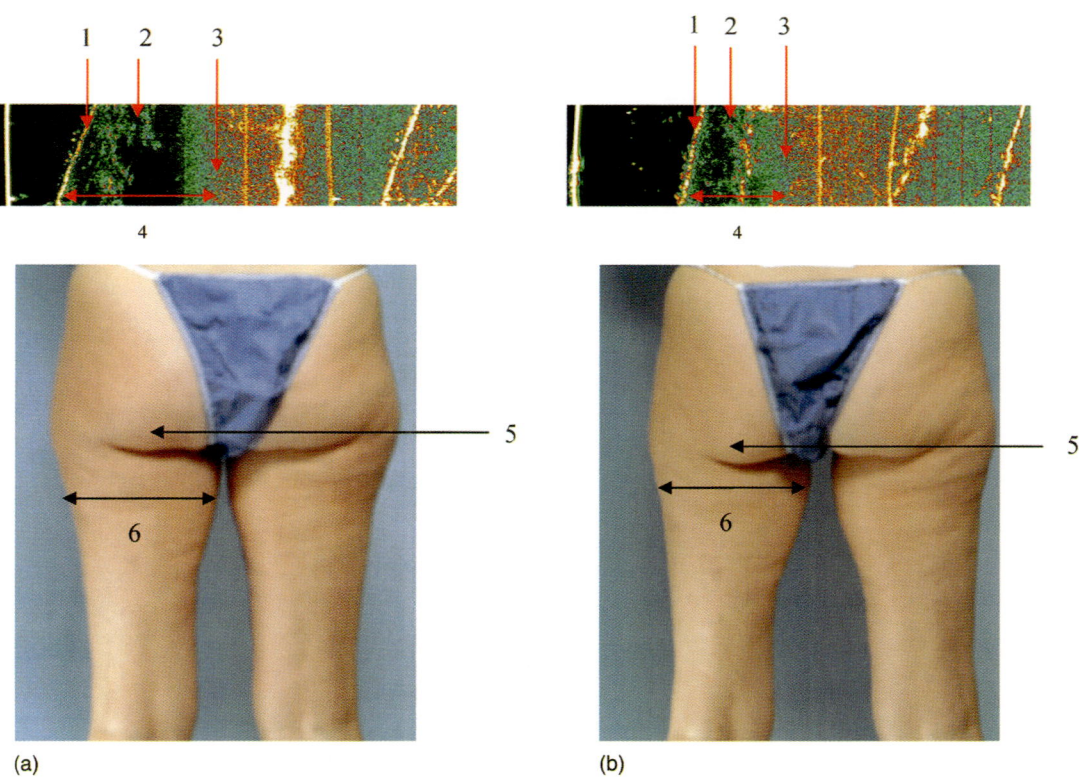

Figure 19.2 (a) Pre-treatment, posterior side of the left thigh of a 49-year-old woman and ultrasound image. (b) Three months after treatment. 1:Epidermis; 2: Hypoechogenic area with herniations; 3: Hyperechogenic area: hypodermis boundary ; 4: Dermis thickness; 5: Reduction in gluteal fold; 6: Reduction in thigh circumference.

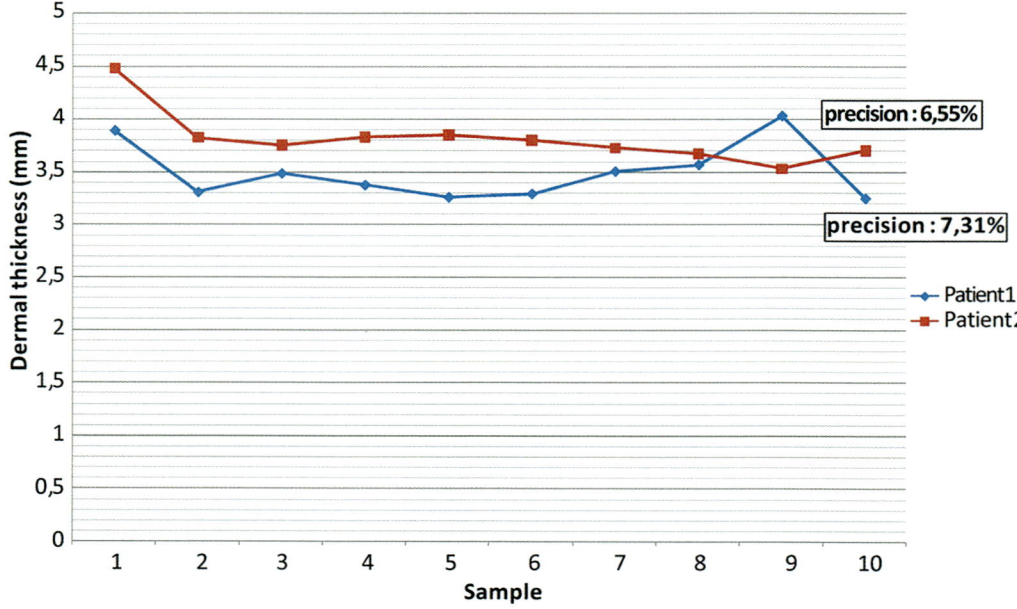

Figure 19.3 Precision measurements: dermal thickness.

Weight loss, diet and exercise have been cited to improve cellulite but, if cellulite increases with weight gain, weight loss is not sufficient to eliminate cellulite. And benefits attributed to the various treatments should be more thoroughly analysed. These techniques may indeed provide some temporary positive results, but none of them has been identified as the technique of choice in the armamentarium against cellulite.

The 1064 nm laser wavelength emitted by the Nd:YAG laser has been widely used to rejuvenate collagen in the treatment of skin aging, mainly on the face [36,44]. This wavelength penetrates several millimeters into the skin and can produce significant bulk heating of the deep dermis. It is currently accepted that these changes may stimulate fibroblasts to produce new collagen.

As it has been recently demonstrated that the heat shock protein (HSP) 47 and 72 are significantly increased in the skin after fractional resurfacing [45], a possible mechanism of action could involve the stimulation of the production of Type I collagen mediated through these HSPs.

Cellulite is a combination of hormonal factors, gender-related dimorphism in the skin architecture, and inflammatory phenomena. It is characterized by altered connective tissue septae that isolate adipose lobules in the hypodermis as seen on MRI [13] and high resolution ultrasound images [14,37]. This results in subsequent herniation of the adipose lobules, deemed to be responsible for the orange peel aspect. The protrusion of fat into the dermis is a characteristic of female anatomy [28,29] and appears as low-density hypoechogenic areas among denser dermal tissue.

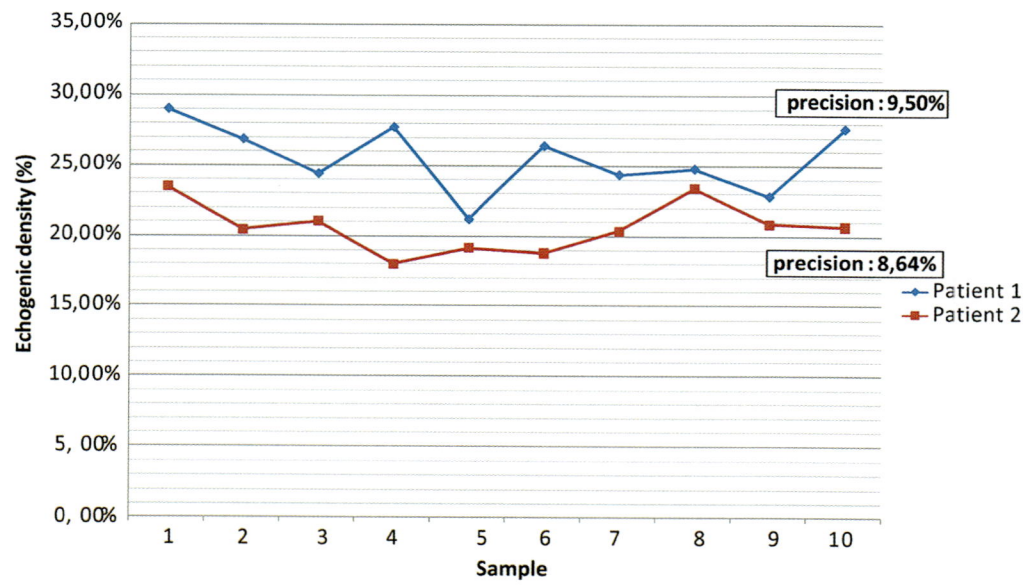

Figure 19.4 Precision measurements: dermal echogenic density.

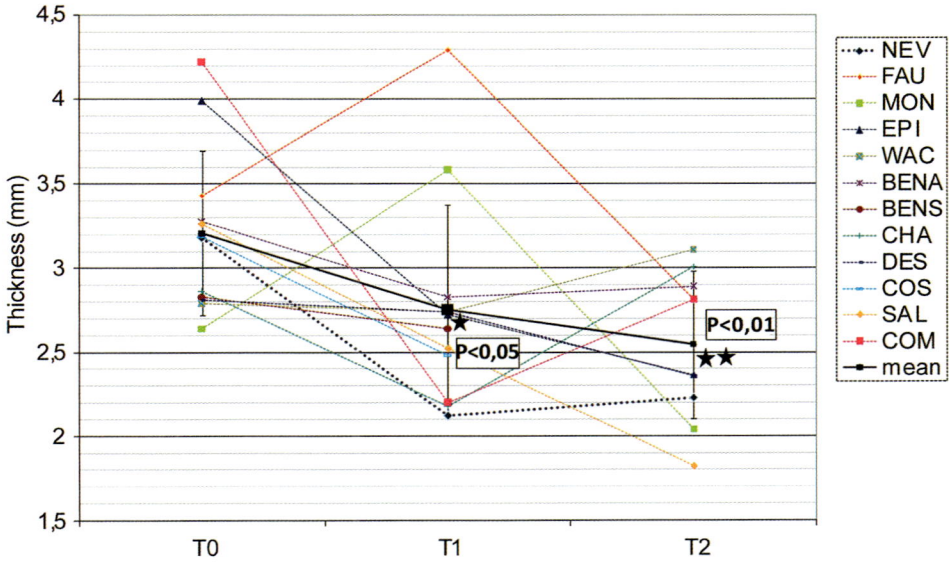

Figure 19.5 Patient measurements: dermal thickness.

The rationale for using the Nd:YAG wavelength to treat cellulite was based on the understanding of this etiopathogenic condition, trying to achieve the same effect on the connective tissue septae as is achieved on the collagen in aging skin.

The exact target of the Nd:YAG radiation is still a subject of discussion. No highly specific chromophore has been described for the 1064 nm wavelength. This lack of specificity may be responsible for the penetration depth, resulting in the bulk heating of the whole skin in the irradiated area. Selective photothermolysis of lipids has been described recently in the infrared spectrum [32]. However, the absorption coefficient of the Nd:YAG wavelength by lipids is not sufficient for this to be a possible mechanism of action.

Notwithstanding the incomplete knowledge of the molecular effects, the present study highlights a potential clinical benefit of the 1064 nm wavelength treatment on cellulite. The reported results are encouraging although the determination of the number of treatments and their time intervals require further study for optimization. The results of this study differ from another study [46] which used the same device and this may be related to treatment parameters and/or technique. We used the highest fluence with this particular device (30 J/cm²), a large spot size (18 mm) and a relatively long pulse duration (30 ms), in order to increase the penetration in the depth of the skin. In our opinion, clinical improvement is clearly related to the effect on deep structures. Other factors include the number and duration of sessions, their frequency, the number of pulses, the overlapping or pulse stacking and the cooling.

Other wavelengths are worth exploring, especially those with a higher lipid absorption coefficient, in an attempt to create a selective photothermolysis process. The validation of new treatments

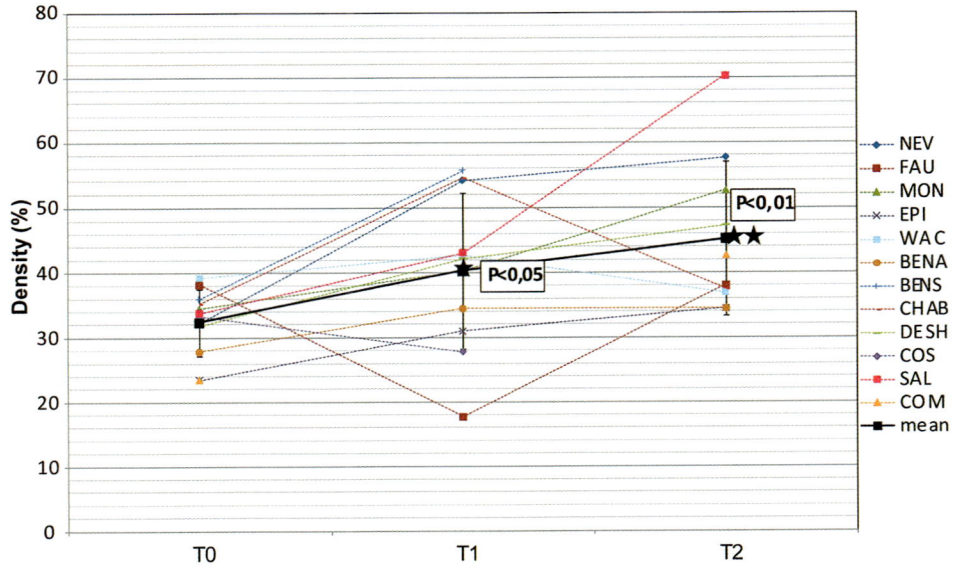

Figure 19.6 Patient measurements: dermal echogenic density.

requires objective means of measurement such as MRI and ultrasound imaging to confirm clinical subjective improvement.

The inability to reach a significant correlation between the ultrasound parameters and the satisfaction grade may be interpreted as the sign of a lag between the improvement in quantitative parameters and the improvement in clinical appearance; it points out more certainly to the subjective value of satisfaction indexes.

In this study, ultrasound imaging coupled with the operator's independent quantitative measurements proved to be a useful tool to evaluate the effects of the treatment on the skin. However, the design of the protocol did not permit an assessment of whether echographic changes were early predictors of future clinical benefits. The 20 MHz frequency probe was the best choice to show the epidermis line and more importantly the depth of the dermis where the whole cellulite formation process takes place. The sensitivity of the ultrasound equipment software was set for optimal dermis imaging and never modified throughout the study. Although the acquisition of the echographic image of the skin requires some degree of training, the accurate results obtained with different operators and with the repositioning of the probe showed that the reliability of measurements was acceptable. The interpretation of the images and the visual determination of the limit between the dermis and the hypodermis are certainly the most critical sources of variability in the performance of quantitative measurements. The development of image-processing tools that define the shape of the image based on the ultrasound energy recorded in each pixel helps to overcome this limitation.

Conclusion

This clinical study is, to the best of our knowledge, the first assessment study using ultrasound measurements to quantitatively measure the efficacy of a laser treatment for cellulite. These results demonstrate that skin ultrasound imaging is a non-invasive, effective, reproducible and accurate examination that can be used in future research on the effect of laser treatments for cellulite. The results of the present study have yet to be completed in an attempt to identify potentially responsive and non-responsive patients and to define the best treatment protocol.

Acknowledgments

This study was supported, in part, by a grant from Candela Corp. This chapter was originally published in *Journal of Cosmetic and Laser Therapy*, 11 (2009) 34-44 and is reproduced from there by permission.

REFERENCES

1. Ph Bitter. Non invasive rejuvenation of photoaged skin using serial full-face intense pulsed light treatments. Dermatol Surg 26:835–43, 2000.
2. DJ Goldberg. New collagen formation after dermal remodeling with an intense pulsed light source. J Cutan Laser Ther 2:59–61, 2000.
3. TS Alster, JR Lupton. Are all infrared lasers equally effective in skin rejuvenation? Semin Cutan Med Surg 21:274–9, 2002.
4. EL Tanzi, CM Williams, TS Alster. Treatment of facial rhytides with a non ablative 1450 nm diode laser: a control clinical and histological study. Dermatol Surg 29:124–8, 2003.
5. MA Trelles. Combined non ablative skin rejuvenation with the 595 and 1450 nm lasers. Dermatol Surg 30:1292–98, 2004.
6. TS Jeffrey. Multicenter study of the safety and efficacy of a 585 nm pulsed dye laser for the non ablative treatment of facial rhytides. Dermatol Surg 31:1–9, 2005.
7. Nürnberger F, Müller G. So-called cellulite: an invented disease. J Dermatol Surg Oncol 4: 221–9, 1978.
8. C Scherwitz, O Braun-Falco. So-called cellulite. J Dermatol Surg Oncol 4:230–4, 1978.
9. ZD Draelos. In search of answers regarding cellulite. Cosmet Dermatol 14:55–8, 2001.
10. ABR Rossi, AL Vergnanini. Cellulite: a review. J Eur Acad Dermatol Venereol 14:251–62, 2000.
11. M Rosenbaum, V Prieto, J Hellmer et al. An exploratory investigation of the morphology and biochemistry of cellulite. Plast Reconstr Surg 101:1934–9, 1998.
12. F Mirrashed, JC Sharp, V Krause et al. Pilot study of dermal and subcutaneous fat structures by MRI in individuals who differ in gender, BMI, and cellulite grading. Skin Res Technol 10:161–8, 2004.
13. B Querleux, C Cornillon, O Jolivet et al. Anatomy and physiology of subcutaneous adipose tissue by in vivo magnetic resonance imaging and spectroscopy: Relationship with sex and presence of cellulite. Skin Res Technol 8:118–24, 2002.
14. GW Lucassen, WLN Van der Sluys, JJ Van herk et al. The effectiveness of massage treatment on cellulite as monitored by ultrasound imaging. Skin Res Technol 3:154–60, 1997.
15. D Quaglino, G Bergamini, F Boraldi et al. Ultrastructural and morphometrical evaluation on normal human dermal connective tissue – the influence of age, sex, and body region. J Br Dermatol 134:1013–22, 1996.
16. AM Kligman, A Pagnoni, T Stoudemayer. Topical retinol improves cellulite. Journal of Dermatological Treatment 10:119–25, 1999.
17. C Bertin, H Zunino, JC Pittet et al. A double blind evaluation of the activity of an anti-cellulite product containing retinol, caffeine and ruscogenine by a combination of several non-invasive methods. J Cosmet Sci 52:199–210, 2001.
18. WP Coleman, CW Hanke, TH Alt et al. Liposuction Cosmetic Surgery of the Skin: Principles and Practice. BC Decker Inc: Philadelphia, PA; 213–38, 1991.
19. DM Hexsel, R Mazzuco. Subcision: a treatment for cellulite. J Int Dermatol 39:539–44, 2000.
20. M Gasparotti. Superficial liposuction: a new application of the technique for aged and flaccid skin. Aesthet Plast Surg 16:141–53, 1992.
21. N Collis, LA Elliot, C Sharpe et al. Cellulite treatment: a myth or reality: a prospective randomized, controlled trial of two therapies, endermologie and aminophylline cream. Plast reconstr Surg 104:1110–14, 1999.
22. AM Rotunda, H Suzuki, RL Moy et al. Detergent effects of sodium deoxycholate are a major feature of an injectable phosphatidylcholine formulation used for localized fat dissolution. Dermatol Surg 30:1001–7, 2004.
23. TS Alster, EL Tanzi. Cellulite treatment using a novel combination of radiofrequency, infrared light and mechanical tissue manipulation device. J Cosmet Laser Ther 7:81–5, 2005.

24. NS Sadick, RS Mulholland. A prospective clinical study to evaluate the efficacy and safety of cellulite treatment using the combination of optical and RF energies for subcutaneous tissue heating. J Cosmet Laser Ther 6:187–90, 2004.

25. M Kulick. Evaluation of the combination of radiofrequency, infrared energy and mechanical rollers with suction to improve skin surface irregularities (cellulite) in a limited treatment area. J Cosmet Laser Ther 8: 185–90, 2006.

26. SB Curri. Cellulite and fatty tissue microcirculation. Cosmet Toilet 108:51–158, 1993.

27. T Lotti, I Ghersetich, C Grappone et al. Proteoglycans in so-called cellulite. J Int Dermatol 29:272–4, 1990.

28. GE Piérard, JL Nizet, C Pierard-Franchimont. Cellulite: from standing fat herniation to hypodermal stretch marks. J Am Dermatopathol 22:34–7, 2000.

29. MM Avram. Cellulite a review of its physiology and treatment. J Cosmet Laser Ther 6:181–85, 2004.

30. DJ Goldberg, S Silapunt. Histologic Evaluation of a Q-Switched Nd: YAG Laser in the Nonablative Treatments of Wrinkles. Dermatologic Surgery 27:744–46, 2001.

31. SH Dayan, AJ Vartanian, G Menaker et al. Nonablative Laser Resurfacing using the Long-Pulse (1064 nm) Nd: YAG Laser. Archives of Facial Plastic Surgery 5 (4):310–15, 2003.

32. RR Anderson, W Farinelli, H Laubach et al. Selective photothermolysis of lipid-rich tissues: a free electron laser study. Lasers Surg Med 38:913–19, 2006.

33. JZ Chen, MR Armenakas, LJ Bernstein et al. Objective Evaluation of Non-Ablative Subsurface Remodeling with The Altus Coolglide Vantage Excel Laser, American Society for Laser Medicine and Surgery Abstracts Twenty-Third Meeting Anaheim, CA: Abstract # 53, 2003.

34. CD Schmults, DJ Goldberg. Non-ablative Facial Remodeling: Clinical and Ultrastructural Changes After Treatment with a New 300 μsec, 1064 nm Nd: YAG Laser. American Society for Laser Medicine and Surgery Abstracts Twenty-Third Meeting Anaheim, CA: Abstract # 63, 2003.

35. JM Kenkel, J Hoopman, S Brown. Treatment of Flushing, Vascular and Pigmented Lesions Using Long Pulse Nd: YAG. American Society for Laser Medicine and Surgery Abstracts Twenty-Third Meeting Anaheim, CA: Abstract # 240, 2003.

36. DJ Key. Single-treatment skin tightening by radiofrequency and long-pulsed, 1064 nm Nd: Yag laser compared. Lasers Surg Med 39:169–75, 2007.

37. R Bousquet-Rouaud. Non ablative 1450 nm diode laser for photorejuvenation: preliminary results of ultrasound measurements. European Society for Laser Dermatology. Fourteenth Congress London. 2005 (abstr).

38. R Bousquet-Rouaud. Ultrasound, a new objective method to assess laser in cellulite. European Society for Laser Dermatology. Fourteenth Congress London. 2005 (abstr).

39. J Serra. Image Analysis and Mathematical Morphology, Vol 1, Academic Press, London 1982.

40. JW Tukey. Exploratory Data Analysis, Addison Wesley, Reading, MA; 1977.

41. LG Roberts. Machine Perception of three dimensional solids, in Optical and Electro-optical Information Processing, JT Tippett et al (Eds) MIT Press, Cambridge, MA; 1965, 159–97.

42. WK Pratt. Digital Image Processing: PIKS inside, 3rd edition, John Willey & Sons Inc: 2001, 433–36.

43. T Pavlidis. Algorithms for Graphics and Image Processing, Computer Science Press Rockville, MD; 1982.

44. MB Taylor, I Prokopenko. Split-face comparison of radiofrequency versus long-pulse Nd: Yag treatment of facial laxity. J Cosmet Laser Ther 8:17–22, 2006.

45. B Hantash, V Bedi, B Kapadia et al. In vivo histological evaluation of a novel ablative fractional resurfacing device. Lasers Surg Med 39:96–107, 2007.

46. A Truitt, A Echague, C Zachary, KM Kelly. Evaluation of the Candela 1064 nm Nd: Yag laser for cellulite and skin tightening. American Society for Laser Medicine and Surgery. 2007 (abstr. 63).

Appendix 1

In order to automatically analyze the ultrasound images, the procedure was as follows:

- The image was extracted from the ultrasound machine as a jpg file which resulted in a 1024 × 224 pixel image (Fig. 19.7).

- The colour image was converted into a 256 grey scale representation.

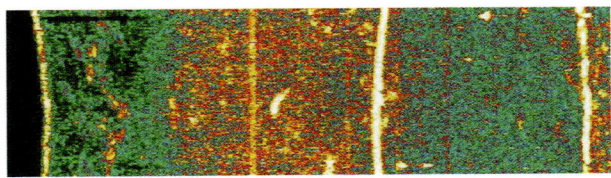

Figure 19.7 Jpg image obtained on the ultrasound machine.

Figure 19.8 Image obtained after the thresholding.

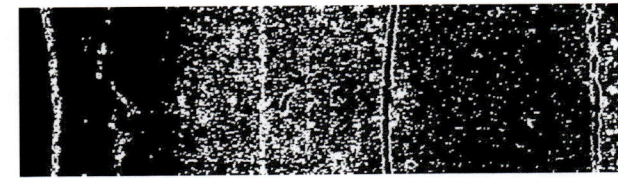

Figure 19.9 Image after dilation.

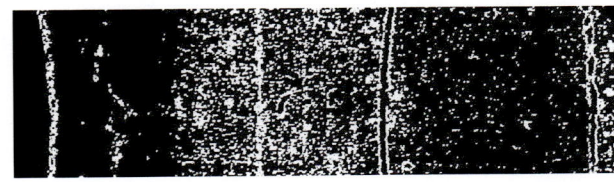

Figure 19.10 Image after median filtering.

143

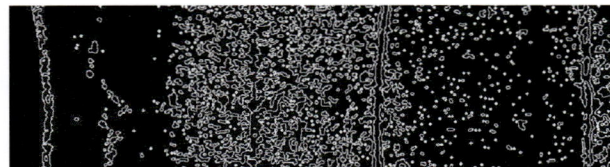

Figure 19.11 Image after the Roberts cross difference operator.

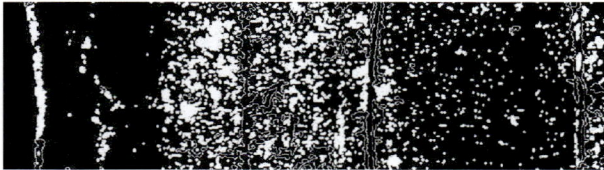

Figure 19.12 Image after closing of holes.

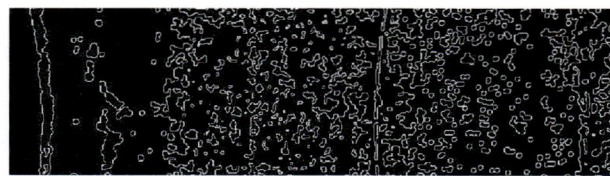

Figure 19.13 Image after last Roberts cross difference operator.

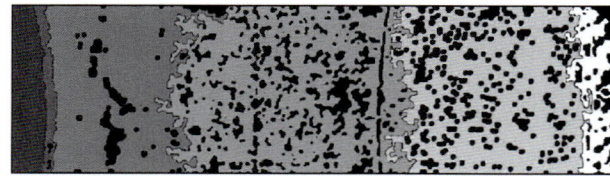

Figure 19.14 Image after split and merge algorithms.

Figure 19.15 Final image.

- Medium high intensity pixels (grey scale between 170 and 200) were selected and their value set to 255 (maximum grey scale) while all others were reduced to zero. This resulted in a binary black and white image (Fig. 19.8).

- A dilation operator was performed (40) using as the structuring element a square image made of 8 pixels at 255 and 1 pixel at 0. This enlarged areas of foreground pixels and reduced the holes within these areas (Fig. 19.9).

- A median filter was applied (41) once with a 3 × 3 window in order to eliminate impulse elements from the image and the "pepper and salt" noise (Fig. 19.10).

- The Roberts cross difference operator was applied (42) in its square root form. This gradient allows a preliminary edge detection (Fig. 19.11).

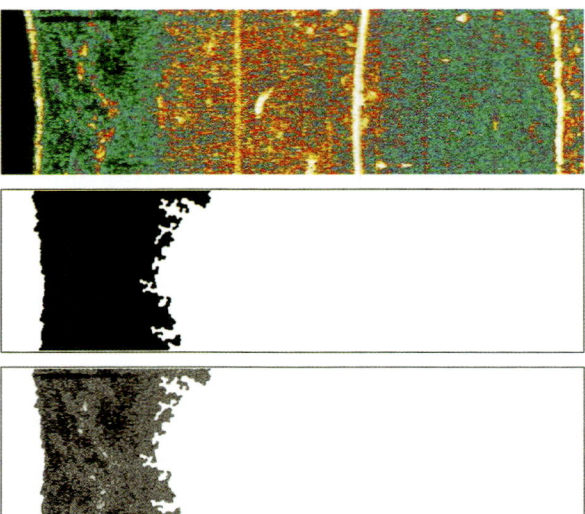

Figure 19.16 Comparison between original and final images.

- Holes were closed (43) using the same structuring element as used in the dilation above (Fig. 19.12).

- A dilation was successively applied, a median filter six times and a Roberts cross difference operator, as described above (Fig. 19.13).

- A split and merge algorithm was applied (44) in order to reintroduce a differentiation of grey scales in the image and to eliminate remaining artefacts between the epidermis and the hypodermic boundary that had been obtained, by filtering pixels with low grey scale (Fig. 19.14).

- The previous operation was repeated until the space between the epidermis and the hypodermic boundary was cleared of any artefact and was brought to a zero grey scale level, while the rest of the image obtained appears at 255 grey scale levels (Fig. 19.15).

The black area on the image that was so obtained at the end of this process was the zone of interest i.e. the space between the epidermis and the hypodermic boundary.

This area was characterized by the number of pixels at zero grey scale (black) multiplied by the area of 1 pixel:

$$\frac{12 \text{ mm} \times 13 \text{mm}}{1024 \times 224} = 6.8 \times 10^{-4} \text{mm}^2$$

The resulting surface was divided by the number of pixel lines (224) to determine the average depth of the dermis.

Echogenicity was obtained from the images in the format of the ultrasound machine using the following procedure:

- The processed image was superimposed onto the original ultrasound image.
- The resulting shape of the zone of interest was copied manually onto the ultrasound image (Fig. 19.16).
- Segment pixels above 40 grey scale were considered to have medium to high echogenicity.
- The segmented area and the total area of the zone of interest were provided as calculated by the ultrasound machine.
- The ratio of the segmented area to the total area was calculated, expressed as a density of echogenicity.

20 Dermoelectroporation and Biodermogenesi®
Pier Antonio Bacci

Cellulitis represents today an unaesthetic condition that requires a precise diagnosis and a precise therapeutical strategy characterised by an integrated treatment with various methodologies.

The aim of the treatment is the best use of the various methodologies and their therapeutic characteristics with the purpose of improving both the aesthetic aspect of the orange peel, the appearance of the unattractive dimpled skin or "dimpled fat", and the istho-pathological alterations that plotted them.

The scientific theory of cellulite is that the skin's underlying support called fibrous septae do not hold the skin together evenly and this uneven support causes the irregular bulging and dimples. The skin is tethered down by string-like tissues that pull it inward, toward the interior of the body.

The tension of these strings pulls sections of fat in along with them.

Cellulite has been compared to the dimples in a mattress that are caused by the strings that hold the "tucks" down. In some regions, such as the back part of the thigh and in the inferior part of the buttock, because of the position, treatment can be difficult.

In fact, it's possible to notice fibrous tissue, with evident lipodisthrophy characterized by little water, little degenerated fat and confined fibrous nodules and with fibrous strings where the microcirculation has altered and the thermography points out a low gradient of oxygen vascularisation, that is "cold cellulites".

A relaxed tissue and lipodisthrophy could have been plotted instead in the arms and in the inside area of the thigh, with elegant skin, a little bedewed but not fibrous.

It is necessary, in the first case, to vascularise, to activate the metabolism and to induce the arrival of water and trophic substances, in the second case it is necessary to increase the tone and the trophism of the tissue without water loss which would provoke further yelding.

Of extreme utility the new "dermoelectroporation" is shown for its characteristics of transdermal introduction of nutritional drugs and as a metabolic activator [1].

The progress of medicine in these last decades, particularly those of molecular biology have allowed us to understand many physiopathological trials and their relationships with the anatomical structures and methabolic functions, up to the control of the genetic structures, certainly opening new perspectives to medicine.

The enormous consequential impulse from the adoption of the biomolecular strategies, in partnership to the best understanding of the genetic phenomenons have opened the road to new methodologies. Among these we find dermoelectroporation® [2–6].

This new methodology is a patented and powered drug delivery system that is indicated for the local administration of ionic drug solutions into the body for medical purposes and can be used, in particular cases, as an alternative to injections.

What's "dermoelectroporation"?

The skin has an exchange function with the outside environment, which is also used as a means of pharmacological introduction [7].

Endermic diffusion is a passive phenomenon; in fact the skin behaves like a passive membrane. Penetration of the substances takes place in two stages characterized by:

1. Dormancy stage, in which the dermic layer is charged, usually electrically
2. Flow stage, in which the flow becomes constant

Dermoelectroporation treatment is a method that enables absorption using equipment that generates special electric pulses allowing the opening of special "electric gates" promoting the passage of substances of adequate size.

In 1970 a group of American dermatologists discovered that by applying an intense electric impulse for a short time at an adequate wavelength, the consequence was a change in polarization of the cellular membrane which could be used to promote a kind of cellular "pulsation".

In fact, after the initial pulse, the polarity is slowly reversed, avoiding electrolysis, and this opens intercellular channels through which substances can pass.

Once they are formed, these channels stay open for a relatively long time, several seconds.

This method was named electroporation treatment and was used, with special techniques, in the transdermic treatment of melanoma.

Electroporation with high voltage is the only system, known until now, to introduce trasdermally the substances of high molecular weight. Over 4000 published scientific reports demonstrate the activity and possibilities of the method [8].

Despite the very similar name, "Dermoelectroporation" is different, because the new method works with lower voltages in comparison to "electroporation".

In the apparatus used for medical and aesthetic purposes (Transderm Ionto® by Mattioli Engineering), dermoelectroporation treatment is applied by a discharge given by an electric inductor charged at a controlled current value and then discharged with a typical kind of reversible exponential voltage wave.

Why does the new method work well only after dermabrasion of the horny layer?

The answer could be that the high voltage in the classical electroporation produces part poration of the horny layer, part poration of the derma (with the residual energy after having perforated the horny layer).

Dermoelectroporation eliminates the need for the high voltage because the horny layer is eliminated with the dermabrasion and so the voltage to porate the derma is lower.

It works like the high voltage electroporation, but replaces the dangerous and hardly controllable effect of the high voltage on the horny layer with the safer dermabrasion.

The smaller energy is used only in order to open watery channels in the derma.

"Transderm® methodology"

It is a methodology that enables transdermal absorption using an apparatus that generates pulses able to open "intercellular gates" used for the passage of substances of suitable dimension avoiding damage to the cellular membranes and of the genoma.

In the apparatus used in our clinical and aesthetical goals (defined Trasnderm® by the producer Mattioli Engineering of Florence) the electric activity of electroporation is given by a discharge sent by an electric inductor loaded with a current value able to produce discharge tensions up to 100 volts and therefore unloaded with a typical reversing exponential waveform (Fig. 20.1).

In contact with the skin an intense ion flux develops that allows to directly charge the skin to a value proportional to the voltage applied.

In this way a temporary perturbation of the normal value of the potential of the cellular membrane occurs and this determines an increase of the permeability; this is dermoelectroporation.

Such situation remains for a limited time, because of the mechanisms of electrolitic conductivity, the potential on the membrane to reach again its equilibrium state.

The technical innovation of the instrument is the use of a transformer to control the current and therefore the ion flux.

The Transderm® realizes a sequence of impulses of opposite polarity to avoid the phenomenon of electrolysis on the electrodes and electrolysis of the drug solution.

Dermoelectroporation, by providing a continuous reversed polarity current, controlling the average pulse value, and varying the pulse shape according to the skin's specific electrical impedance, promotes the transdermal delivery of drugs as in classical iontophoresis, despite the fact that the average current is zero.

Moreover, macromolecules are also transdermally delivered for the first time from an iontophoretic device.

The absence of temporary pH change allows the use of microdermabrasion before D.E.P. application.

Pre-treatment with microdermabrasion promotes the transdermal delivery rate and ensures repeatability as a result of the standardization of the thickness and permeability of the stratum corneum.

The pulse shapes operates at a much lower energy and penetrate even under high skin impedance conditions.

Possibility of use

Dermatological studies show as the intradermal or subcutaneous use of collagen, jaluronic or elastin is the natural trial of regeneration or production shown here, while it is known plotted regeneration can be stimulated using the substances of base that constitute the precursors of such substances.

All of this has opened a new frontier in the anti-aging protocols of regeneration and of rejuvenation reducing, in the meantime, the use of the needles and bloodier methodologies.

Our experience is particularly on the face where we have had good results using the protocol named "Bioresurfacing" that signifies a treatment procedure aimed at rejuvenating the face by non-surgical, "soft", out-patient treatment means [9–11].

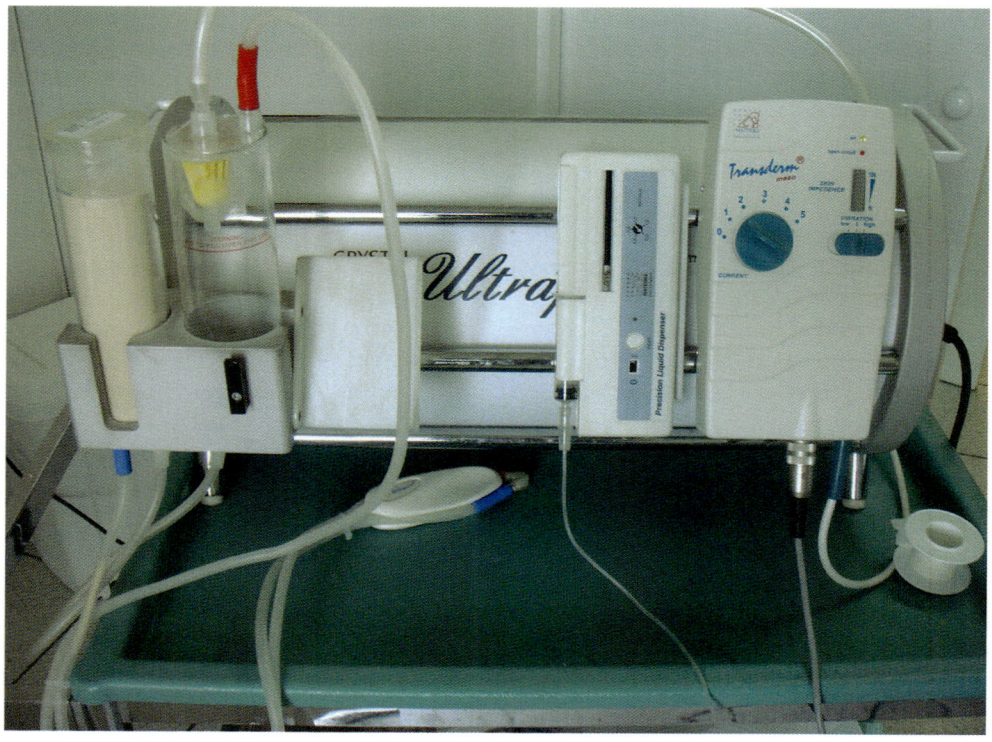

Figure 20.1 This instrument contains in the same structure two probes for microdermobrasion and dermoelectroporation, and one electronic pump to distribute equally different subtstances.

This procedure is suitable in subjects exhibiting the effects of acne, initial stages of skin aging without tissue yield, and upkeep of aesthetic surgery.

The treatment requires bimonthly or monthly sessions – a total of four to eight – of a procedure consisting first of superficial microdermabrasion performed with corundum crystals, intended for the removal of the corneus layer and for vascularization.

The treatment is aimed at improving the outer appearance by stimulating reconstitution of new collagenous and matrix tissue, but also reducing fibrosis in the difficult areas.

Skin smoothing performed by very superficial microdermabrasion with corundum powder crystals, being made aseptic by means of non-alcoholic detergents, the skin is smoothed without being traumatized. At the end of the session, the crystals remaining on the skin are used to perform a final regularizing "gommage" with the fingers, and then the skin is washed with physiological solution (Fig. 20.2).

These crystals are then used with a manual massage to promote further mechanical smoothing of the skin.

Immediately afterwards, active substances such as collagen, jaluronic acid, amino acids and elastin or, better, their precursors are introduced by means of the dermoelectroporation treatment, this new method for this purpose, consisting of a device that exploits an electric wave characterized by the possibility of creating the opening of "intercellular gates" that allow the passage of the molecules.

Over the clean skin a sterile gauze pad is applied and on it is poured a sterile solution of glicin, praline, lysine and glucoamminoglycan (so the precursors of the collagen and elastin and jaluronic acid) whose transdermic introduction is helped by the dermoelectroporation treatment. The procedure usually lasts 5 minutes per area, until the substances are absorbed. To care for a little area with fibrosis and sclerotic septum we can use a particular probe normally used to care for irregulaties of the lips (Fig. 20.3).

The equipment for dermoelectroporation treatment also makes use of a vibrating action that stimulates the Merkel corpuscles to greater connective restructuring of the tissue itself.

The cellulitis asks for integrated treatments according to the various pathologies. There exist however zones of extreme

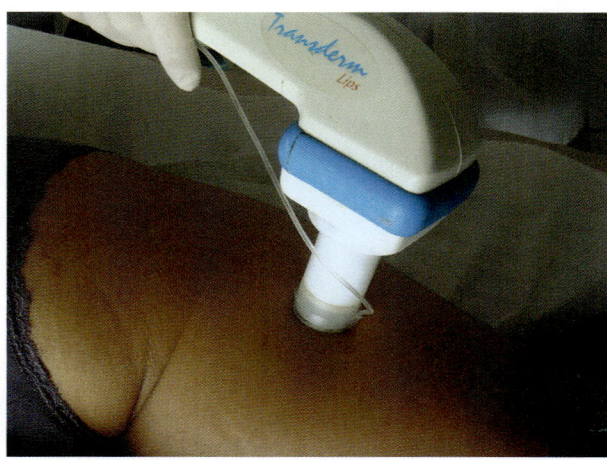

Figure 20.3 This slide shows the second phase of dermoelectroporation to introduce nutritional subtances.

difficulty such as the back part of the thigh, that have shown notable improvements using, as extension of the normal protocols, a new I manipulate of dermoelectroporation purposely conceived and improved.

University of Florence experimental studies have shown the passage of trains of bovine collagen type 1, a big molecule of 0,8 micron, in the skin of rape using the methodology Transderm® [12,13].

It's interesting to notice that as the molecules enter precise zones of the skin using some watery channels, "the watery electropores" they arrive in depth [14,15]. The big molecules, such as collagen, have not altered.

Biodermogenesi®

This new Italian method is aimed to care for the alterations of the skin structure characterised by fibrosis and reduction of the microcirculation (Fig. 20.4).

This new methodology presents four phases of treatment. In the first phase a very superficial mechanical peeling is done to stimulate a mechanical activation of the micro-circulation of the skin, with the second phase using electric power to bring nutrition to the tissue and cells using the active ingredients as precursors of elastic and collagen. In the third phase, by the magnetic field, we bring the blood moderately to the surface and we contemporaneously favour a cellular mitosis, particularly to the fibrose tissues. In the fourth phase we activate a lymphatic drainage to reabsorb toxins and water produced with the driven mitosis, at the same time we restore the normal pH and hydro-lipid film of the skin.

The third phase of this treatment is, with no doubt, the most important one. The situation created from the continuous and repetitive ionic migration, guaranteed by the higher activity driven from sodium and potassium, realises a good cellular nutrition and a toxin elimination. Thanks to the attrition generated by the moving ions and to the better blood flux, with consequential increasing of the oxygenation of the treated area, we can improve the tissular temperature of 2–3 degrees centigrade favoring tissue regeneration by an increase of the cellular mitosis by 300%, thanks also to the flux of blood and oxygen.

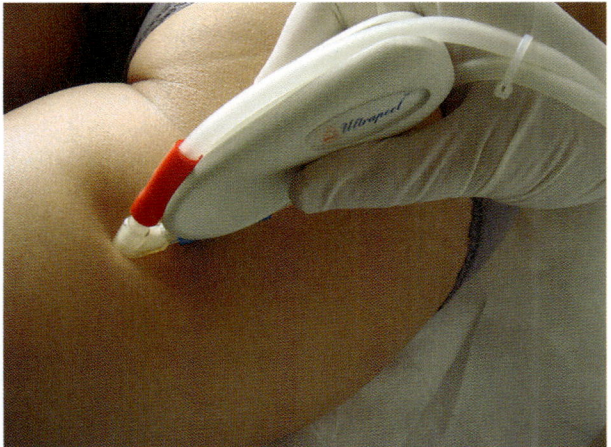

Figure 20.2 This slide shows the first phase of microdermabrasion using corundum crystals.

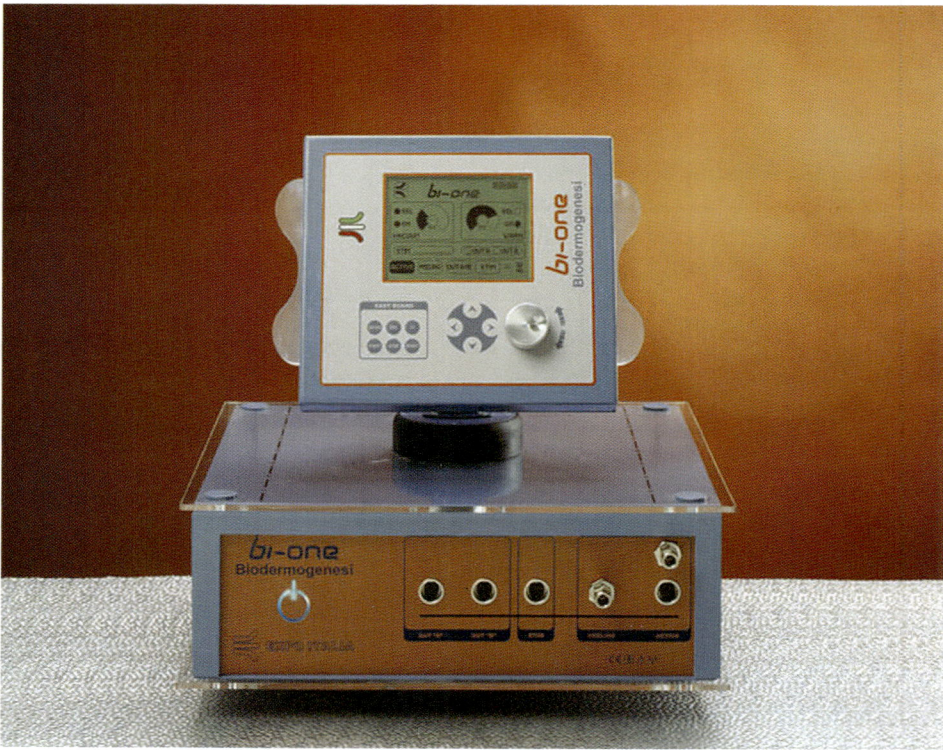

Figure 20.4 This instrument contains two probes for use of magnetic fields.

This instrument produces energy with a variable and constant intensity of frequency, measuring through the feedback, the quantity of energy that can be actually efficacious.

This exclusive stimulation interacts with the sodium and potassium pumping, which are real biological vehicles able to transport inside the cellular membrane all precursors for intracutaneous nutrition. This synergy permits the derma to expand, encouraging a progressive renovation of the capillary calibre (Fig. 20.5).

Clinical studies and biopsies enable us to see the change of the skin structure about extracellular matrix and collagen tissue. We can see also an interesting increase of reticular layer demonstrating a new metabolism of the skin thanks to the better microcirculation [16,17] (Figs. 20.6 and 20.7).

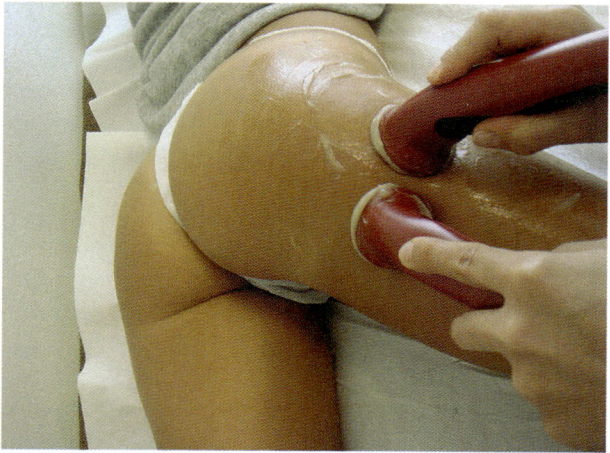

Figure 20.5 Two probes provide magnetic fields to increase temperature and microcirculation.

The regenerative process of the Biodermogenesi™ is determined with the production of collagen and elastic fibers in order to permit a stability of the obtained result. The elastic collagen starts to take its specific action inside the skin which gives the correct support that permits the blood supply of capillary and reactivates the fibroblast (Figs. 20.8 and 20.9).

The reactivation of cell production, a superior vascularisation and restart of the lymphatic circulation system are able to guarantee a superior hydration of the tissue that has a much more compact and turgid look. Using this strategy in the difficult area, as an internal face of the thigh of a young girl with stretch marks and cellulitis, we can have a real improvement of the visibility of the red marks with reduction of the scars and the orange peel skin at the same time.

Biodermogenesi is a revolutionary method for cellulitis because it uses a sophisticated device emitting radiofrequencies and magnetic fields together, providing us with the possibility of reducing the cellulitic nodules without causing damage to the vascular structure, muscles, bones and internal organs. The adipose cellulites which are effected by this treatment deflate with liberating lipids and triglycerides which then will be eliminated physiologically from the organism, but above all liberate the energy.

Here is the innovation: this energy is used from the other handful of magnetic fields which is used at the same moment and has the capacity to restore the tissue, avoiding breakdown and treating the orange peel skin.

Each Biotermogenesi session is about 40 minutes for 10–20 cycles of a treatment (Fig. 20.10).

The new method takes the advantage of uniting the magnetic fields and shock waves in a way to induce a progressive reduction of the adipose tissue and progressive repair of the tissue with the

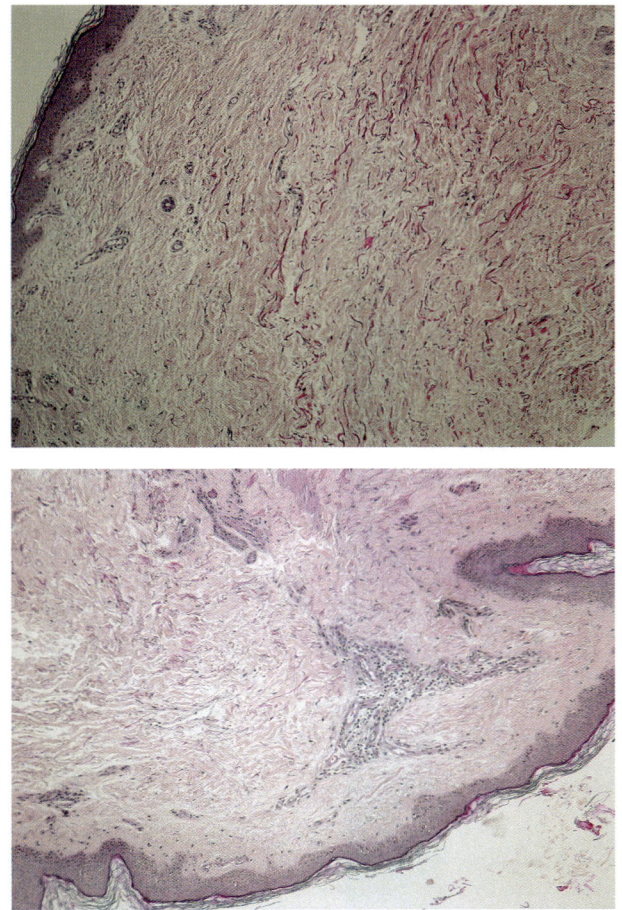

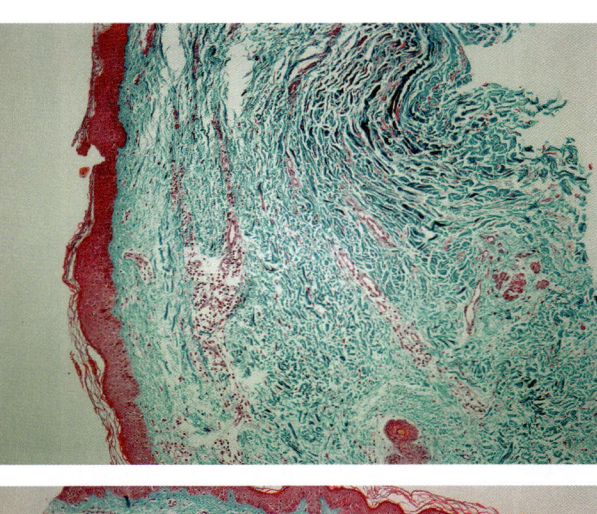

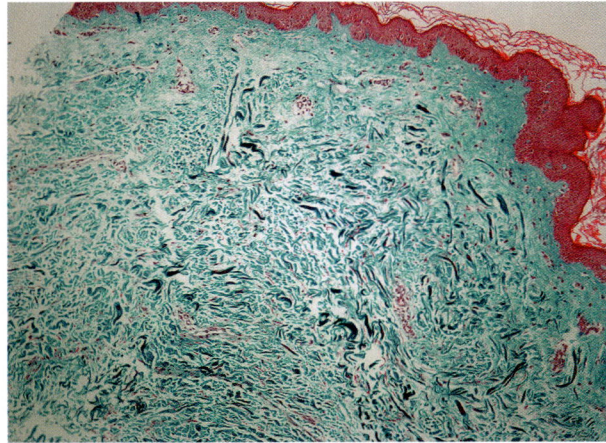

Figures 20.6–7 These biopsies, before and after, show the improvement of the skin with fibrose cellulite and stretch marks only using the Biodermogenesi, we can see the increase of reticular fibers after treatments.

Figures 20.8–9 These biopsies, before and after, show the improvement of the same are with the reduction of pericapillar flogosis, an improvement of reticular dermal layer and regularisation of the collagen.

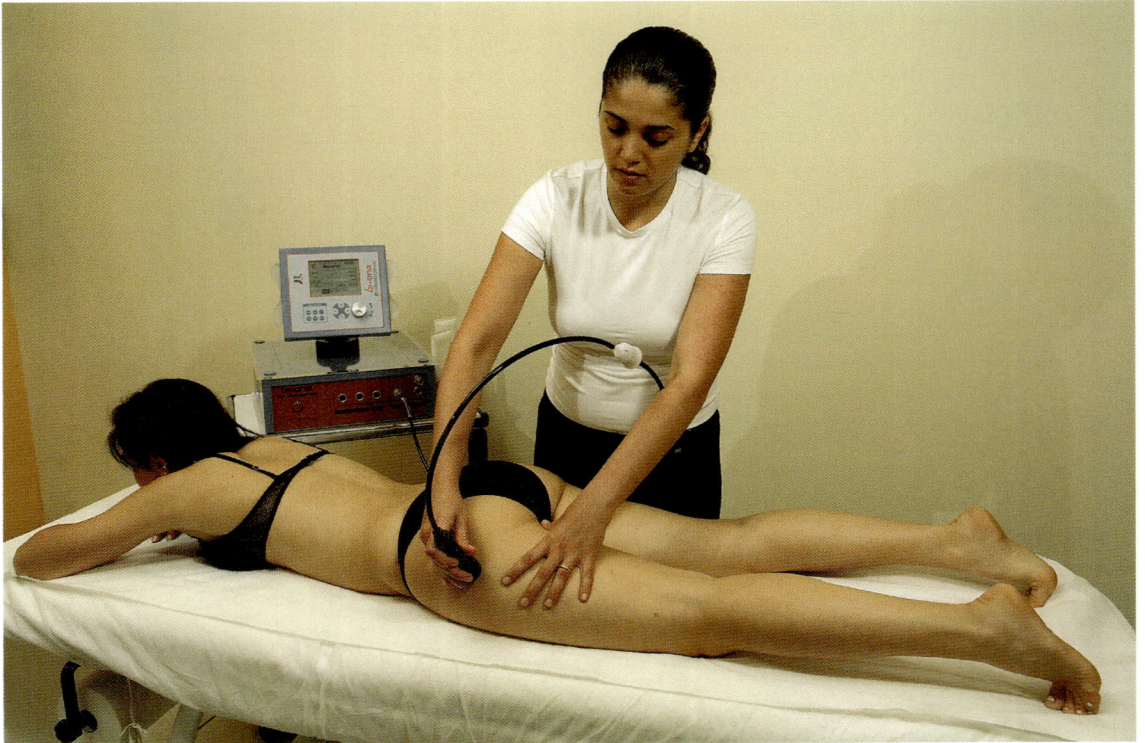

Figure 20.10 The application of Biodermogenesi.

cellulite. For the first time a method of work is studied that on the same device is reacting on two levels contemporaneously using the energies that are compatible biologically, first fighting against adiposity for reduction then transforming part of the same adipose tissue in to an energy which is necessary for the repair of the skin with the cellulite.

The utilisation of this method will become a must in the treatment of all kinds of cellulite, for different reasons classified in four clinical groups, each of them needs a different personalised treatment.

Dermoelectroporation and Biodermogenesi

We cannot have miracles, and this integrated protocol does not substitute liposculpture but it can be a good integration of the surgical moment and an interesting solution for non-surgical patients.

The experience of using the two combined therapies gave very interesting results on more than 100 treated patients, 30 patients done with the single handful confirmed the positive results especially those who followed a complete combined treatment.

There are several stages in attaining this end:

1. Traction of the strings, lymphatic drainage and vascularization performed with Endermologie®.
2. Skin smoothing performed by very superficial microdermabrasion with corundum powder crystals (Ultrapeel Transderm® by Mattioli Engineering).
3. Electric and pharmacological stimulation, using the dermoelectroporation treatment with Transderm®.
4. After that we can apply a session of Biodermogenesi (by Expo Italia®) to improve the cellular activity and adipose methabolism using magnetic field.

The treatment is usually performed once or twice a week for 10–15 times, and then a maintenance treatment every 21 days.

Certainly, DermoElectroPoration and Biodermogenesi are not the panacea for cellulite but it is an interesting integrated and non-invasive treatment, as a valid weapon for the treatment of the adipose and fibrose cellulite in the difficult areas, as posterior area of the thigh, buttock and for painful cellulite [22–24].

Surely, however, it represents a new frontier in the knowledge of the physiopathology and in the treatment of that great world of the "interstitial matrix" and it certainly represents an open window in the future.

REFERENCES

1. PA Bacci, Dermoelectroporation: clinical observations, in Reserved File Mattioli Engineering – Florence, (2002–2003)
2. CT Costello, AH Jeske, Iontophoresis: applications in trandermal medication delivery. Phys Ther 75:554–63, 1995.
3. C Curdy, YN Kalia, RH Guy, Non invasive assessment of the effects of iontophoresis on human skin in vivo. J.Pharm 53(6):769–77, Jun 2001.
4. A Jadoul, J Bouwstra, VV Prest. Effects of iontophoresis and electroporation on the stratum corneum, Review of the basical study. Adv Drug Deliv Rev 4;35(1):89–95, Jan 1999.
5. WE Rhodes, Iontophoretic based trandermal delivery: new advance revitalise an establishment technology. Drug Delivery Tecnology, 1995.
6. AA Shults, TD Strout, P Jordan, B Worthing, Safety, tolerability and efficacy of iontophoresis with lidocaine for dermal anesthesia in ED pediatric patients. J Emerg Nurs 29(4): 289–96, August 2002.
7. FG Albergati, PA Bacci, La matrice extracellulare, Minelli Ed., Arezzo, Italy, 2004.
8. PA Bacci, Cirurgia minimamente invasive con hilos tesores, Amolca, Caracas, 2007: 98–120.
9. PA Bacci, The bioresurfacing and the role of dermoelectroporation on aesthetic medicine of the face, Italian Congress of Aesthetic Medecin, Milan, October 2001. Abstract.
10. PA Bacci, The bioresurfacing and dermoelectroporation, Annual meeting of AACS, Hollywood, January 29th 2004, Abstract book.
11. PA Bacci, The bioresurfacing, 4th World Congress on Cosmetic and Dermatologic Surgery, APACS, February 26–29th, 2004, Manila Philippines, Abstract book.
12. S Pacini, B Peruzzi, M Gulisano et al. Qualitative and quantitative analysis od trandermic delivery of different biological molecules by iontophoresis, Italian Journal of Anatomy and Embriology, September 14–18th, 2003, Vol 18, Suppl. N.2, Book 3; July–September 2003: 127.
13. M Gulisano, S Pacini, S Menchetti et al. Analisi qualitativa e quantitativa sperimentale di ionoforesi, in PA Bacci, S Mariani. "La flebologia in pratica", Alberti & C. Ed, Arezzo –Italy, 2003, 107–11, ISBN 88.87936.595.
14. S Pacini, B Peruzzi, GF Bernabei et al. In vivo evaluation of transdermal delivery of collagen and lidocaine by a novel system of dermoelectroporation, Reserved File Mattioli Engineering – Florence, 2003 (to publied).
15. Asbill, El. Cattan, B Michniak, Enhancement of transdermal drug delivery: chemical and physical approaches. Crit Rev Ther Drug Carr Syst 17(6):621–58, 2000.
16. PA Bacci, La biodermogenesi, Eupraghia, Minelli editore, 1:2–3, 2009.
17. PA Bacci, M Busoni, R La Marca, Studio bioptico dopo trattamento con biodermogenesi – Atti Congresso de Cirurgia y medicina Estetica, Sitges, Barcelona 15 May, 2009.

21 Carboxitherapy
Gustavo Leibaschoff

Carboxitherapy consists of the therapeutic use of carbon dioxide (CO_2) in its gaseous state, either transcutaneous or by subcutaneous injection.

Carbodioxidetherapy (CDT) is the subcutaneous administration of the gas.

This therapy was first performed in Argentina [1] and in France, in the thermal waters station of Royat, near Clermont Ferrand [2]. There a group of cardiologists from the hospital of Clermont Ferrand, began to treat patients with peripheral organic and functional arteriopathies (atherosclerotic, Buerger's disease, Raynaud's disease, etc.). In 1953 the cardiologist Jean Baptiste Romuef, published a paper about his 20 years of experience with the subcutaneous injection of CO_2 [3]. Afterwards, the Parisian cardiologist Jerome Berthier, along with Luigi Parassoni from Gaillard A, started its application on patients with cellulite [4].

The first paper about the use of CDT was published in the Journal of the Argentine Medical Association (1934).

Up to 1983 402,000 patients had been treated in Royat. By 1994, 20,000 patients were treated per year. This number of patients confirms the popularity and perhaps the efficacy of this therapeutic method.

Carbon dioxide (CO_2) is an odorless colorless gas first discovered by Van Helmont, in 1648. The clinical use of CO_2 is not new. Many years ago, in France, Clermont Ferrand used thermal CO_2 (CO_2 99.4%, N 0.558%, O_2 0.021%, plus argon, xenon, and krypton traces) for treating lower limb peripheral arteriopathies, especially the obliterating ones [5].

When administered subcutaneously, CO_2 immediately diffuses at the coetaneous and muscular microcirculatory level.

After the administration of 200 cc of CO_2 in the canine thigh subcutaneous tissue, CO_2 is detected in femoral venous blood in approximately 5 minutes, with a maximum time lag of 30 minutes. This demonstrates the ability of CO_2 to diffuse across fasciae, and reach the underlying muscles [6].

Most of the gas is eliminated through the lungs (expiration), while a smaller portion is converted into carbonic acid in tissues and eliminated through the kidneys.

At the vascular level, CO_2 increases vascular tone and produces active microcirculatory vasodilatation. CO_2-induced vasodilatation results from its direct activity on arteriole smooth muscle cells [7].

In addition, this promotes Bohr's effect, a mechanism that allows tissue CO_2 transfer to lungs and lung O_2 transfer to tissues through the oxy-hemoglobin dissociation curve. When administered through an external route, CO_2 promotes this mechanism, resulting in a higher tissue oxygenation and neoangiogenesis.

Although it is toxic when inhaled (10% in air may cause asphyxia), subcutaneous or intra-abdominal administration of CO_2 has not shown any toxic effects, even at high doses (2–10 liters).

Pharmacodynamics

- Active vasodilatation
- Direct activity on arteriolar smooth muscle fiber
- Sympathicolytic activity
- Increase in arterio-arteriolar sphygmicity
- Increase of oxidative phenomena, with the resulting hydrolysis of triglycerides into fatty acid in the adipose tissue
- Haemorheologic activity
- Improves erythrocyte deformation

Indications

Cosmetic medicine
  Cellulite PEFE [8]
  Localized adiposity
  Skin laxity
  Aging skin of the face [22,23]
  Stretch marks (estriae)
Cosmetic Surgery [11]
  Pre and post lipo [25]
  Complications of lipo
Angiology
  Organic and functional artheriopathies
  Microangiopathies (atherosclerosis, diabetic)
Urology
  Erectile dysfunction
Dermatology
  Psoriasis
Phlebology
  Ulcers

Cosmetic Surgery

In this case I use CO_2 three weeks before liposculpture and continue the treatment 10 days after the surgery, for two months, twice a week (pre- and post-liposculpture) [9].

According to the most recent studies, cellulite has its origins in the ECM (extracellular matrix) and in the microcirculatory alterations, the network of diminutive arteries, veins and lymphatics that crosses the connective tissue.

If this microcirculatory system starts failing, the tissue is not fed efficiently.

Substances start accumulating and forming edemas, nodules, and skin retractions.

The CO_2 reverses this situation when injected in the affected zones through a very thin needle (27 G). It produces vasodilatation [10].

It improves the speed of the microcirculation (increase flow motion).

The tissues receive more oxygen and the toxins are eliminated.

The edema is reduced.

It also favors the lipolisis (reduces the size of the fat cells), and the lipoclasis (the destruction of the fat cells) [13].

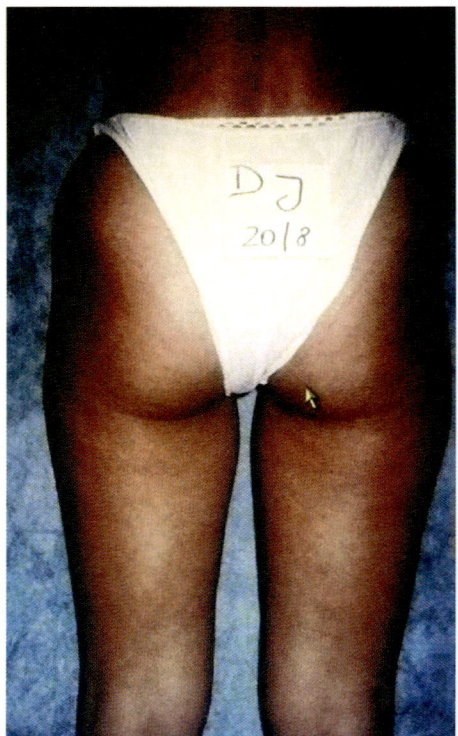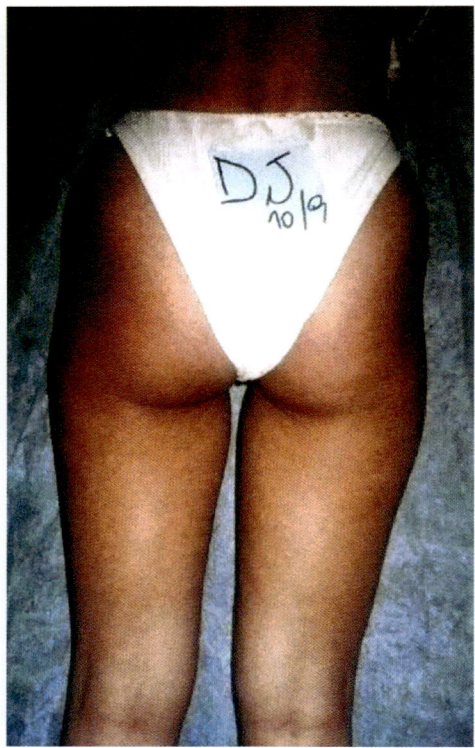

Figure 21.1 Before and after with CO_2, twice a week plus mesotherapy; notice the surface of the skin. (=1E, p. 199, Fig. 2).

Another interesting fact is that Carboxitherapy provides excellent results for patients with longtime cellulite.

It also provides great results for young patients as a preventive method.

Lipodystrophy and cellulite are pathologies in which micro-circulatory disorders resulting in interstitial edema constitute triggering factors that also support the pathological process. Since subcutaneous CO_2 improves capillary blood flow and reduces stasis, Carboxitherapy contributes to the restoration of microvascular-tissue unit exchanges.

Administrated through a subcutaneous route, CO_2 causes subcutaneous microcirculation vasodilatation expressed in an increase of blood flow and the opening of "virtual" capillaries that normally are closed. This seems to occur from dilatation of arteriole smooth muscle cells [12], with an increase in tissue CO_2 that is maintained for a certain post-therapy period [13].

In the case of cellulite and lipolymphedema, Carboxitherapy shows an effective activity. Cellulite and lipolymphedema show microvascular alterations (stasis micro-angiopathy) and histomorphological disorders (adipocyte aggregation and fibrosis) [18].

Carboxitherapy technique produces a lipolysis action by increasing the blood flow in pre-capillary arterioles and also by stimulating the fat cells' beta1-2 adreno-receptors [24].

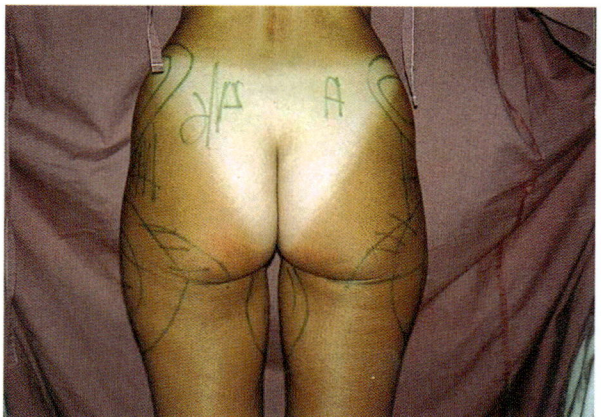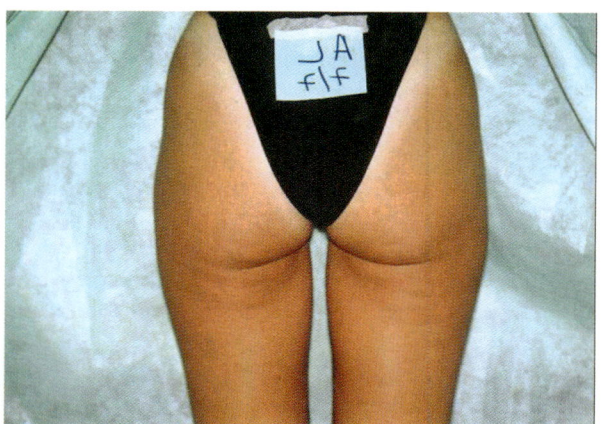

Figure 21.2 Before and after treatment with Carboxitherapy, plue mesotherapy and Endermologie.

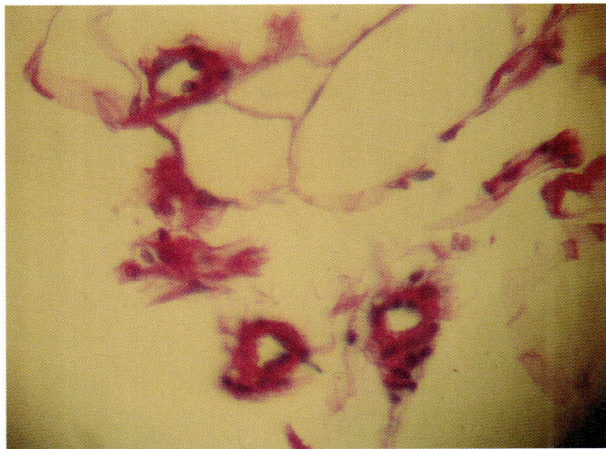

Figure 21.3 The sections show subcutaneous cell tissue with varying degrees of mucinosis, interstitial edema, and proliferation of blood and lymphatic vessels with varying degrees of microangiopathies (grade 1 and 2, according to Handelsman). There is fibrous thickening of the interlobar connective septa and inflammatory perivascular and interstitial infiltrates [25]. Diagnosis: Edematous-fibrosclerotic panniculopathy (cellulite).

The concept of localized adiposity is often misunderstood.

Histological studies showed hypertrophic fat cells (larger size), hyperplasy fat cells (larger number) and always a microcirculatory and lymphatic alteration is reported.

This is why CDT is suggested as an initial treatment in localized obesity, because it will improve the microcirculation and the lymphatic system helping in that way to eliminate the metabolites of the fat cells.

This was also evident in treatments for systemic multiple lipomatosis in which, in combination with surgery, a reduction in adipose masses was observed. Hence, it is evident that Carboxitherapy has good results both in terms of clinical manifestations and histology [14].

Treatment Method
Equipment
Allows CO_2 administration in a controlled manner: flow velocity, injection time, total volume and monitoring of administration dose percentage.

The gas in the canister is administered in sterile conditions, at very low pressure.

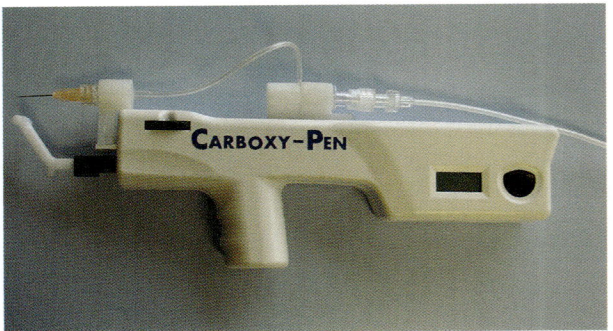

Figure 21.4 Modern device for Carboxitherapy, that allows work without pain and in a safe way.

(a)

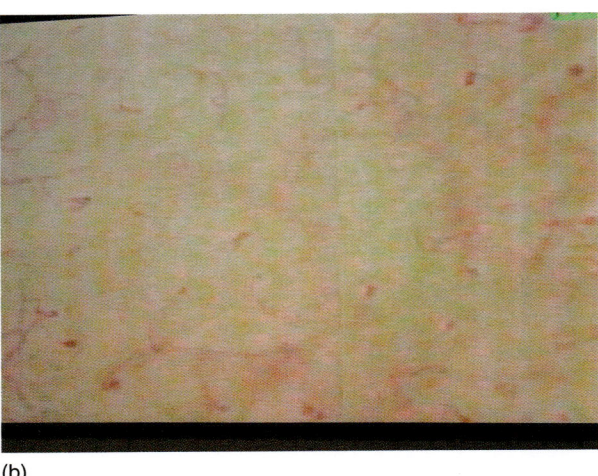

(b)

Figure 21.5 (a) Videocapillaroscopy before the use of CO_2; (b) After administration of subcutaneous CO_2, there is an increase in vertical capillaries (black points) and transverse capillarie.

Inject the gas through a state-of-the-art computerized unit at a constant pressure and volume in a period of time; also allow a perfect control of the amount of gas, from 1 cc to 100 cc.

CO_2 is applied in the subcutaneous through a very fine small needle (27 G, 30 G) and in a different depth accord the aesthetic pathology:

1 mm: In stretch marks, laxity in the face and neck,
2 mm: Detachment in the face and neck (for example, in deep nasolabio fold)
4 mm: Laxity in the body, and in the treatment of cellulite
8–10 mm: Subcutaneous administration in localized adiposity.

The goal for the successful subcutaneous application of CO_2 is injection in different planes, superficial (1 mm), medium (3–4 mm) for collagen stimulation and more uniform surface, and subdermal inside the fat deposit (6–10 mm) for lipolysis.

The Carboxitherapy (CDT) effects start in the microcirculation and can be observed through a videocapilaroscopy (VCP), allowing doctors to demonstrate the action of the technique before results are visualized on the surface [15].

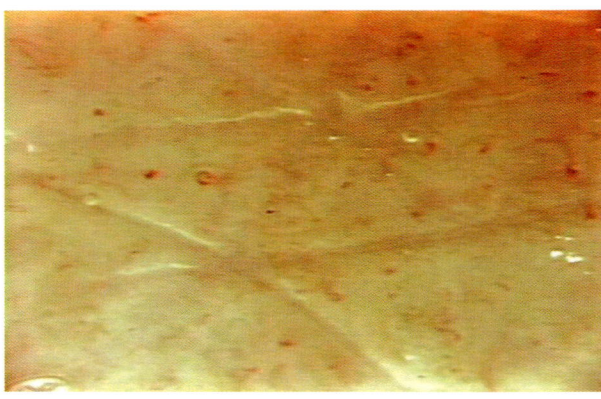 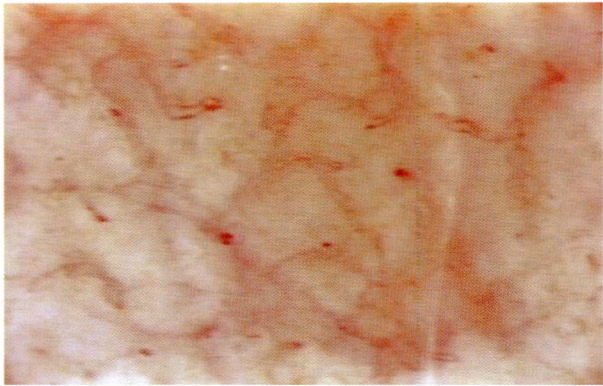

Figure 21.6 Before CO_2, less number of vertical capillaries (VC); after increase the number of VC and the color look more pink (increase of microcirculation).

Until now, the absence of clinical parameters and instruments, for the semiologic characterization and differential diagnosis limited treatment investigation to inspection and palpation.

With the VCP we can see the changes at microcirculatory level and know if we are making the right treatment.

VCP is a non-invasive method that analyzes capillaries through static and dynamic images [16].

Also, the VCP allows the observation of:

- morphology of vascular micro-architecture
- morphology of capillaries
- degree of capillary filling
- type of capillary flow (color)
- assessment of an increase in vascularization
- increase in capillary density
- morphology of the venular system.

One of the most scientific classifications of cellulite was made for the Plastic and Reconstructive Surgery Cathedra of the University of Sienna, headed by Dr. Prof. D´Aniello. They use the clinical, the videocapillaroscopy (VCP), the laser fluxometry and the histopathology for diagnostic classification.

This linkage of the morphologic and biologic allows us also to evaluate evolutionary purposes and prognoses.

A complete system consists of a probe, a lens, a power supply, and a monitor. The handheld probe is comfortable and lightweight. Lenses are easily installed and switched.

The VL-7EX features freeze-frame capability. The VL-7EX video microscope is a high quality, low cost, light weight, and handheld electronic imaging system. Video microscopy allows the medical professional to perform evaluations of skin conditions "live" (microcirculation), while patients view their condition on the screen as the analysis is being performed. With the VL-7EX video microscope, one can see both the surface and sub-surface details in high resolution on a full-color video monitor display.

When used by aesthetic physicians, the Scalar VL-7EX video microscope enhances the client's understanding of the specific characteristics of the microcirculation and features of their skin.

Scalar VL-7EX video microscopes add efficiency and depth to analyses of skin (microcirculation). Effective treatment and services performed can be verified with before and after comparisons that are achieved by archiving video images to printers or VCRs attached to the instruments.

Gustavo Leibaschoff, MD, and Cosmetic Surgeon Luis Coll, MD (Universitary Dermatologist UBA) conducted development and study about the cellulite, Carboxitherapy (Carboxy-Pen™) and videocapilaroscopy in 15 patients with cellulite syndrome (EFP).

The images obtained in the prospective study by VCP showed that immediately after the first session using Carboxitherapy in different doses, 150 cc and 50 cc vertical capillaries significantly increase, $35.2 +/-3.3\%$ per mm^2 in the area of injection.

After a week of the Carboxitherapy session the images showed a decrease of 8.2% of vertical capillaries compared with the previous images post-injection.

Contraindications of CDT

Recent or acute myocardial infarction
Inestable angina
Congestive heart failure
Severe high blood pressure
Acute thrombophlebitis
Gangrene
Localized infections
Epilepsy
Respiratory failure
Renal failure
Pregnancy

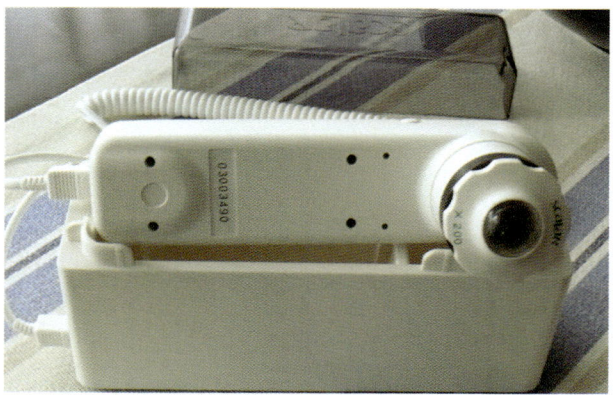

Figure 21.7 Scalar VL-7EX video visualization systems enhance skin analysis.

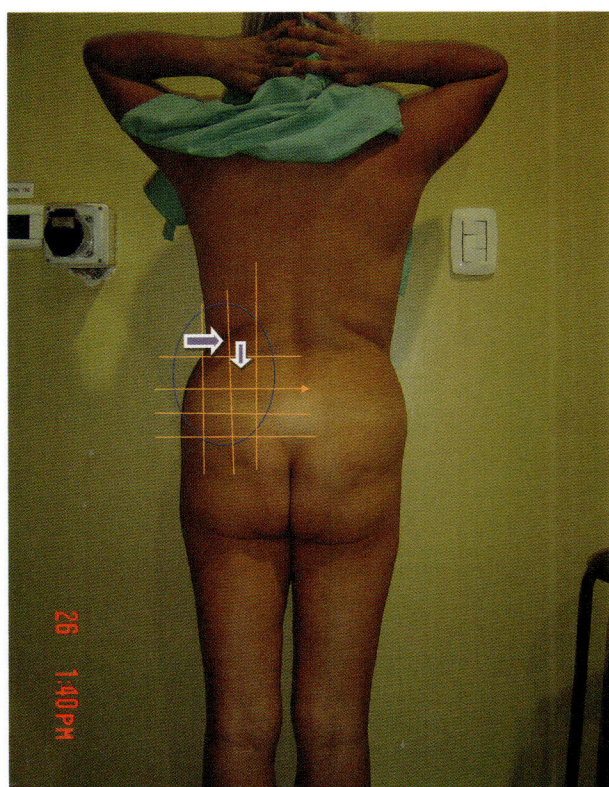

Figure 21.8 In each quadrant inject 50 cc (follow blue arrow).

Side Effects of CDT

Local burning or oppressive pain, fleeting, at the injection site are related to flow velocity and patient's pain threshold.

The Carboxy-Pen™ device uses an special regulator allowing a progressive control of the flow pressure of the gas injection with fewer less side effects.

Limb heaviness sensation (no longer than 2 hours), is related to dose (more than 300 cc in each limb).

Rubor at the injection site, during 30 minutes.

Echymosis (try to avoid vessels and varicose veins).

Subcutaneous crepitation, of variable duration (no longer than 30 minutes).

Protocol in Cellulite

Subcutaneous injection using volumes between 100–200 cc per limb. Initial flow may vary between 10–50 cc/min [17].

It is advisable to make punctures in different directions (downward-upward and upward-downward) with a 27 G or 30 G needle.

Divide the area into four to six quadrants per limb (see the diagram below).

The first session it is suggested to inject no more of 10–20 cc per quadrant and then in the following sessions increase up to 50 cc per quadrant.

Accompany with manual massage (move fingers as in piano playing over subcutaneous emphysema areas) in order to contribute to gas diffusion, to control emphysema and to reduce patient's possible discomfort.

Frequency of Sessions

On a daily basis

Ideal for patients staying at thermal centers or patients receiving one-week treatment. Generally, two or three cycles per year are suggested.

Two or three sessions per week

It is the more widespread frequency and the most recommended, particularly if symptoms and an important microcirculatory stasis are present. Also used for achieving lipolytic effects (to reduce localized obesities).

One session per week

An alternative for patients with aesthetic problems, showing no symptoms. At least 15 sessions should be performed.

CDT has its use in facial treatment as well, in the laxity of the skin, in the periocular area to decrease dark circles, to increase the firmness of the skin and reduce the hyperpigmentation.

In the skin rejuvenation before the mesotherapy, CDT increases the aesthetic results.

For a full facial treatment, the total of CO_2 is around 10 cc. In the forehead several punctures (six to eight weekly), 1 mm depth, 1 cc of CO_2. In the temporal and preauricular area (close to the hair line) one puncture in each area, weekly, 1 mm depth, 1 cc of CO_2.

Over crow's feet one puncture in each small line, weekly, 1 mm depth, 1 cc of CO_2.

In the superior eyelid, one puncture, monthly, 2 mm depth for detach, 1–2 cc of CO_2. The same for the inferior eyelid.

Over the Nasogenian fold first one puncture monthly, 2 mm depth for detach, 1 cc of CO_2 and 2 superficial punctures, 1 mm depth in the line of the Nasogenian fold, monthly, 1 cc of CO_2 each.

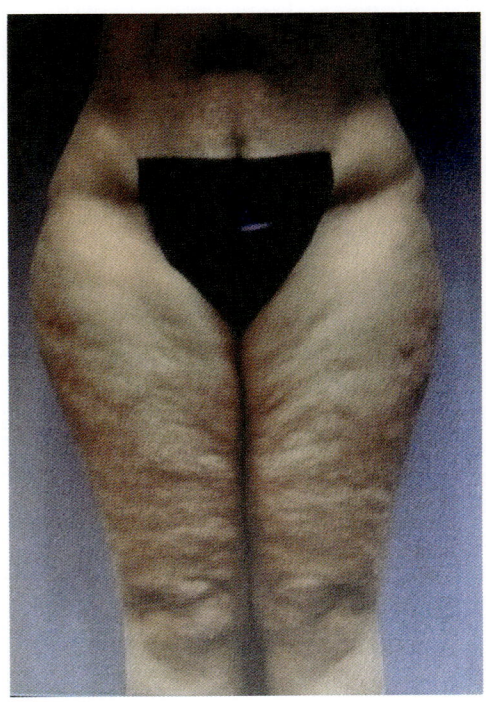

Figure 21.9 Before liposculpture.

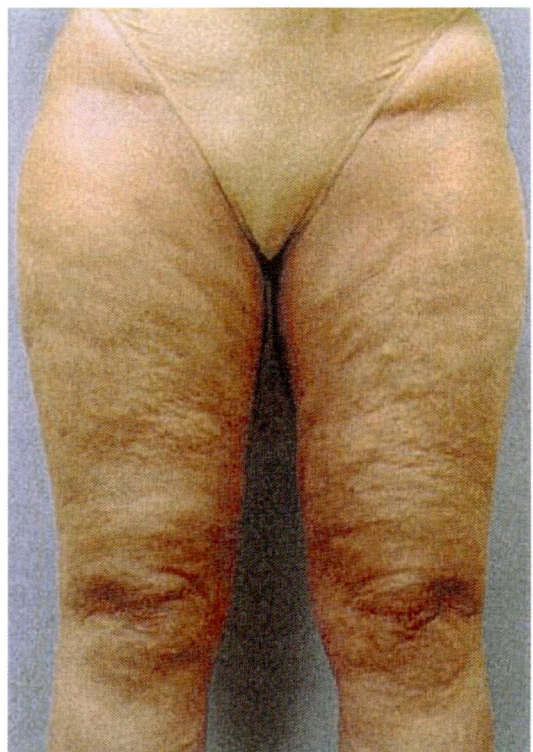 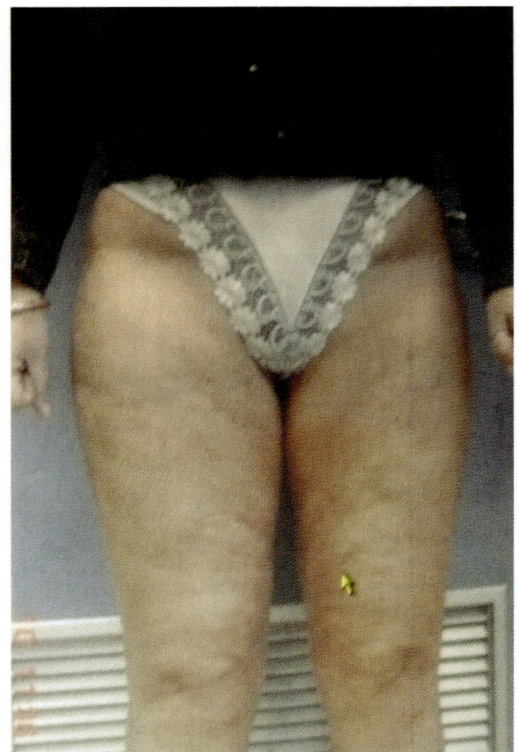

Figure 21.10 After liposuction and after 20 sessions of CO_2 300 cc each leg.

In the neck, if there is only laxity of the skin, three punctures, one below the lateral jaw angle (both sides), one below the chin, 2 mm depth for detach, 1–2 cc of CO_2 in each puncture every 15 days. With localized obesity in the neck, a subcutaneous puncture 6 mm depth, below the chin, 5–10 cc of CO_2 every 15 days.

For the revitalization of the chest, several punctures (six to eight) with a regular distribution, 1 mm depth, 1 cc of CO_2, weekly.

The eyelid treatment with Carboxitherapy used once weekly typically begins to show an improvement in eyelid pigmentation after one to three weeks, the texture after two to four weeks and the eyelid contour in three to five weeks.

When Carboxitherapy is performed less frequently the results occur more gradually.

The treatments continue for two to three months and need to be repeated after six to 12 months depending on the case [22].

Stretch Marks

The first results with the use of CDT are seen after a few sessions [21]. The quality of the skin is important in the treatment of the stretch marks. There will be a better result if there is a soft skin texture, a good firmness of the skin and a homogeneous color of the stretch marks (more pink).

One session every 15 days for three to four months.

The technique is a combination of a single deep puncture (6 mm) injecting CO_2 200 cc and multiple superficial (1 mm) punctures injecting CO_2 5 cc in each stretch mark path.

Conclusions

It's a useful tool for the treatment of cellulite, localized adiposities, stretch marks, skin laxity, etc.

Easy application with no significant or adverse side effects.

Possible association to other types of procedure (mesotherapy, radiofrequency, etc.) [20].

Device: It's important to have a device that allows a progressive control of the flow, slow or fast, small or larger amount of gas (1 cc to 100 cc) according to treatment needs. These are the conditions to obtain a painless application.

REFERENCES

1. Mariano Castex, A Di Cio. El anhidrico carbonico y el carbogeno en el tratamiento de las arteriopatias perifericas. Boletines de la academia nacional de medicina de Buenos, Buenos Aires; 1934.
2. M Castex, A Di cio, GA Lista. Mal perforante plantar con calcificacion arterial - Resultados del tratamiento con carbogeno. Revista de la Asociación Medica Argentina; DICIEMBRE 30 DE 1934.
3. F Romeuf. Etude sur l'injection sous cutanee de gaz thermaux de Royat. Clermont J B Imp Moderne, 15 rue du Port 31. Mars 1940.
4. A Gaillard. Interet de la technique des perfusions de gaz dans le traitment thermal des arteriopathies. Clemont Ferrand Thermal Royat 1988.
5. CA Petit. Guide thermal de Royat 12 eme (ed.) 1880–1898, Clermont Ferrand; 1980.
6. J Berthier. Arteriopathie diabetique et thermalisme. Reunion de l'Association Nationale de Formation Continue en Medicine Thermale, Paris; 17 decembre 1993.
7. C Colin, D Lagneaux, J Lecomte. Sur l'action vasodilatatrice du dioxyde de carbone injecte sous forme gazeuse

dans le tegument del'homme. Presse Thermale Climatique 116(4):255–58, 1979 France.

8. C Brandi. Rol del CO_2 como complemento de la lipoplastia. International School of Aesthetic Medicine. 8° Course of Aesthetic Medicine, Dpto. Of Plastic & Aesthetic Surgery University of Siena; 28–29/11/2003 – Italy.

9. E Savin, O Bailliart, P Bonin et al. Vasomotor effects of transcutaneous CO_2 in Stage II peripheral occlusive arterial disease. Angiology 46(9):786–91, 1995.

10. BR Hartman, E Bassenge, M Pittier. Effect of Carbon Dioxide enriched water on the cutaneous microcirculation and oxygen tension in the skin of the foot. Angiology 48(11):957–63, Nov 1997.

11. C Brandi, L Grimaldi, C D'aniello et al. Role of carbossiterapy in plastic surgery - Strategies for prevention :The role of medical sciences and nutrition - European Congress The Ageing Society - Salsomaggiore Terme; October 27–29 2000 – Italy.

12. T Ito, JL Moore. Topical application of CO_2 increase skin blood flow. J Invest Dermato 93:259, 1989.

13. C Brandi, C D'aniello, l Grimaldi, P Lattarulo. Carbon dioxide therapy in the treatment of localized adiposities: clinical study and histopathological correlations. Aesthetic Plastic Surgery vol. 25(3):May – June, 2001.

14. C D'Aniello, C Brandi, PA Bacci, P Lattarulo. The role of carbon dioxide in Symmetric Multiple Lipomatosis therapeutic strategy. Unita operativa di Chirugia Plastica, Universita degli Studi di Siena RIV. ITAL. CHIR. PLASTICA 31:265–69, 1999 – Siena.

15. A Bollinger, B Fagrell. Cinical Capillaroscopy 1990.

16. C Albergati, P Lattarulo, S Curri. Relationship between dosis and the microcirculatory answer in patients with Cellulite Syndrome, after the injection of CO_2. XVII Congreso Nacional de Medicina Estetica Roma; 1997.

17. C Brandi, L Grimaldi, B Bosi et al. The role of carbon dioxide therapy as a complement of liposuction. Caiazzo Unit of Plastic Surgery – University Study of Siena The xvi. Mondial congress of isaps abstract book, 2002 / MAY, 2002 - 07- 26 -29 - ISTANBUL – TURKEY.

18. S Curri, T Ryan. Microangiopatia de estasis 1989.

19. PG Stavropoulos, CC Zouboulis, C Trautmann, CE Orfanos. Symmetric lipomatoses in female patients. Dermatology 194(1):26–31, 1997.

20. G Leibaschoff. Cellulite: Treatment and clinic therapeutic approach. Am J Cosm Surg 1997.

21. V Campos. CO_2 insuflation for gynoid lipodystrophy treatment: Brazilian experience in Cellulite. J Am Academy of Dermatology 2007, February 2007.

22. T Jevaoun. Treatment of the laxity of the eyelid with Carboxitherapy (CDT). Hospital General of Bonsucesso, Brasil.

23. JC Tavares Ferreira et al. Increase in collagen turnover induced by intradermal injection of carbon dioxide in rats. Journal of Drugs in Dermatology, 2008.

24. M Lafontan, C Sengenes, J Galitzky. Recent developments on lipolysis regulation in humans and discovery of a new lipolytic pathway. M Berlan, I De Gliszezinski, F Crampes et al. International journal of obesity and related metabolic disorders: journal of the International Association for the Study of Obesity 24(Suppl 4):S47–52, 2000.

25. G Leibaschoff, A Diz, MC Sluga et al. A double-blind, prospective, clinical, surgical, histopathological and ultrasound study comparing the effectiveness and safety of liposuction performed using Laserlipolysis and Internal Ultrasound Lipoplasty method, and assessing the evolution in patients. Congress of the Australasian College of Cosmetic Surgery, Gold Coast, Australia; May, 2008.

22 TriPollar™ Radiofrequency
Woraphong Manuskiatti

Introduction

Radiofrequency (RF) energy is a wavelength situated in the range of electromagnetic rays. Propagation of RF through the cutaneous tissue rapidly oscillates electromagnetic fields causing a movement of charged ions within the tissue which subsequently creates an electrical current generating heat proportional to the dermis' and subcutaneous tissues' electrical resistance. The application of RF has been extensively used in surgery for hemostasis and tissue ablation (electro-surgery) [1–3], but more recently RF has been applied as a means of shrinking redundant or lax connective tissues through the mechanism of collagen denaturation [4–6]. Collagen molecules are produced by fibroblasts which synthesize three polypeptide chains that wrap around one another in a triple helix. The phenomenon of thermal shrinkage of collagen begins with denaturation of the triple helix of the collagen fibers. When collagen is heated, the heat-labile intramolecular cross-links are broken, and the protein undergoes a transition from a highly organized crystalline structure to a random, gel-like state (denaturation). Collagen shrinkage occurs through the cumulative effect of the "unwinding" of the triple helix, due to the destruction of the heat-labile intramolecular cross-links, and the residual tension of the heat-stable intermolecular cross-links. Heated fibroblasts are also implicated in new collagen formation and collagen remodeling which also contribute to the final cosmetic outcome. The precise heat-induced behavior of connective tissues and the extent of tissue shrinkage are dependent on several factors which include the maximum temperature reached, exposure time, tissue hydration and tissue age [7].

RF energy can be delivered to cutaneous tissue through either a single-electrode tip and a grounding plate (mono-polar—the first generation RF technology) [6,8] or a two-electrode applicator (bi-polar—the second generation RF technology) [9,10]. Less electrical current is required with a bi-polar RF than with a mono-polar one for achieving a similar tissue response, because the current penetrates through a much smaller volume of tissue. When a mono-polar RF energy is applied for volumetric heating of the skin, the RF current will find the path with the least electrical resistance to flow in the body (i.e. vascular and lymphatic systems), so the benefit of heating the adipose tissue, which has a higher electrical resistance, is controversial. In contrast, with a bipolar RF, the electrical current propagation is limited to the area between the two electrodes, and the depth of penetration under the skin is estimated to be approximately half the distance between the electrodes. Therefore, the depth of penetration is constant and cannot be changed for various body areas or different skin conditions. Moreover, mono- and bipolar RF configurations must use a cooling device in order to prevent epidermal overheating and the potential for burn injuries, thus reducing the efficacy of the treatment (Table 22.1).

Developed in 2006, TriPollar™ RF is the third generation RF technology employing a multiple-electrode configuration (Figs. 22.1–22.2). TriPollar technology is based on the use of three or more electrodes to deliver focused RF current into the skin, thus generating heat through resistance in both the dermal and subcutaneous layers. The depth of heat penetration is approximately the average distance between the three electrodes. One acts as a positive pole while the other two act as negative poles. The current flowing through the common, positive pole is twice that which flows through each of the negative poles. To avoid overheating of this common pole and of the tissue in contact with this pole, a sequence of electrical modulation is applied so that each electrode, in turn, acts as the common pole. Due to its design, no active cooling of the electrodes or the skin is required.

Mechanisms of Action

The radiofrequency device is used to deliver selective and focused electro-heating to the dermis and subdermal layers of the skin, causing instant collagen contraction and subsequent remodeling [7,11]. An immediate tightening effect is visible on the skin following each treatment due to collagen fibers shrinking [8,12]. Thermal injury of the extracellular matrix initiates a cascade of wound healing phases including inflammation, proliferation, and collagen remodeling. The latter two phases of wound healing are thought to be the most important mechanisms responsible for the outcome of the treatment. These effects are more pronounced a few weeks to months following the treatment when the migration of fibroblasts into the inflammatory area initiates the production of new collagen fibers [13,14].

Table 22.1 Summary of current radiofrequency technology

Technology	Penetration depth	Required power	Pain level	Cooling device	Clinical outcome
Monopolar	Deep and uncontrolled 5–20 mm	High power (200–350 W)	Very painful	Always required	After 5–6 months
Bi-polar	Superficial and constant 1–5 mm	Medium power (10–200)	Painful	Sometimes necessary	After days-weeks
TriPollar	Dermal and subcutaneous layers 20 mm	Low power (5–30 W)	Warm massage-like sensation	No cooling needed	Some temporary immediate result. Long-term outcome noted after weeks

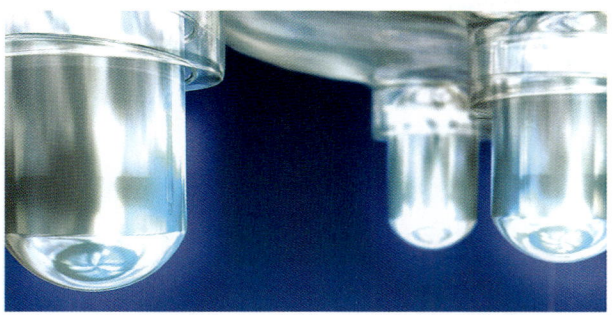

Figure 22.1. TriPollar radiofrequency applicator. The three-electrode configuration of TriPollar RF is aimed to deliver focused RF current into the skin tissue. (Courtesy Pollogen Ltd., Tel Aviv, Israel).

Moreover, simultaneously heating the superficial and deep layers of the skin may enhance local blood circulation and drainage of the free fatty acids to the lymphatic system. This is confirmed by findings of a previous study on the effect of TriPollar™ RF in *ex vivo* human skin harvested from a post-abdominoplasty skin sample and maintained in survival conditions [15]. Following a single treatment at 25 watts (W) to a skin model, a significant increase in glycerol release by the skin was observed, indicating an increase of tissue lipolytic activity (Fig. 22.3). In addition, following TriPollar™ RF treatment, neocollagenesis was demonstrated with a statistically significant repair of altered collagen in skin that was experimentally aged using UV radiation, with a tendency towards increasing collagen synthesis (Fig. 22.4). The histological analysis of the subcutaneous layer after the TriPollar™ treatment demonstrated elongated and irregular-shaped adipocytes with shrunken and partially ruptured cell walls. No tissue necrosis or carbonization of the hypodermis was observed (Fig. 22.5). Similar to the aforementioned study, a recent histological examination of a skin biopsy taken after seven TriPollar™ RF treatments revealed an increase of 49% in dermal thickness, focal thickening of collagen fibers and focal shrinkage of fat cells [16].

Indications

The TriPollar™ RF system is currently used for

- Treatment of skin laxity (Fig. 22.6)
- Improvement of skin texture (Fig. 22.7)
- Treatment of cellulite (Fig. 22.8) and body contouring (Fig. 22.9)
- Localized fat reduction
- Improvement of striae appearance (Fig. 22.10)

Contraindications

There are several contraindications to using TriPollar™ RF device, including

- Having an implant in the treatment area, or an active implant (including pacemaker) anywhere in the body
- History of bleeding coagulopathies or use of anticoagulants

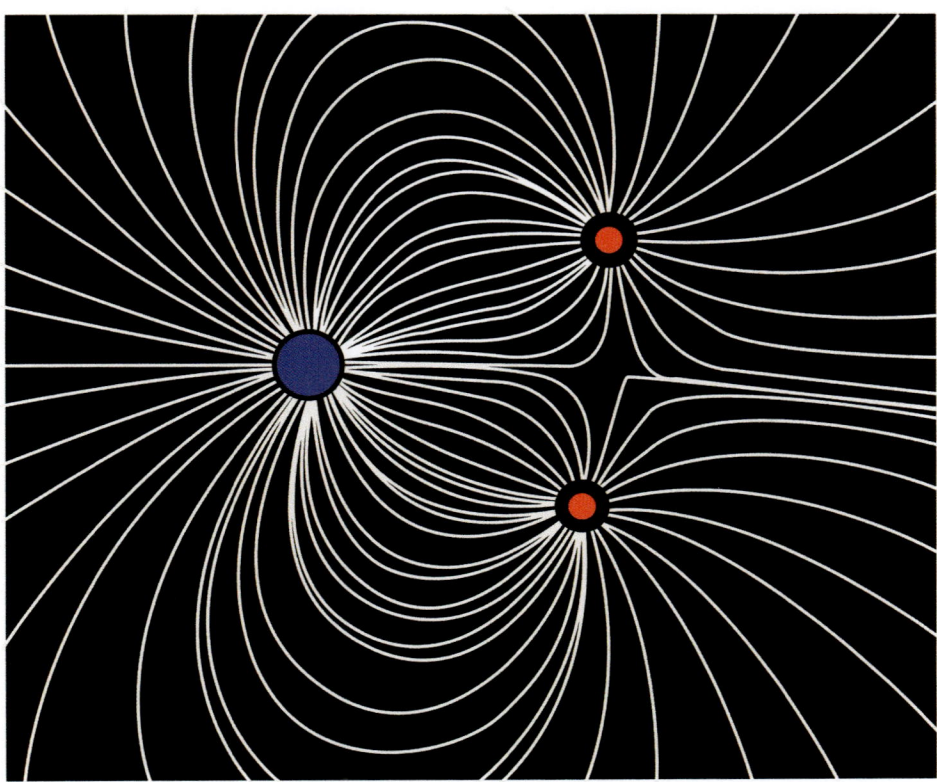

Figure 22.2 TriPollar electrode configuration. One electrode acts as a positive pole while the other two act as negative poles. The current flowing through the common, positive pole is twice that which flows through each of the negative poles. (Courtesy Pollogen Ltd., Tel Aviv, Israel).

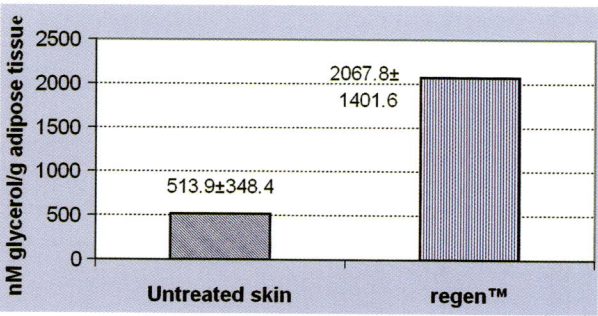

Figure 22.3 Evaluation of the lipolytic effect following a TriPollar™ RF treatment. A significant increase of glycerol release of the treated skin is demonstrated. (Modified from Boisnic S. Evaluation du dispositif de radiofréquence tripolaire Regen™ en utilisant un modèle experimental de peau humaine. Nouv Dermatol. 2008;28:331–332.)

- Expectation of pregnancy, pregnant, having given birth less than three months prior, postpartum or nursing
- Having significant concurrent skin conditions, including infections, herpes simplex, open lacerations/abrasions or any inflammatory skin conditions affecting the areas to be treated
- Having or undergoing any form of treatment for active cancer, having a history of skin cancer or any other localized cancer in the areas to be treated, or having pre-cancerous lesions at the treatment areas
- Undergoing invasive or ablative procedures in the areas to be treated such as: liposuction, plastic surgery, any other surgery in the treatment area, laser resurfacing or deep chemical peeling during the course of the treatment, or before complete healing has occurred
- Taking medications, herbal preparations, food supplements or vitamins that might cause fragile skin or impaired skin healing such as prolonged steroid therapy, NSAIDs, warfarin, heparin, ginkgo, ginseng, garlic, etc.

System Overview

The Regen™ system (Pollogen Ltd., Tel Aviv, Israel) was the first system based on the TriPollar RF technology delivering energy at a frequency of 1 MHz and having a maximum power of 30 watts. Two applicators of different sizes are available for treatment of different anatomical sites including the face, neck, arms, abdomen, buttocks and thighs (Fig 22.11). Recently, the second generation of TriPollar RF—Apollo™ system with a maximum power of 50 watts has been launched (Fig. 22.12). Three sizes of applicators, large, medium and small, for the body, arms, neck, and face, respectively, are available.

Treatment Technique

Prior to treatment, remove all jewelry, including necklaces, bracelets, watches, rings, etc. Clean the treatment area with soap and water and dry completely. Take pre-treatment photographs and circumference measurements at specific reference points, as a baseline assessment. Prepare the patient in a comfortable position for treatment. After that, set the appropriate treatment parameters for the specified treatment area. Then, lubricate the treatment area with a thin layer of glycerin oil. Glycerin oil acts as a lubricant. In addition, glycerin has high electrical resistance, thus 'forcing' the

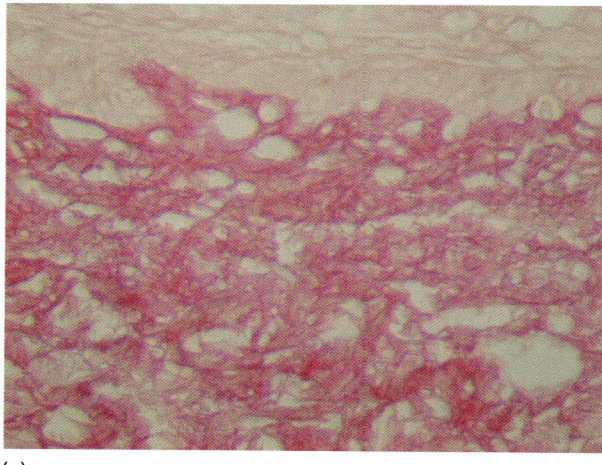

(a)

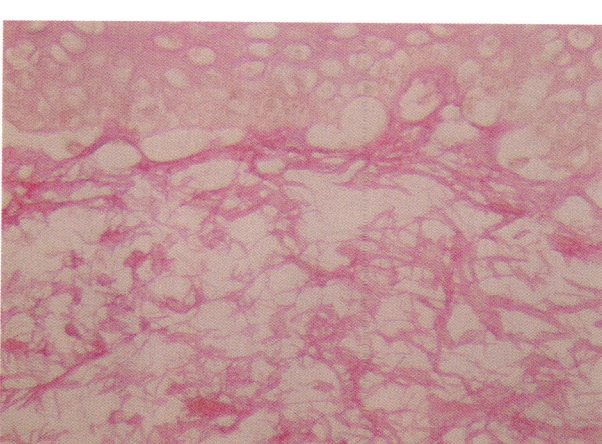

(b)

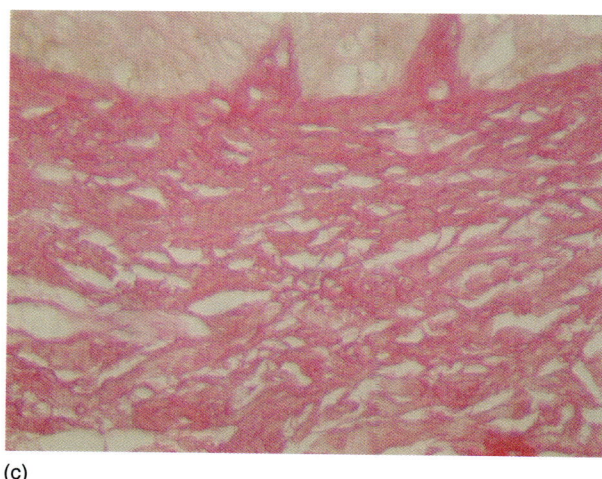

(c)

Figure 22.4 Histological examination. (a) Untreated skin; (b) Ultraviolet (UV)-irradiated skin; (c) UV-irradiated skin follow by TriPollar™ RF treatment. Note the new collagen production induced by RF treatment. (Courtesy Sylvie Boisnic, M.D.)

electrical current to enter more deeply into the skin. Position the TriPollar™ applicator suitable for the treatment area on the skin and press the foot switch to begin treatment. During treatment, place the applicator on the area to be treated, with slight pressure and maneuver in linear or circular massaging movements, depending on the area. Both the patient and operator should

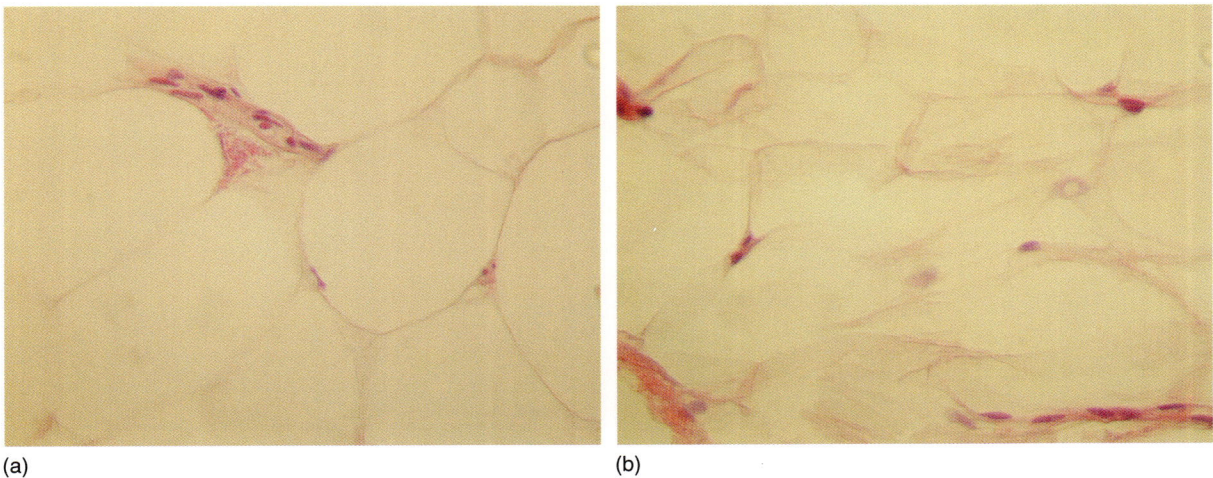

(a)   (b)

Figure 22.5 Histological finding of adipocytes in the subcutaneous layer after the TriPollar™ treatment demonstrates modifications in the shape (inhomogeneity: elongated, irregular) of the membrane (shrunken and some have partial ruptures of the cell wall). No tissue necrosis or carbonization of the hypodermis layer was observed. (Courtesy Sylvie Boisnic, M.D.)

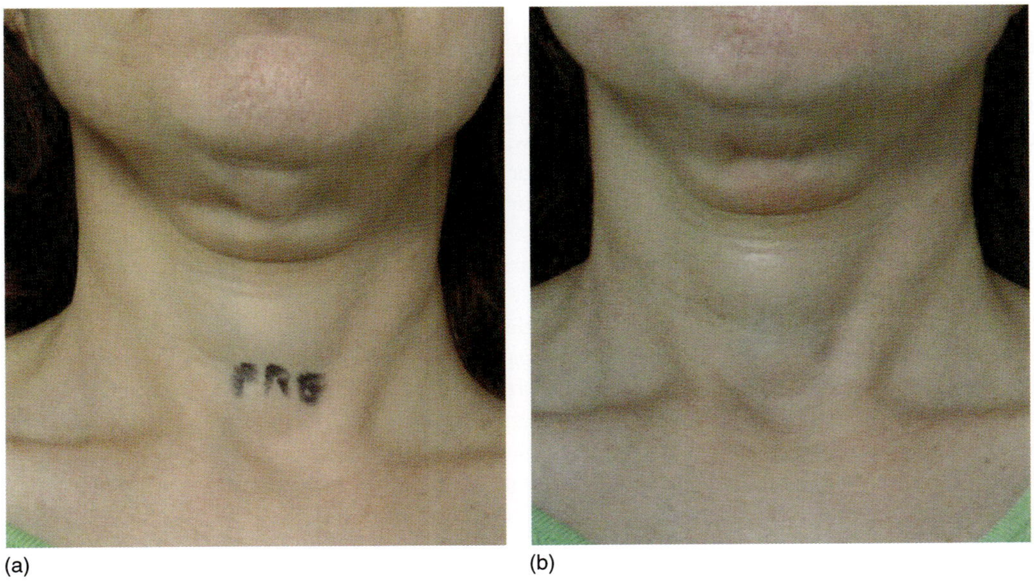

(a)   (b)

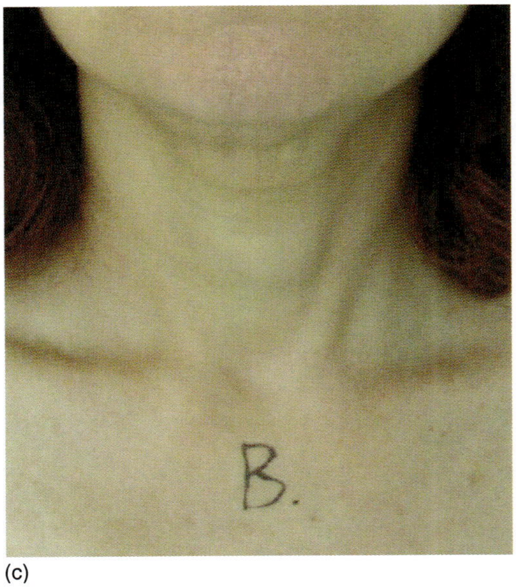

(c)

Figure 22.6 Submental and neck skin, before treatment (a); immediately after TriPollar™ treatment (b); after six treatments (c). (Courtesy Alex Levenberg, M.D.)

161

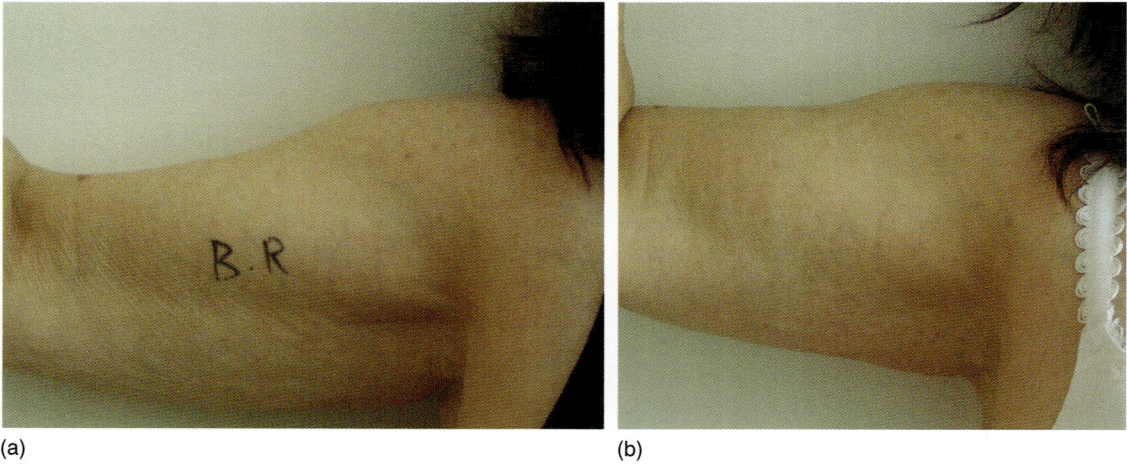

(a) (b)

Figure 22.7 Arm skin, (a) before treatment; (b) after seven TriPollar™ treatments. Note the progressive skin tightening and improvement of skin texture. (Courtesy Alex Levenberg, M.D.)

monitor in real-time the treatment effects. The operator should constantly monitor skin tightness, warmth and erythema, while periodically measuring skin temperature using a non-contact IR thermometer. Shortly after commencing treatment there will be a noticeable tightening of the skin in most patients. Additionally, approximately three quarters of the way through the treatment, erythema should be visible (Fig. 22.13) and the skin should be warm to the touch. Measured skin temperature should be maintained between 40°C–42°C for safety reasons. The erythema usually disappears within 2–3 hours after completion of the treatment.

Treatment Regimen

Treatments shall be given once a week for a period of six to eight weeks [17,18]. A previous study demonstrated that the treatment effects appeared to be sustained as long as one and a half months after the treatment was discontinued [17]. However, monthly maintenance treatments are recommended to further enhance the clinical results achieved.

Initial Studies

Recent studies have demonstrated that TriPollar™ RF treatment is an effective and safe procedure for circumference reduction and cellulite treatment. Manuskiatti and colleagues [18] performed eight weekly treatments of TriPollar™ RF on 39 healthy females with cellulite measured as Nurnberger–Muller cellulite scale II or above. The study subjects were evaluated both quantitatively by measuring body weight, circumference and thickness of the superficial subcutaneous tissue, and qualitatively by photographic assessment and patient satisfaction questionnaire.

According to the study, significant reduction of circumferential measurements of the abdomen and thigh was observed, comparing between the baseline and one month following the final treatment visit, and were reduced 3.50 ± 4.61 cm with a maximum reduction of 14.4 cm, and 1.71 ± 2.20 cm with a maximum reduction of 9.1 cm, respectively. Reduction of circumference measurements of the arm (maximum reduction of 1 cm) and buttock (maximum reduction of 5.2 cm) areas comparing between baseline and one month following the final treatment visit was not

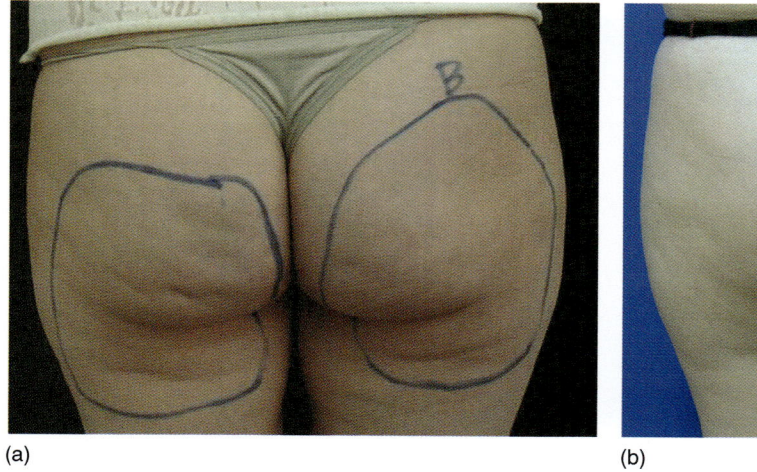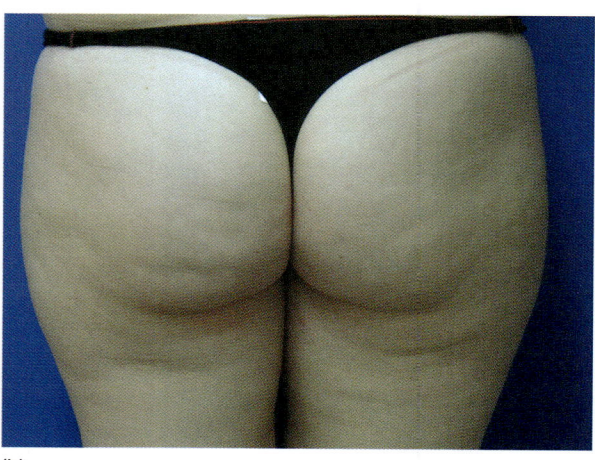

(a) (b)

Figure 22.8 Cellulite on the buttock, (a) before treatment; (b) after five TriPollar™ treatments. (Courtesy Pollogen Ltd., Tel Aviv, Israel).

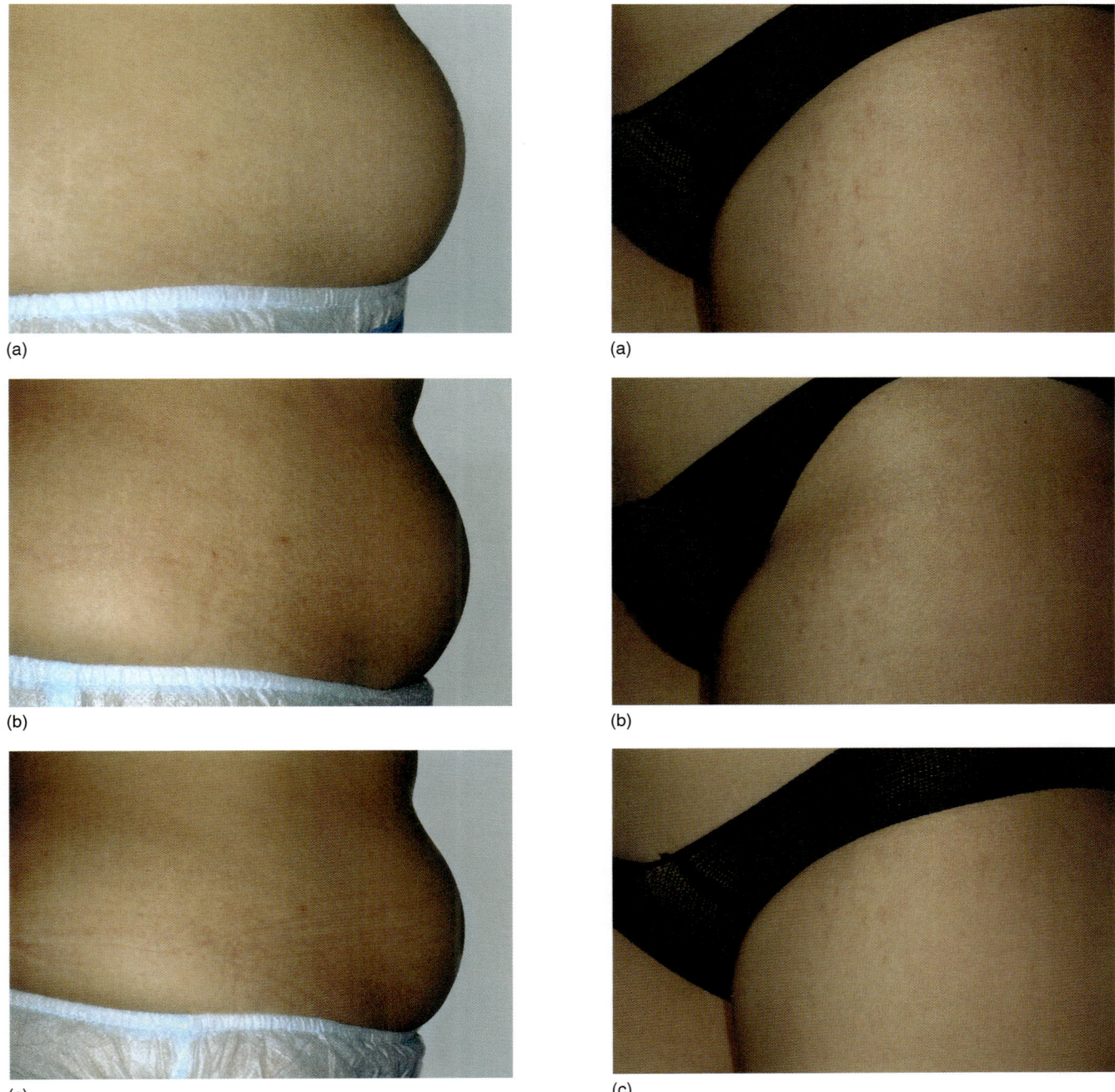

(a)

(b)

(c)

(a)

(b)

(c)

Figure 22.9 Body contouring. (a) before treatment; (b) four weeks after eight weekly TriPollar™ treatments with 9 cm reduction of the abdominal circumference; (c) eight weeks after treatment.

Figure 22.10 Striae rubra (a) before TriPollar™ treatment; (b) one month after six weekly treatments; (c) three months after six treatments. Note the progressive improvement at the longer follow-up period.

statistically significant. Evaluation of circumference measurement at one month after the series of treatments was stopped, confirmed that a significant circumference reduction was sustained (less than 1% reduction in efficacy was noticed). Quartile grading scores correlating to approximately 50% improvement in overall cellulite appearance were observed.

As is consistent with reports from prior studies on RF-induced skin tightening [5,6,19], initial studies using the TriPollar™ RF device [17,18] also noted considerable variability in the treatment outcomes, with some subjects achieving marked improvement and others showing minimal improvement or unchanged from

baseline. While the reasons underlying this variability remain unclear, further studies are warranted to fully elucidate this issue. However, we observe that the baseline severity of cellulite and skin laxity affects the degree of improvement. When there is less irregular skin surface and/or skin laxity, there will be better response to the treatment.

Ultrasound measurements of the distance between the epidermis and the superficial fascia revealed a distance reduction of 0.61 ± 2.1 mm, representing an average reduction of 10.5% in the thickness of superficial adipose tissue with a maximum reduction of 39% at the thigh region (Fig. 22.14), and a distance

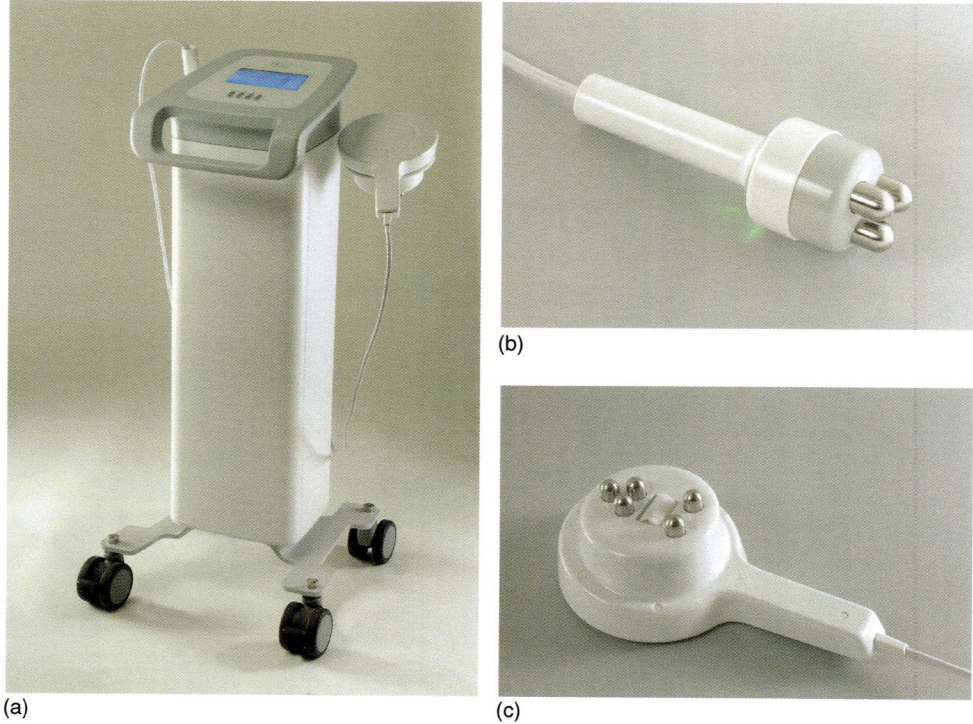

Figure 22.11 Regen™ system having a maximum power of 30 W (a) and two sizes of applicators for the treatment of different anatomical sites including a small applicator for treatment of the face and neck (b), and a larger applicator for the treatment of the arms, abdomen, buttocks and thighs (c). (Courtesy Pollogen Ltd., Tel Aviv, Israel).

reduction at the abdomen region of 0.34 ± 2.2 mm, representing an average reduction of 4% in the thickness of adipose tissue, with a maximum reduction of 31%. However, this reduction of superficial subcutaneous thickness was found to be statistically significant only at the thigh region when compared to the baseline.

Given the proven efficacy in induction of collagen remodeling [15,20,21], TriPollar™ RF has recently been used to successfully improve stretch marks' appearance [17]. Seventeen females with striae distensae were enrolled for six weekly treatment sessions of 40–45 minutes each. Treatment evaluations, including standardized photographs and a UVA-light video camera were made at baseline, and at one and six weeks after the final treatment. In addition, the subjects were asked to rate their overall satisfaction at the last follow-up visit.

The result of the study indicated that TriPollar™ RF offered a beneficial effect on improvement of striate appearance. Evaluation performed at one week after a series of six weekly treatments noted 41.2% and 11.8% of the subjects having 25%–50% and 51%–75% improvement of their striae, respectively. Compared to the one-week follow-up visit, at six weeks after the last treatment, a higher percentage of the subjects were rated to have improvement of their striae including 26.5% showing 51%–75% improvement and 5.9% showing >75% improvement. None of the subjects was rated as having no improvement. According to the satisfaction survey, 12% (2/17), 23% (4/17), and 65% (11/17) of the study subjects reported their satisfaction with the overall improvement as slightly satisfied, satisfied, and very satisfied, respectively. In terms of treatment complications, there were no adverse effects, such as postoperative purpura, bullae, crusts, ulcerations, or dyschromia observed.

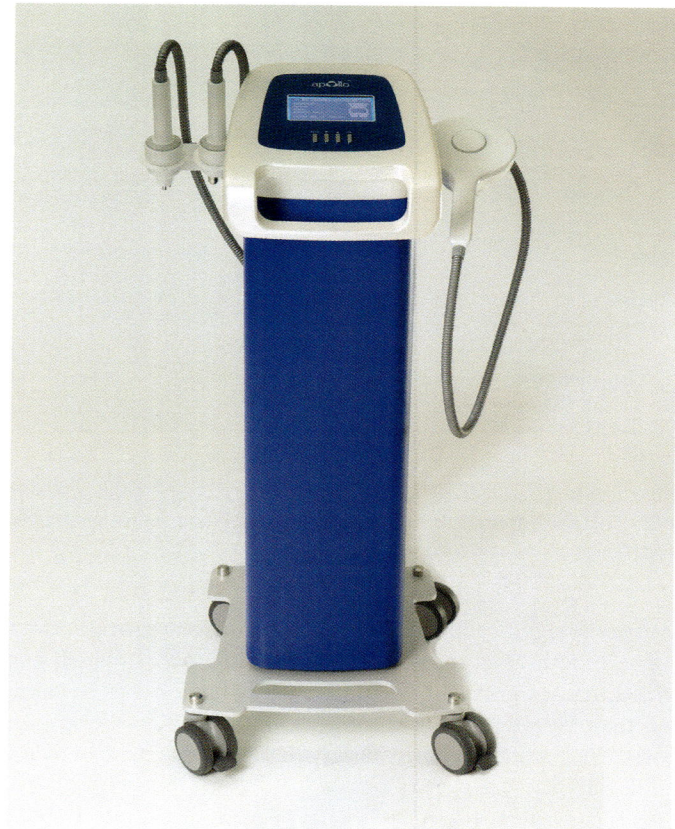

Figure 22.12 Apollo™ system with a maximum power of 50 W and available with three sizes of applicators, including large, medium and small applicators for the body, arms and neck, and face, respectively (Courtesy Pollogen Ltd., Tel Aviv, Israel).

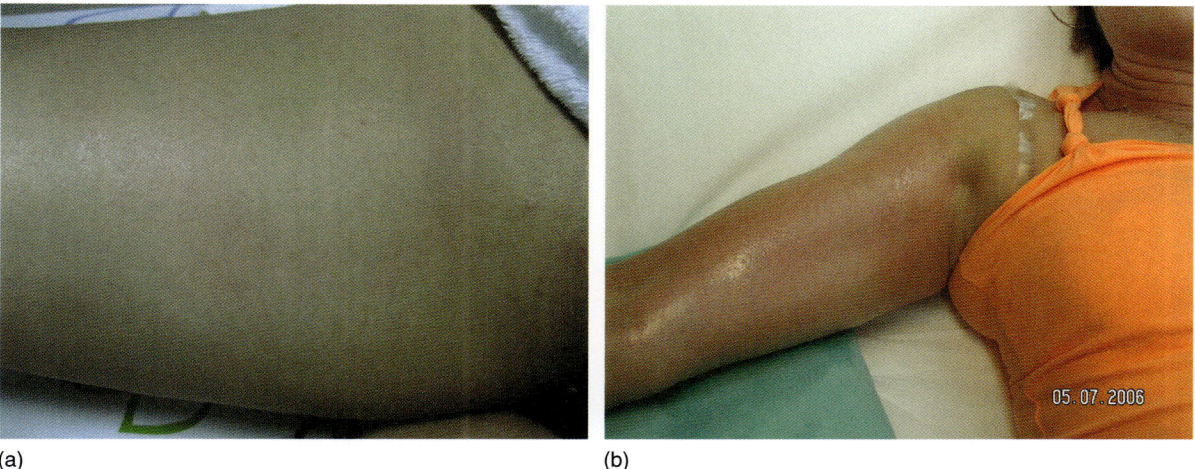

(a)   (b)

Figure 22.13 Endpoint of treatment is erythema and the skin is warm to the touch. (a) Erythema in a skin phototype V patient at a skin surface temperature of 40°C; (b) erythema in skin phototype II patient at the same surface temperature. Note the difference in the degree of redness. (Courtesy Alex Levenberg, M.D.)

Scanned images from a UVA camera did not reveal significant differences in the striae surface smoothness at one- and six-week follow-ups, compared with that of baseline. However, the sample size of this study may be too small to detect an objective improvement of skin surface smoothness, compared with that of baseline (Fig. 22.15). Moreover, at the six-week follow-up visit, there was an increase in the number of patients showing higher improvement scores as compared to that of the one-week follow-up visit. This suggests that the improvement is a long-term process and there may be advantages if the clinical follow-up can extend beyond six weeks, as more favorable changes may be noted with a prolonged follow-up period (Fig. 22.10).

that the treated skin became warm to the touch and erythema, immediately after the treatment. The erythema was reported to disappear within 2–3 hours after completion of the treatment session by all subjects. Treatment was well tolerated with minimal to no discomfort. The sensation most often described was a mild heating with occasional pinching. Another study using such a device to treat 17 patients for a total of 102 treatment sessions found that the procedure was well tolerated in all study subjects [17]. The subject's reported feeling during the treatment was described as comfortable in 29.4% (5/17) of the subjects, very comfortable in 64.7% (11/17), and extremely comfortable in 5.9% (1/17).

Treatment Tolerability

Our early study [18] evaluating the use of the TriPollar™ RF device in 39 females who underwent 656 treatment sessions, has noted

Side Effects

Experience in our recent study using the Regen™ system for circumference reduction and cellulite treatment noted that the

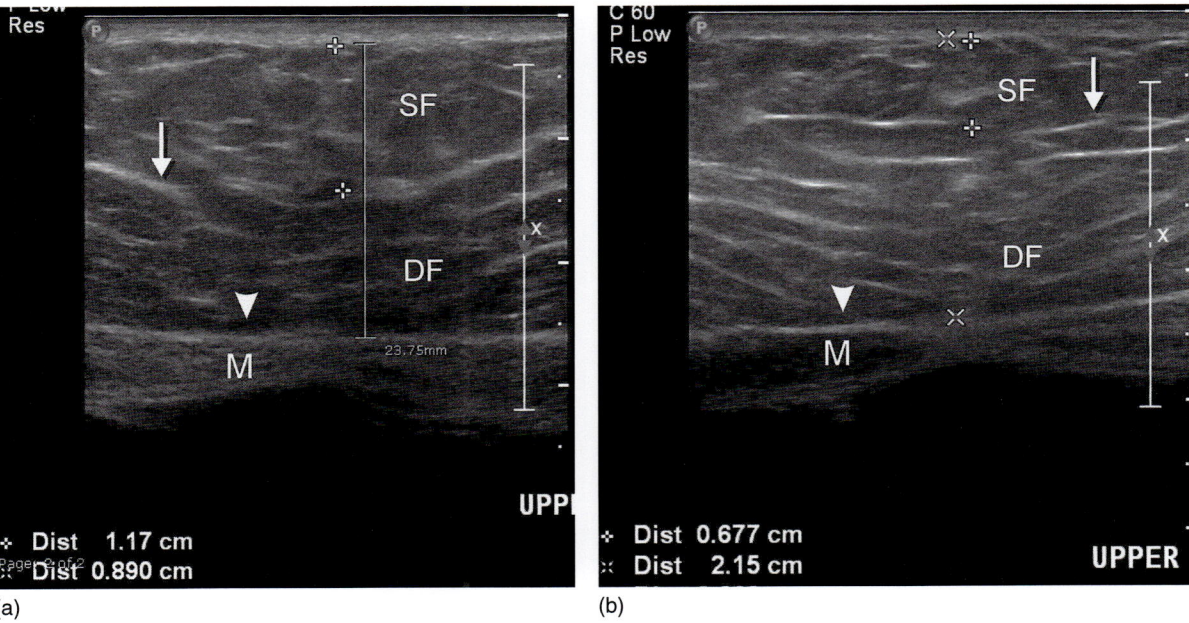

(a)   (b)

Figure 22.14 Ultrasound measurement of a thigh region. (a) Before treatment, the thickness of the superficial fat layer is 1.17 cm; (b) after eight TriPollar™ treatments, the thickness is 0.68 cm; SF, superficial fat layer; DF, deep fat layer; M, muscle; ↓, superficial fascia; ▯ deep fascia.

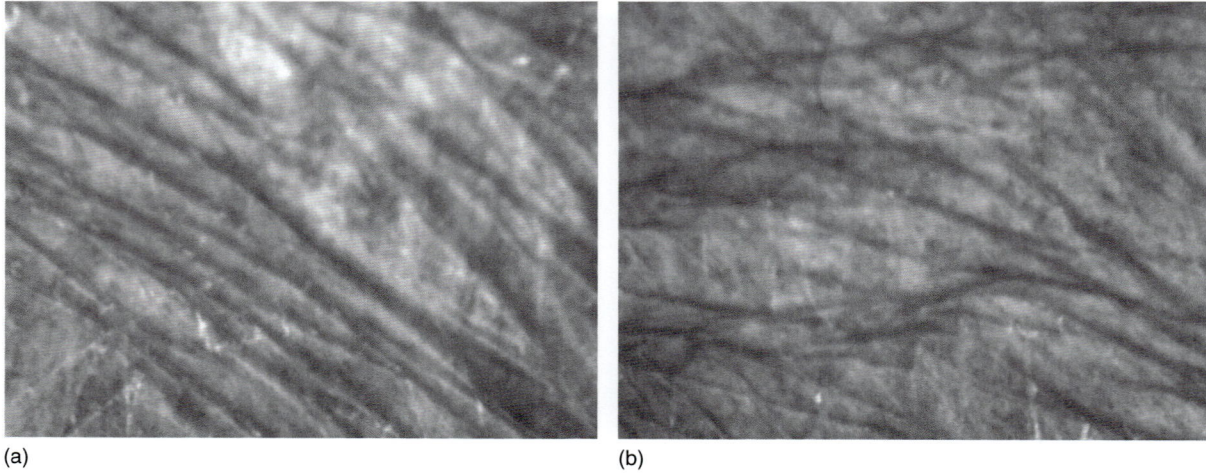

(a)   (b)

Figure 22.15 Images from a UVA-light video camera (Visioscan® VC 98, Courage-Khazaka, Köln, Germany) showing striae surface smoothness before treatment (a); (b) six weeks after six TriPollar™ treatments. Note the improvement of surface irregularity.

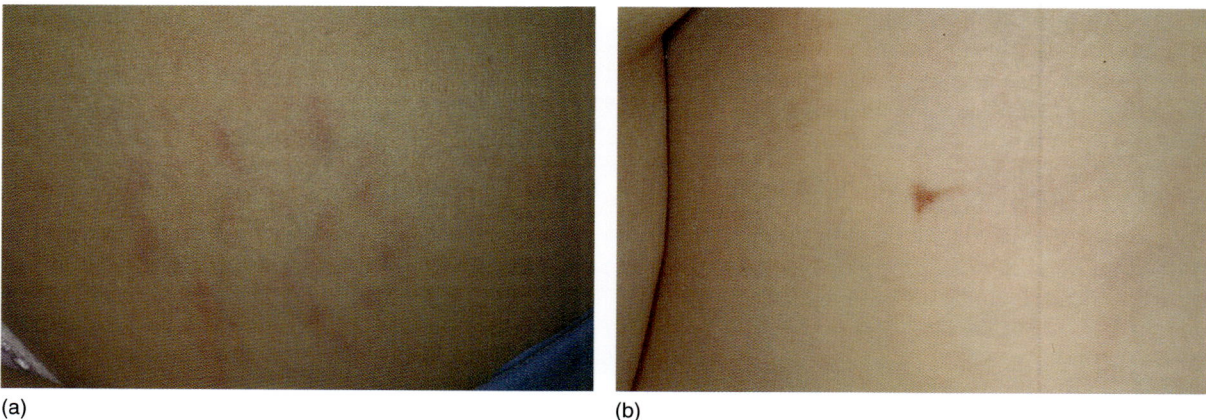

(a)   (b)

Figure 22.16 Side effects of TriPollar™ RF treatment. (a) bruise; (b) primary degree burn.

adverse effects in a series of 656 treatment sessions included erythematous papules, papular urticaria, primary degree burn, blister and bruising, observed in 0.3% (2/656), 0.15% (1/656), 0.15% (1.656), 0.15% (1/656), and 0.15% (1/656) of 656 treatment sessions, respectively (Figs. 22.16) [18]. We suspect that the reason for these adverse effects may be a result of individual reactions to RF heating and/or improper treatment skill of the treatment provider, including a too-slow movement of the electrode and an inadequate amount of glycerin oil used. All of the side effects were mild, asymptomatic and self-limited within one week except the primary degree burns and blisters, which cleared after a week course of topical corticosteroids.

Conclusions

The TriPollar™ RF device is a multi-polar RF system which can safely and effectively be used for skin tightening and circumference reduction, particularly on the body and facial areas, as well as for the treatment of cellulite, reduction of localized fat and improvement of striae appearance. Application of this treatment modality is simple, non-invasive and safe on all skin types. Qualitative as well as quantitative assessments have been documented and the outcome from previous research studies has shown that the improvements are maintained as a long-term effect.

REFERENCES

1. B Chehrazi, WF Collins, Jr. A comparison of effects of bipolar and monopolar electrocoagulation in brain. J Neurosurg 54:197–203, 1981.
2. OG Anfinsen, K Gjesdal, F Brosstad et al. The activation of platelet function, coagulation, and fibrinolysis during radiofrequency catheter ablation in heparinized patients. J Cardiovasc Electrophysiol 10:503–12, 1999.
3. A Michelucci, E Antonucci, AA Conti et al. Electrophysiologic procedures and activation of the hemostatic system. Am Heart J 138:128–32, 1999.
4. TS Alster, E Tanzi. Improvement of neck and cheek laxity with a nonablative radiofrequency device: a lifting experience. Dermatol Surg 30:503–7, 2004.
5. BS Biesman, K Pope. Monopolar radiofrequency treatment of the eyelids: a safety evaluation. Dermatol Surg 33:794–801, 2007.

6. R Fitzpatrick, R Geronemus, D Goldberg et al. Multicenter study of noninvasive radiofrequency for periorbital tissue tightening. Lasers Surg Med 33:232–42, 2003.

7. BD Zelickson, D Kist, E Bernstein et al. Histological and ultrastructural evaluation of the effects of a radiofrequency-based nonablative dermal remodeling device: a pilot study. Arch Dermatol 140:204–9, 2004.

8. JS Dover, B Zelickson. Results of a survey of 5,700 patient monopolar radiofrequency facial skin tightening treatments: assessment of a low-energy multiple-pass technique leading to a clinical end point algorithm. Dermatol Surg 33:900–7, 2007.

9. G Montesi, S Calvieri, A Balzani et al. Bipolar radiofrequency in the treatment of dermatologic imperfections: clinicopathological and immunohistochemical aspects. J Drugs Dermatol 6:890–6, 2007.

10. CS Yu, CK Yeung, SY Shek et al. Combined infrared light and bipolar radiofrequency for skin tightening in Asians. Lasers Surg Med 39:471–5, 2007.

11. SP Arnoczky, A Aksan. Thermal modification of connective tissues: basic science considerations and clinical implications. J Am Acad Orthop Surg 8:305–13, 2000.

12. LG Jacobson, M Alexiades-Armenakas, L Bernstein et al. Treatment of nasolabial folds and jowls with a noninvasive radiofrequency device. Arch Dermatol 139:1371–2, 2003.

13. AJ Singer, RA Clark. Cutaneous wound healing. N Engl J Med 341:738–46, 1999.

14. C Sussman, BM Bates-Jensen. Wound Healing Physiology: Acute and Chronic. In: C Sussman and BM Bates-Jensen (eds). Wound Care. Philadelphia: Lippincott Williams & Wilkins; p. 21–51.

15. S Boisnic. Evaluation du dispositif de radiofréquence tripolaire Regen™ en utilisant un modèle experimental de peau humaine. Nouv Dermatol 28:331–2, 2008.

16. H Kaplan, A Gat. Clinical and histological results following TriPollar radiofrequency skin treatments. J Cosmet Laser Ther 11:78–84, 2009.

17. W Manuskiatti, E Boonthaweeyuwat, S Varothai. Treatment of striae distensae with a TriPollar radiofrequency device: a pilot study. J Dermotolg Treat 20:359–64, 2009.

18. W Manuskiatti, C Wachirakaphan, N Lektrakul et al. Circumference Reduction and Cellulite Treatment with a TriPollar Radiofrequency Device: A Pilot Study. J Eur Acad Dermatol Venereol 23:820–7, 2009.

19. RA Weiss, MA Weiss, G Munavalli et al. Monopolar radiofrequency facial tightening: a retrospective analysis of efficacy and safety in over 600 treatments. J Drugs Dermatol 5:707–12, 2006.

20. M Emilia del Pino, RH Rosado, A Azuela et al. Effect of controlled volumetric tissue heating with radiofrequency on cellulite and the subcutaneous tissue of the buttocks and thighs. J Drugs Dermatol 5:714–22, 2006.

21. DJ Goldberg, A Fazeli, AL Berlin. Clinical, laboratory, and MRI analysis of cellulite treatment with a unipolar radiofrequency device. Dermatol Surg 34:204–9, 2008.

23 Cryolipolysis™ for Subcutaneous Fat Layer Reduction
Mathew Avram

Introduction

A recent development in aesthetic procedures has been the introduction of a unique, non-invasive method of fat layer reduction, termed "cryolipolysis". This novel non-invasive technology uses controlled cooling exposure to produce a gradual reduction of the subcutaneous fat layer using natural thermal diffusion without damage to other tissues. This visible fat layer reduction occurs over a period of months with the removal of fat (adipocytes) through the body's natural inflammatory clearing process.

Background

The clinical entity of cold panniculitis, also known as "popsicle panniculitis", serves as the basis for the concept of cryolipolysis. Numerous studies have documented that localized inflammation and subsequent clearance of subcutaneous fat can occur under certain conditions when exposed to cold. Such inflammation has been described most frequently in infants and toddlers [1,2], but has also been seen in adult females who participate in equestrian activities [3]. Case reports have described a clinically evident inflammation in infants [1,2] as confirmed histologically after apparently minor cold exposure, i.e., ice cube application for few minutes. Histological assessment of the exposed areas have demonstrated that perivascular infiltration of histiocytes with a few lymphocytes, most intense at the dermal-subdermal junction with extensions into the adjacent dermis and subcutaneous fat, begins about 24 hours after cold exposure. The changes become more obvious over the course of 72 hours with the appearance of additional inflammatory cells in the subcutaneous fat, rupture of some of the adipose tissue cells, and aggregation of the lipids. There is progression of the inflammatory response for three more days with histiocytes, neutrophils, lymphocytes and other mononuclear cells surrounding the adipocytes [1]. Within a few weeks, panniculitis resolves spontaneously without any persistent tissue damage or scarring, and without evidence of cryoglobulins for any of the infants evaluated.

Case reports also have been documented of panniculitis in women who have been horseback riding in cold and damp conditions [3]. In these cases, the inflammatory reaction in the adipose tissue occurred at the dermal-subcutaneous junction with an infiltrate of lymphocytes and neutrophils, as well as a scattering of mast cells and foamy histiocytes. The infiltrate extends from a perivascular location into adjacent adipose tissue where adipocyte cells are ruptured and small cystic spaces form.

Preclinical Studies

Manstein et al. [4] performed pig studies to investigate the potential for selective damage to subcutaneous fat with controlled application of cooling to the skin surface. Three complementary pig studies have been reported: an initial exploratory study, a dosimetry study, and a safety study to assess the potential impact of such selective damage to subcutaneous fat on serum lipid levels.

The "exploratory" study was designed to determine the feasibility of using cold exposure to the skin to remove subcutaneous fat. A slightly convex, circular copper plate was pressed firmly against the pig's skin surface and chilled by circulating cold antifreeze solution at $-7°C$ through a heat exchanger chamber attached to the copper plate. The cold exposure was repeated at multiple sites on the pig, with exposure time varying from 5 to 21 minutes. The pig was observed for three point five months for evidence of local fat loss. The amount of fat loss at each test site was estimated relative to neighboring unexposed fat at the margins of the test site.

No apparent skin injury or scar was documented in any of the test areas. There was a slight increase in pigmentation at the one week follow-up for some of the test sites but there was no hypopigmentation or textural changes. Selective fat loss was evident on gross specimens by a smooth indentation along the surface of the animal of a size and shape similar to that of the cooling device. A reduction of fat in the superficial fat layer was documented at 3.5 months with 80% of the superficial fat layer removed for a total fat loss of 40% from the procedure. Histology demonstrated a marked reduction of fat with a reduced distance between fat septae.

The dosimetry study was performed on four pigs with a prototype device (Zeltiq™ Aesthetics, Pleasanton, CA) that contained a thermoelectric cooling (TEC) element. A variable, preset plate temperature was maintained constant during each cold exposure by electronic regulation according to temperature sensors embedded within the cooling plate. Test sites were exposed to either a flat configuration with the device applicator pressed firmly against the skin surface or a folded configuration with the skin fold captured between two cooling plates. The cooling temperature ranged from $-1°C$ to $-7°C$ for 10 minutes. The pigs were sacrificed at selected time points from immediately to 28 days after cold exposure. Test sites and surrounding areas were photographed and examined clinically. Histological analyses of the test sites were also completed using deep tissue vertical sections (skin, fat, underlying muscle) stained with hematoxylin and eosin to assess the level of fat damage and to assess for any damage to surrounding tissue and /or structures.

There was no injury to the epidermis or dermis at any of the test sites during the dosimetry study. At day after exposure, adipocytes appeared normal initially, but inflammation of the subcutaneous fat was noted as localized clusters of mixed neutrophil and mononuclear cell inflammatory infiltrate in a predominately lobular pattern presented. The inflammation increased for a period of 30 days following exposure with evidence of phagocytosis. Lipid-laden mononuclear inflammatory cells became more numerous.

Concomitantly, the average size of the adipocytes appeared reduced, with a wider range of adipocyte sizes noted. The degree of the inflammatory response was dependent on the temperature used. Fat damage was significantly greater at lower temperatures and increased significantly over time when compared to an unexposed control.

The lipid level study included six pigs for which a 15% area of the skin surface was exposed to cooling with a prototype cooling device that included a flat copper plate cooled by a thermoelectric cooling (TEC) element. Test sites were exposed to temperatures that ranged between −5°C and −8°C for 10 minutes. Blood samples were obtained after a 12-hour fast prior to treatment, within one hour and one day, one week, and one, two, and three months post-treatment. The lipid levels over time following cold exposure demonstrated no significant change other than a temporary decrease in serum triglycerides immediately following the cold exposure, which can likely be attributed to fasting prior to and during general anesthesia.

These preclinical studies demonstrated that non-invasive, selective, localized damage to subcutaneous fat without epidermal or dermal injury can be achieved. Selective effects on the subcutaneous fat were evident after exposure to cooling on the skin surface with a range of temperatures and exposure times with both histological assessment and gross observation. Further, there was no increase in lipid levels.

The findings from these studies were further supported by additional animal studies that demonstrated no significant change in lipid levels or liver function after cryolipolysis [5]. Four pigs were treated and survived for 90 days. Three pigs received a single treatment; one pig received multiple treatments staged at 90, 60, 30, 14, seven, and three days and immediately prior to sacrifice. Approximately 25–30% of the total body surface area was treated in each animal. Fat layer reduction was evident by ultrasound measurements (Fig. 23.1) and gross pathology (Fig. 23.2). Lipid levels were completed (on the single treatment animals) at baseline prior to treatment and at one day, one week, and one, two, and three months after treatment. Serum lipids levels remained within normal variation throughout the 90-day evaluation period.

Erythema was observed immediately post-treatment in the pigs' skin and resolved within 30 minutes. The skin was cold to the touch, firm though not hard, following treatment. There was

no evidence of swelling, purpura, or scar at any follow-up visit or on the day of necropsy. Histologic analysis correlated to clinical observation, showing no damage to the dermis or epidermis in any of the areas treated. In addition, there was no damage observed in neighboring appendageal structures, such as hair follicles or sweat glands. See Fig. 23.3.

These pig studies showed that the inflammatory response observed with controlled, selective cooling was consistent with the clinical and histologic findings seen with cold panniculitis in infants and female horseback riders. These animal studies also establish the selective, localized effects of cryolipolysis to significantly reduce subcutaneous fat without causing damage to the overlying skin and the lack of effect on serum lipid levels in the animal model.

Mechanisms of Action of Cryolipolysis

Histologic analysis at various time periods after cold exposure demonstrates that cryolipolysis results in the death of adipocytes that are subsequently removed by phagocytosis [4,5]. Immediately post-treatment, there are no changes in the subcutaneous fat; no inflammatory cells are present and the cell membranes of the adipocytes are intact. Within three days of treatment, however, an inflammatory process stimulated by adipocyte apoptosis is noted, as reflected by an influx of inflammatory cells. The inflammation appears to peak at approximately 14 days following treatment when the adipocytes are surrounded by histiocytes, neutrophils, lymphocytes, and other mononuclear cells. Between 14 and 30 days after treatment, macrophages and other phagocytes surround, envelope and digest the contents of dead cells as part of the body's normal injury recovery response to remove the unwanted material from the body. The adipocytes become smaller and irregularly shaped as they are slowly digested by the macrophages surrounding them. Subsequently, the inflammatory response subsides and the adipocyte volume decreases with a thickening of the interlobular septae occurring by 60 days. The inflammatory process declines further by 90 days. The lobules previously containing fat cells are decreased in size with the septae eventually constituting a majority of the tissue volume. See Fig. 23.4.

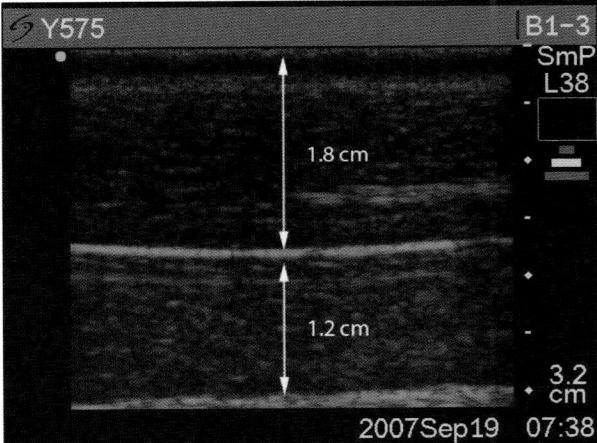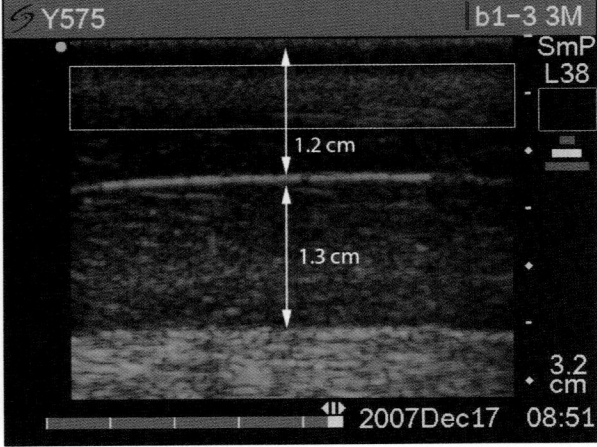

Figure 23.1 Reduction of fat layer as documented with ultrasound measurements in an animal model. The image on the left was obtained prior to treatment; the image on the right was obtained three months after treatment [5].

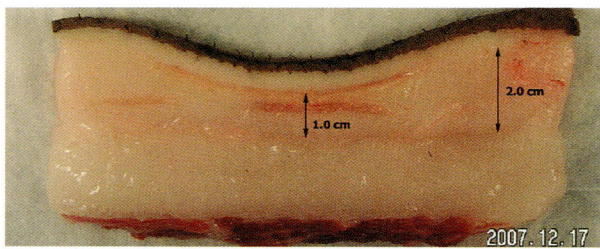

Figure 23.2 Fat layer reduction as seen with gross pathology in an animal model three months after treatment [5].

The extravasated lipids remain trapped within the subcutaneous tissue until digestion and clearance by an inflammatory process. This resorption takes place over a period of more than 90 days, resulting in a gradual displacement of the lipids. Histology shows a clear reduction in fat layer thickness results. The results are also easily visible on gross pathology sections at 90 days.

The mechanisms governing the apoptosis and subsequent elimination of adipocytes are not fully understood. Initial studies have been performed in an attempt to identify a possible pathway. [6]. Pig adipocytes were isolated, cultured and exposed to temperatures ranging from −2°C to 28°C and 5% CO_2 for one hour. Following exposure, the cells were returned to normal culture conditions (5% CO_2 and 37°C) for a recovery period of either 2 or 24 hours. Assays were performed to identify the extent of necrotic cell death and apoptotic cell death indicated that adipocytes cooled to −2, 0 and 2°C were all necrotically damaged regardless of recovery

time, as were most of the adipocytes cooled to 7°C. Adipocytes cooled to temperatures between 14°C and 28°C displayed no necrotic injury. In fact, all fat cells showed approximately the same extent of apoptotic injury after 48 hours of recovery. The results at higher temperatures suggest that the mechanism of action responsible for adipocyte death is based on an event that triggers apoptosis, although further studies are needed to determine the exact cause of the apoptotic injury.

Thus, preclinical studies have confirmed that the phenomenon of cold-induced panniculitis can be replicated in experimental porcine models. The mechanism for this process, however, is not completely understood.

Clinical Studies

Cryolipolysis is performed as an outpatient procedure with the Zeltiq System (Zeltiq Aesthetics, Pleasanton, CA). The device consists of a control unit with a cooling applicator that is applied to the area of treatment. Tissue is drawn into a cup-shaped applicator with a moderate vacuum to optimally position the tissue between two cooling panels. The selected heat extraction rate (i.e., cooling) is modulated by thermoelectric cooling elements and controlled by thermistors that monitor the heat flux out of the tissue.

A coupling gel is applied to the skin surface before placement of the applicator on the treatment area to ensure consistent thermal contact. The applicator is positioned on the skin with the use of a moderate vacuum. Treatment with the cold exposure, which includes a predetermined energy extraction rate expressed as a cooling intensity factor (CIF) and duration of up to 60 minutes, is initiated. At the conclusion of the treatment time, the system automatically discontinues the cold exposure and the applicator is removed by release of the vacuum. Additional application sites may be treated to ensure that the entire area of desired reduction is appropriately exposed to cooling.

Clinical evaluation of cryolipolysis has shown that selective removal of fat is achieved in humans as well. A multi-center, prospective, non-randomized clinical study performed by Dover et al. [7] evaluated the use of cryolipolysis for fat layer reduction of the flanks (i.e., love handles) and back (i.e., back fat pads). Preprogrammed treatment protocols were utilized to control the rate of heat extraction and duration of treatment for 32 patients. A contralateral, untreated area was maintained as a control to confirm actual efficacy. Efficacy was assessed by three assessment techniques: ultrasound measurement of fat layer reduction, comparison of pre- and post-treatment photographs, and physician assessment. These assessments confirmed that cryolipolysis results in a visible contour change in a majority of subjects, with the best cosmetic results noted in those patients presenting with modest discrete fat bulges. See Figs 23.5 and 23.6. Ultrasound measurements taken on a subset of 10 subjects demonstrated a fat layer reduction in 100% of these subjects with an average reduction of 22.4% at four months post-treatment. There were no device-related adverse events reported, confirming the safety of this treatment.

Further safety studies have also been performed to assess whether cryolipolysis is associated with an alteration in local sensory function or nerve fibers, or an elevation in lipid levels or liver function values as a result of cold exposure. Coleman et al. [8] documented the results of neural assessments and Riopelle

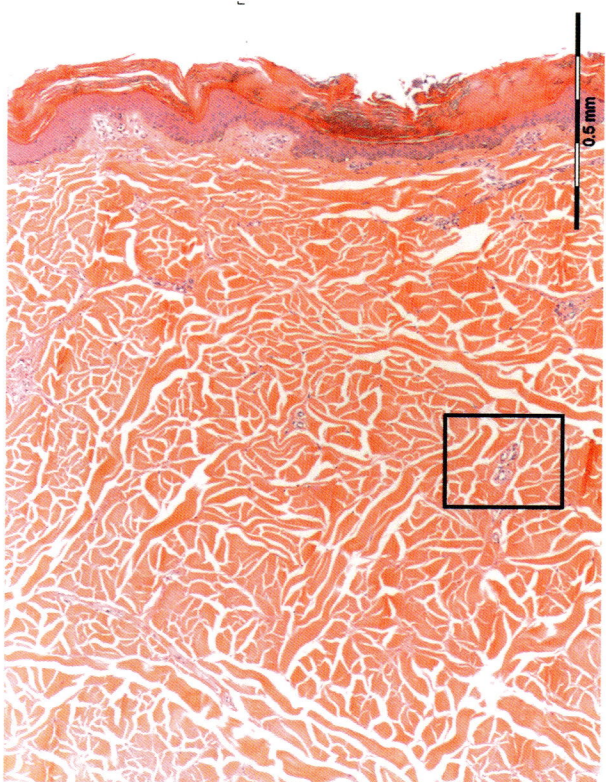

Figure 23.3 Tissue section showing dermis or epidermis in an animal model three months after treatment. Tissue is intact; there is no evidence of damage following treatment [5].

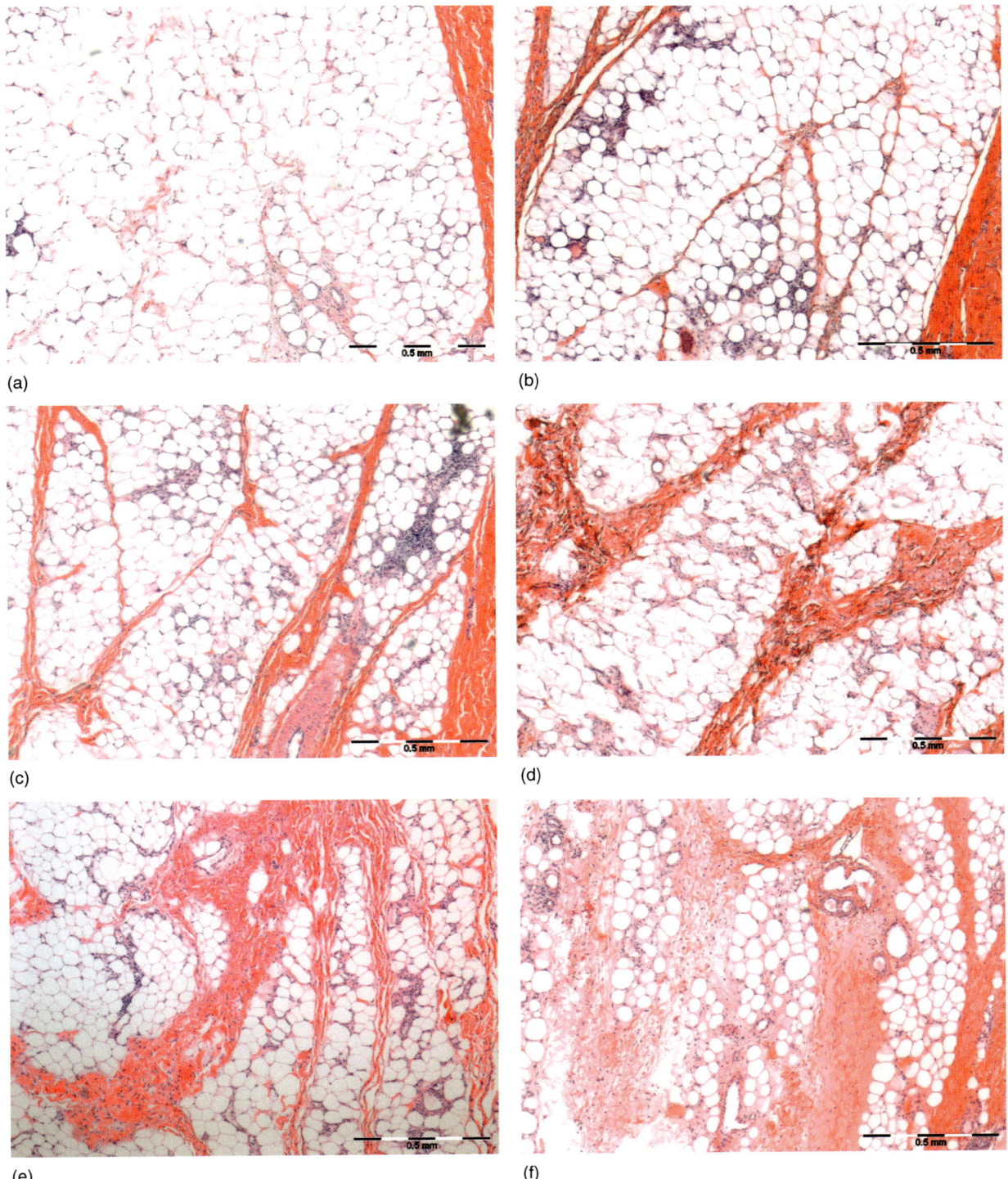

Figure 23.4 Histological sequence of inflammatory response following treatment at three days (a), seven days (b), 14 days (c), 30 days (d), 60 days (e), and 90 days (f) after treatment [5].

et al. [9] assessed lipid levels and liver function tests for 90 days post-treatment.

Ten subjects were treated with a prototype cooling device (Zeltiq Aesthetics, Pleasanton, CA) during the Coleman study to determine if fat reduction in humans caused by cold exposure is associated with local sensory function or nerve fiber changes. Fat reduction was assessed in nine of 10 subjects via ultrasound prior to treatment and at follow-up. Sensory function was assessed by neurologist evaluation (n = 9) and nerve staining was completed on tissue obtained with a biopsy from one subject. Treatment resulted in a normalized fat layer reduction of 25.5% at six months post-treatment. Transient reduction in sensation occurred in six of the nine subjects assessed by neurologic evaluation. Sensation returned within seven weeks post-treatment (with a mean of 3.6 weeks). Biopsies also showed no long-term change in nerve fiber structure.

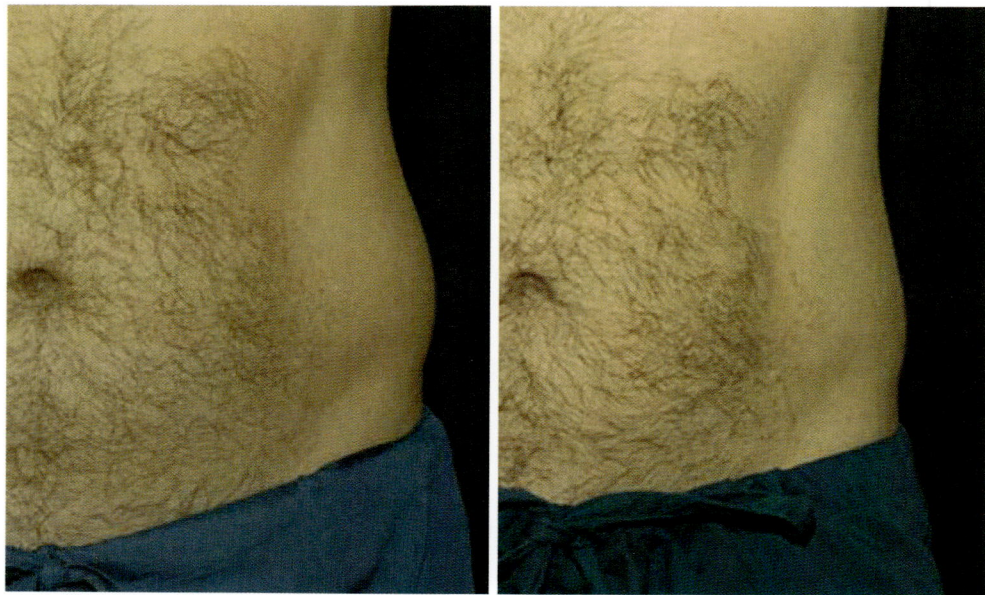

Figure 23.5 Reduction of love handle. Image on left was taken prior to procedure; image on right was taken four months following the procedure [7].

Ten subjects with discrete fat bulges ("love handles") were treated with the Zeltiq prototype cooling device during the Riopelle study to determine if a cosmetically significant fat layer reduction was associated with a meaningful change in lipid profile and liver function tests. High frequency ultrasound imaging was used to objectively measure fat layer reduction and photographs were taken pre-treatment and at follow-up visits. Lipid profiles and liver function tests were obtained on all subjects prior to treatment and at baseline, one, four, eight and 12 weeks post-treatment, which ensured that they were assessed through the 90 days after treatment normally associated with peak lipid resorption. Pre-treatment and six-month post-treatment ultrasound images provided objective evidence of fat layer reduction in eight out of ten subjects. No clinically significant changes or abnormal values were identified for either lipid levels or liver function tests over the 90-day follow-up period.

These clinical studies demonstrate that selective cryolipolysis results in reductions in subcutaneous fat without damage to the surrounding tissues. Ultrasound images and photographic reviews demonstrate fat layer reduction, with the greatest cosmetic improvement observed in subjects with modest fat bulges. Analysis of lipid levels, neurological response, and the lack of device-related adverse events demonstrate the safety of cryolipolysis. Further clinical evaluation is required, however, to more fully understand the potential application to other parts of the body and the optimal treatment parameters for each. Additional studies would also be beneficial to assess whether cryolipolysis poses a unique risk to patients with rare

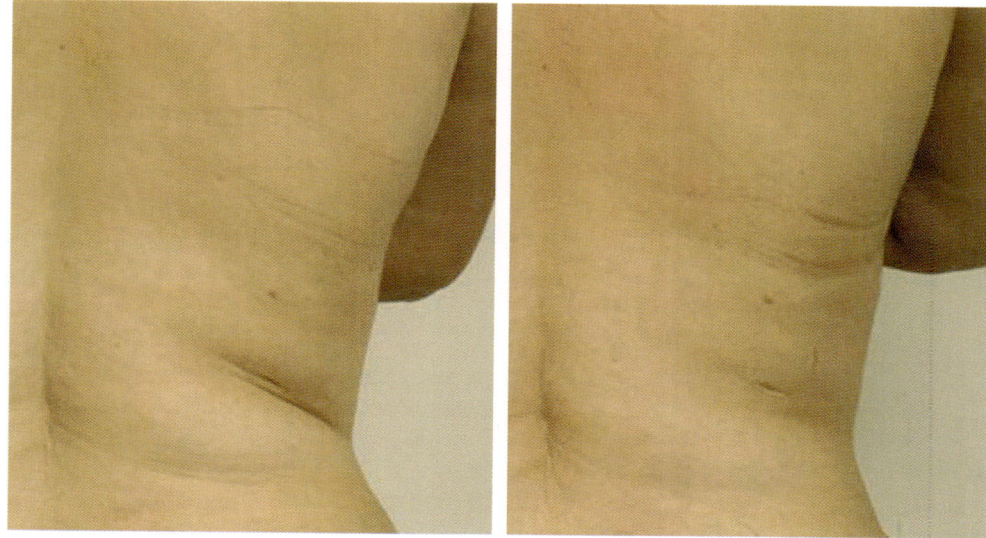

Figure 23.6 Reduction of back fat. Image on left was taken prior to procedure; image on right was taken four months following the procedure.

conditions such as cryoglobulinemia, paryoxysmal cold hemoglobinuria, or cold urticaria.

Discussion

Cryolipolysis is a unique technology that has produced effective non-invasive, selective fat removal. Both human and animal studies confirm the clinical findings of cold-induced panniculitis and subsequent fat layer reduction. Histology findings confirm the selective removal of fat tissue in both humans and animals. This reduction is not immediate, but rather gradually occurs over a period of months. Notably the mechanism of action for cryolipolysis is not yet completely understood. Importantly, it has not produced any significant adverse side effects in studies to date, no laboratory abnormalities have been noted with lipid levels or liver function tests, and any observed effects have been minor and temporary.

At this time, it is unknown whether cryolipolysis is significantly effective for improvement of the appearance of cellulite. Although effective for fat removal, it is not yet known whether cold application to the skin would have an impact on the architectural features of the subcutaneous fat and dermis that produce cellulite. Studies are awaited.

Given the clinical efficacy of this device, it will be most effective for fat layer reduction in confined anatomical areas. At this point, there is no evidence to suggest it can remove fat from large areas on a scale seen with liposuction procedures. Further studies will more fully characterize the clinical potential of this technology.

Importantly, however, cryolipolysis is a relatively rapid, non-invasive means of removing fat in a safe manner. It requires no pain management, no tumescent or other anesthesia. Moreover, there is no "downtime" associated with this procedure from work or social activities. It has the potential to provide safe, effective treatments of localized fat accumulation in a safe and gradual manner.

Conlusion

Cryolipolysis is a unique technique that has demonstrated efficacy for non-invasive, selective fat removal.

REFERENCES

1. H Rotman Cold Panniculitis in Children. Arch Derm 94: 720–21, 1966.
2. WC Duncan, RG Free man CL Heaton. Cold Panniculitis. Arch Derm 722–24, 1966.
3. BE Beachman, PH Cooper, CS Buchanan, PE Weary. Equestrian Cold Panniculitis in Women. Arch Derm 1025–27, 1980.
4. D Manstein, H Laubach, K Watanabe et al. Selective Cryolysis: A Novel Method of Non-Invasive Fat Removal. Lasers Surg Med 40:595–604, 2009.
5. B Zelickson, BM Egbert, J Preciado et al. In press. Derm Surg, accepted manuscript.
6. J Preciado, J Allison. The Effect of Cold Exposure on Adipocytes: Examining a Novel Method for the Noninvasive Removal of Rat. Oral presentation at the Society for Cryobiology Annual International Conference, 21 July 2008.
7. J Dover, J Burns, S Coleman et al. A Prospective Clinical Study of Noninvasive Cryolypolysis for Subcutaneous Fat Layer Reduction – Interim Report of Available Subject Data. ASLMS, April 2009.
8. SR Coleman, K Sachdeva, BM Egbert et al. Clinical Efficacy of Noninvasive Cryolipolysis and Its Effects on Peripheral Nerves. Aesth Plast Surg 2009 March 19 (epub ahead of print).
9. J Riopelle, MY Tsai, B Kovack. Lipid and Liver Function Effects of the Cryolipolysis Procedure in a Study of Male Love Handle Reduction. ASLMS, April 2009.

24 Subcision®
Doris Hexsel, Rosemarie Mazzuco, and Mariana Soirefmann

Introduction

Subcision® is a simple surgical technique, originally described by Orentreich and Orentreich [1], in which subcutaneous (SQ) fibrous septa are cut; this both diminishes the traction exerted on the skin and creates hematomas which in turn promotes the formation of new connective tissue. Therefore, it acts as an autologous and physiologic filler [2]. In 1997, the present authors described the effectiveness of Subcision® for the treatment of high degree cellulite (Figs. 24.1 and 24.2) and in 2000, the same authors presented a detailed step-by-step guide to the procedure, based on the use of Subcision® in 232 female patients [3].

Indications and Action Mechanisms

Subcision® can be used in the treatment of all conditions where there are SQ septa pulling the skin surface. These include wrinkles and folds, depressed scars [4] and lesions [5], as well as cellulite [2]. Subcision® can also be used to correct other skin relief alterations, such those that appear after liposuction (Figs. 24.3 and 24.4), trauma, or inflammatory diseases, and those appearing in the donor areas of the fat grafts [1,3] on the face [5] and also on the body [5]. Subcision® has also been reported for the treatment of acne scars [6], stretch marks [7] and auricular deformities in rabbits [8].

In case of cellulite, Subcision® is useful for the treatment of high degree cellulite, such as grade two and three, in which the depressed lesions are visible when the patient is in the standing position and with relaxed gluteus muscles (see Fig. 24.11) [3].

Two action mechanisms were initially described by Orentreich and Orentreich: the cutting of subcutaneous fibrous septa which releases the tension exerted on the skin; and the formation of new connective tissue which results from the creation of hematomas [1]. The surgical movements cut the septa and nearby vessels, giving rise to hematomas, the size of which depends on the size of the cut vessels, the extension of the treated lesion, the post-operative care, and the integrity of the blood coagulation mechanisms. These aspects directly determine the proportion of the filling effect in the treated area [3]. In the treatment of cellulite, a third action mechanism is involved: the redistribution of the traction and tension forces between fat lobes, which contributes to the improvement of the relief of the treated areas [3].

The number of the Subcisions® necessary to correct a defect depends on the size, depth and location of the defect, as well as on the degree (or quantity) of new collagen formation. Most cases can be treated by one or two procedures, with a minimum interval of two months between them.

Contraindications for Subcision®

Orentreich and Orentreich described the following contra-indications for Subcision®, divided into two categories:

1. Absolute: Active infection in or immediately adjacent to the area to be treated as well as in the case of scars like "ice pick" acne scars.
2. Relative: coagulation disorders, atrophic scars, history of hypertrophic scars or keloids.

   Hexsel and Mazzuco, described other contraindications when using this technique to treat large areas, such as the use of medicines or the existence of diseases which may interfere with blood coagulation or with anesthetics and medicines which can alter the expected or desired post-operative evolution [3].

Other contraindications were published, including pregnancy, first degree of cellulite, cottage cheese or orange peel lesions, severe illnesses, and patients who will be unable to follow post-operatory recommendations or with unrealistic expectations [9].

Pre-Operative Consultation

For Subcision®, previous medical evaluation is important, not only for adequate patient selection but also to prepare the patients for the procedure.

The pre-operative care is, basically, the same as any other out-patient surgical procedure. Some items should be checked, such as the tendency to develop keloids or allergic reactions and the medicines that patients are taking.

Some medicines should be avoided in the pre-op period: anti-coagulant agents, drugs which interfere with platelet aggregation, beta-blockers, immunosuppressant agents, neuroleptic agents, oral isotretinoin and iron. These, as well as the smoking habit, are relative contraindications to the procedure.

Contraindications for this procedure include local infections and diseases, as well as presence of risk factors for trombophilia.

Laboratory exams should be requested at this time. They should include a coagulogram and any other exam required according to the patient's needs [2,3].

Prophylactic antibiotic therapy with Ciprofloxacin 500 mg is recommended twice a day.

Surgical Technique

The surgical procedure includes the follow steps:

1. ***Skin Marking:*** The skin relief depressions should be marked prior to the procedure. This should be done while observing the patient standing in an upright position, with relaxed muscles [3] (Fig. 24.5). The light source should be perpendicular to the skin surface, in order to better observe the skin relief alterations [5]. Slight lesions, such as those evident only when the muscles are contracted, should not be treated due to the risk of becoming raised [2,3]. It is recommended to choose lesions up to 30 millimeters (mm) in diameter or only part of larger

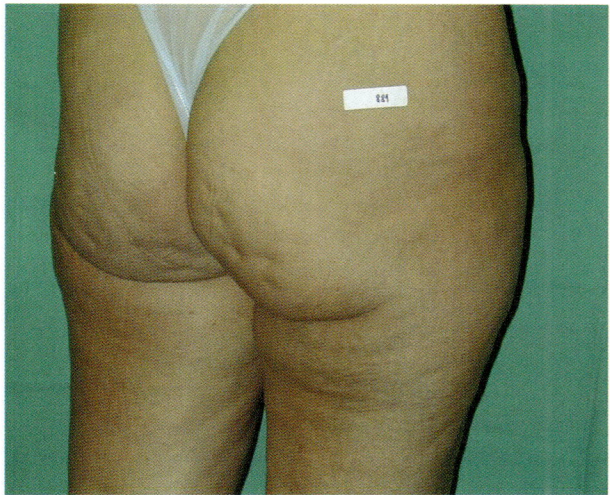

Figure 24.1 Sixty-two year old female presenting cellulite on the buttocks.

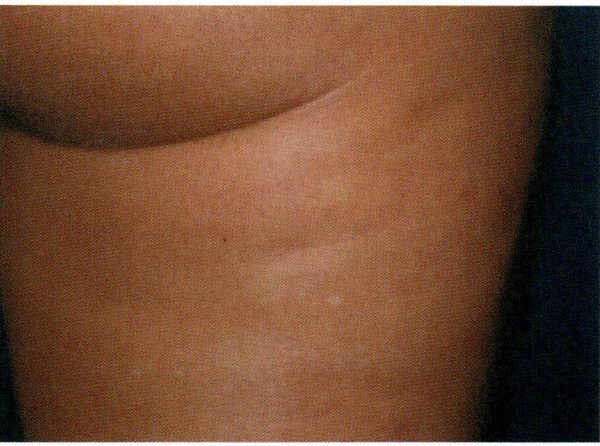

Figure 24.3 Liposuction sequela on the upper part of the thighs.

lesions not exceeding this measurement [3], to avoid the creation of large hematomas and the formation of extensive dissection planes, increasing the risk of complications that may arise as a result of these situations [10].

2. *Antisepsis:* Antisepsis should be rigorous and widespread, in all the large surgical areas [2]. The most frequently used antiseptic is iodized alcohol, and in patients that are allergic to iodine, chlorexidine or the antiseptic adopted by each establishment. It is recommended that the procedure be carried out in a surgical room and that sterile clothes and fields are used.

3. *Anesthesia:* Infiltrated local anesthesia is given with the patient lying down (Fig. 24.6). The needle should be inserted 1 to 2 cm beneath the marked skin and the anesthetic injected while withdrawing the needle, into the subcutaneous level. Upon completing the injection, an anesthetic button is left at the site where the Subcision® needle will be placed. General anesthesia and blocks (rachidian and epidural) are not recommended, as they increase the surgical burden and because of the necessity of using a vasodilator at the site. The latter offers several advantages, it permits the identification of the

extension of the anesthetized area, can indicate the presence of large vessels in the area and limits the size of the hematomas, reducing bleeding, as well as increasing the safe dose and duration of the anesthetic [2]. Two percent (2%) lidocaine with epinephrine or norepinephrine 1:200.000 is preferred [2]. Tumescent anesthesia is also an option, when there are many depressions [11], although as this infiltrates the fat, it may reduce bleeding and consequent hematoma formation, which is wanted in this procedure, and prevent the bed for the hematoma. The recommended dose of 2% lidocaine with vasoconstrictor is from 7.0 mg/kg [12] and the dose of lidocaine per session should not exceed 500 mg [12]. The number of lesions treatable in a single session depends on the dose of anesthetic that can be used for each patient, which is calculated according to the patient's body weight [13,14]. The total anesthetic dose described as safe for lidocaine with vasoconstrictor should not exceed 500 mg [12,15] or 7.0 mg/kg [10].

4. *Cutting the subcutaneous septa:* Following maximum vasoconstriction, apparent due to paleness and piloerection, the procedure can begin. A BD Nokor® calibre 18G needle [3] is preferred, as it has a cutting blade at the point. Other alternatives are a special scalpel, with the same cutting blade at

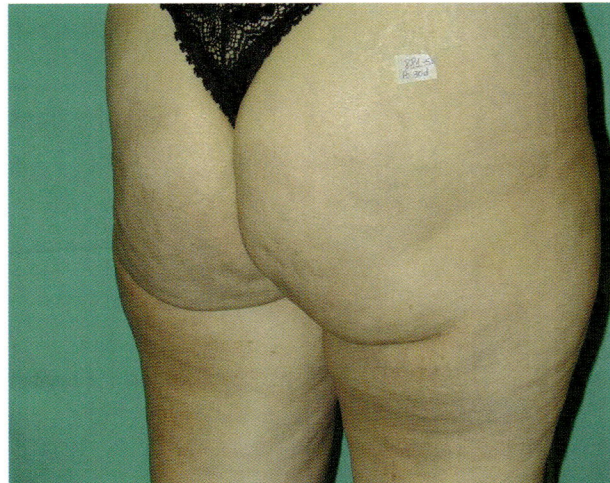

Figure 24.2 Same patient as Fig. 24.1, one month after Subcision®.

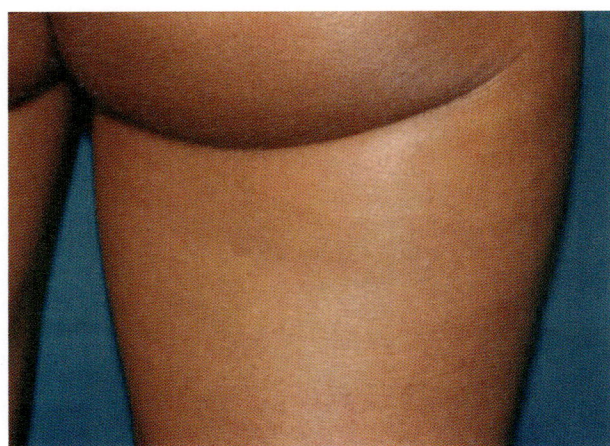

Figure 24.4 Same patient as Fig. 24.3, after Subcision®.

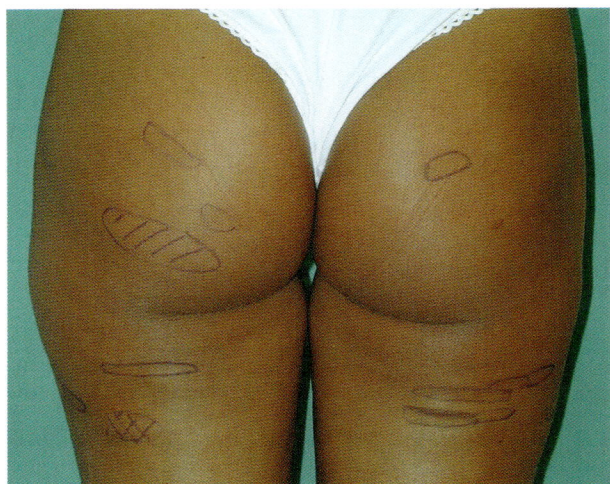

Figure 24.5 Lesions' borders are marked before the procedure. In this case, the raised areas, well indicated for liposuction, are also marked with lines inside the borders.

the point, or a normal or three-beveled needle, as described by Orentreich and Orentreich [1]. The needle should be inserted about 1.5 cm beneath the lesion at the point where the anesthetic button was previously placed (Fig. 24.7). The insertion should be made at an angle of 45° to 90° to the skin surface and then, at a depth of 1.5 to 2 cm below the skin surface the needle should be positioned parallel to the epidermis, with the cutting edge to the left against the septum. The septa are cut on the back stroke of the needle, while maintaining the blade traction against the septa, thus releasing the tension that they exert on the skin. This cutting

technique allows a precise cut of the specific septa pulling the skin down, with a minimum of tissue damage, which assures better post-operative results. A slight pinch test on the treated lesion is useful because it reveals any areas that remain retracted by septa [3,16]. Recently, Al-Khenaizan [4] suggested a simple method to ensure continuous orientation of the Nokor® needle during Subcision®: the hub of the needle is marked with two short straight lines perpendicular to the triangular cutting surface, at the 12 and six o'clock position of the hub. This ensures that the cutting triangular surface is always in the horizontal position, parallel to the skin surface with the cutting edge to the left or the right.

5. *Compression:* Following the cutting of the septa, vigorous compression is required in the treated area for 5 to 10 minutes, sufficient time for the coagulation process, permitting hemostasis and control of the size of the hematomas. The use of sandbags made from washable material is recommended, weighing approximately 5 kg or 10 pounds, wrapped in sterile fabric [3]. Such bags produce a more uniform and efficacious compression than that achieved manually.

6. *Dressings:* The treated areas are covered with sterile adhesive bandages. Additional compression with dressings and compressive clothing (elastic pants or shorts) are also recommended, that should be worn for 30 days.

The following post-operative instructions are given to the patients:

- Use analgesics for the first 48 hours; this period can be extended if pain persists; acetaminophen at a dose of 750 mg every 6 hours is recommended;
- Continue use of the antibiotic until the third day;

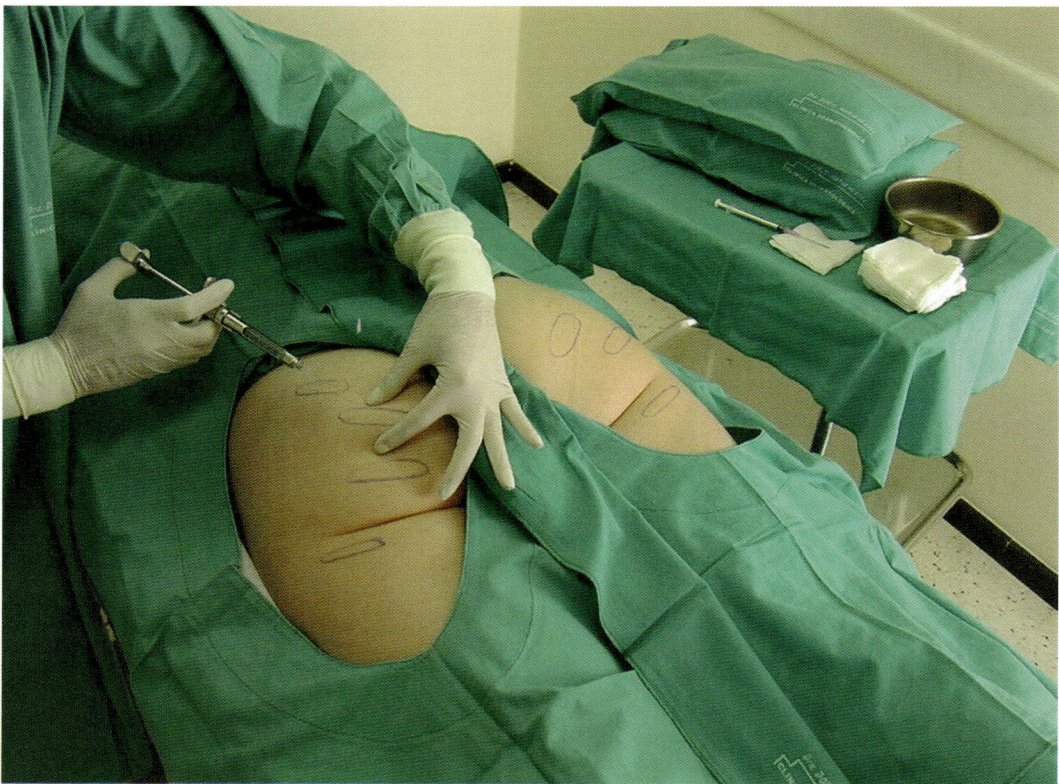

Figure 24.6 After antisepsis of the surgical area, local anesthesia is performed in the surgical room. Sterile sheets are used to protect the surgical area.

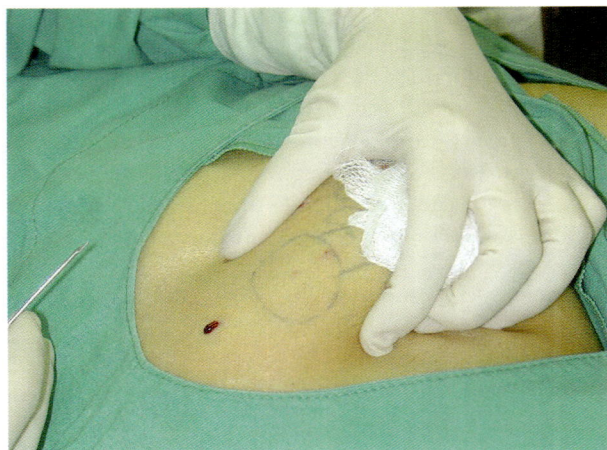

Figure 24.7 A gentle pinch test is performed in order to find residual septa pulling the skin surface.

- Physical exercise only after the third week;
- Use compressive clothing for 30 days.

The Post-Operative Period

The first post-operative evaluation should be made after 72 hours, when the dressings are removed and the antibiotic suspended [3]. Hematomas and hemosiderosis are expected in all the patients in this period. The hematomas should follow a normal evolution of spontaneous reabsorption over a period varying from 10 to 30 days. Hemosiderosis may persist for several months and is directly proportional to the quantity of iron present in the red blood cells.

Complications

According to Orentreich and Orentreich [1], the complications listed below may arise. They are rare and easily dealt.

1. *hematomas and ecchymosis (Fig. 24.8);*
2. *erythema, edema and local discomfort;*
3. *infection;*
4. *alterations to the consistency of the skin and SQ in the treated areas;*

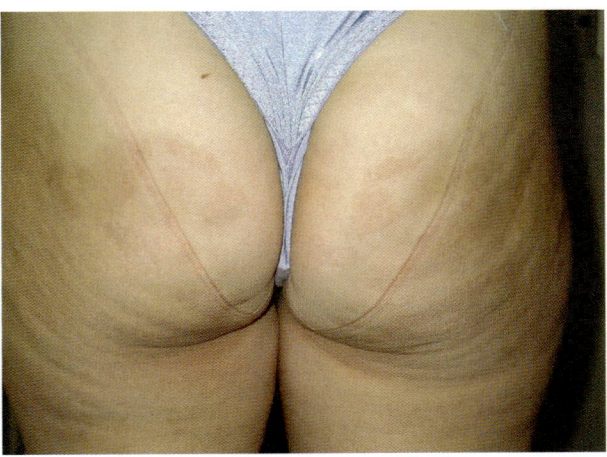

Figure 24.9 Hemosiderosis one month after Subcision®.

5. *alterations to the color of the skin in the treated area;*
6. *sub-optimal response;*
7. *excessive response;*
8. *keloid scars.*

In fact, complications arising from Subcision® [16] for the treatment of cellulite are rare. This is due to the safety of the method and the local anatomy, as usually the areas commonly treated are free of vital structures and large blood vessels.

Other complications include:

9. ***Hemosiderosis*** occurs due to the extravasation of the red blood cells and the deposit of hemosiderin, a pigment that contains iron, decorrent by the degradation of the hemoglobin [17], giving the skin a chestnut pigmentation. It occurs in all treated patients to varying degrees, and its resolution occurs spontaneously within two to 12 months (Fig. 24.9).

10. ***Organized hematomas or seromas*** may occur in some treated areas, but usually clear up spontaneously in a period from one to three months. They are usually painful and hard to the touch.

11. ***False excess response*** is characterized by a raised area of skin at the treated area, appearing as a herniation of the

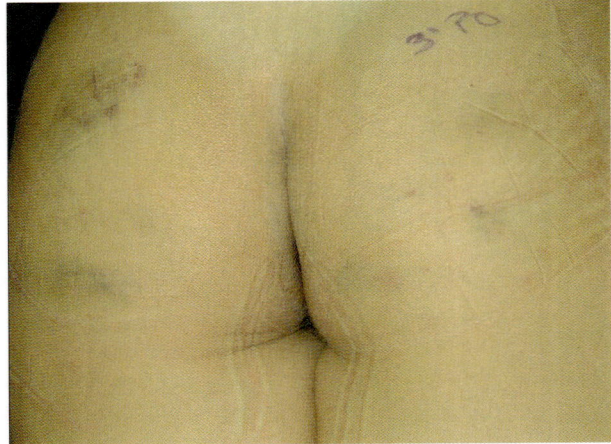

Figure 24.8 Hematomas in the 3rd PO day, in well compressed areas.

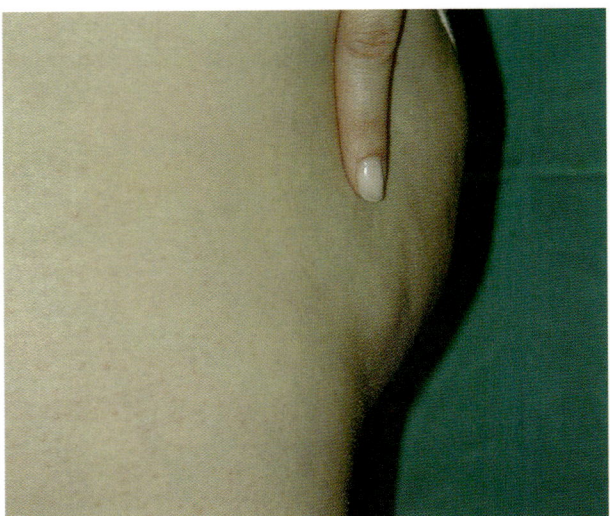

Figure 24.10 False excess response after Subcision®.

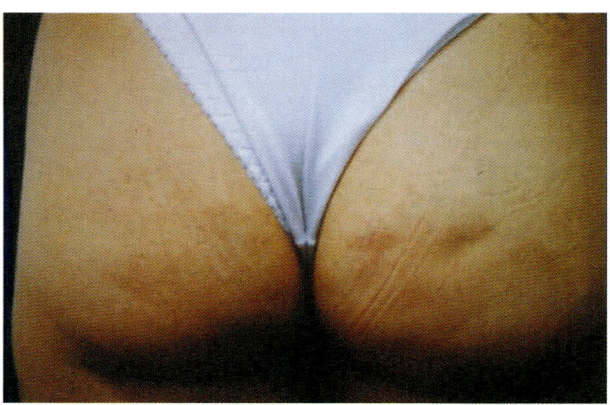

Figure 24.11 Cellulite on the buttocks before treatment.

skin and SQ fat (Fig. 24.10). This does not respond well to corticoid injections and may be due to bad technique (complete Subcision® in extensive areas or excessively superficial) or a lack of post-operative care, such as the non-use of compressive clothing for 30 days following the procedure. Favorable results can be obtained with the use of liposuction with micro-canulas in the affected area. It is important to keep in mind that some septa are not exerting excessive skin retraction. Therefore, they should remain intact [9].

Associated Procedures

Recently, Sasaki published a study comparing Subcision® alone versus Subcision® associated with fillers and other adjacent surgical procedures. The author concluded that the use of Subcision® alone for resistant wrinkles, folds, or scars can result in a satisfactory outcome with minimal complications. Moreover, results may be further optimized with the immediate addition of fillers into the released tract. An adjacent aesthetic surgical procedure may provide additional benefit, but not as much as observed with the usage of fillers. The study did not include cellulite patients [18].

Balighi et al. published a clinical trial regarding the use of Subcision® in acne scars with and without subdermal implant. The authors concluded that Subcision® seems to be a safe method to correct the rolling acne scars with long-term improvement. The subdermal implant led to no significant superior results [19].

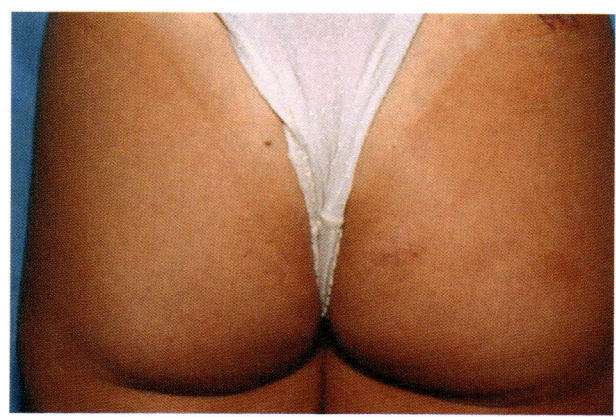

Figure 24.12 Same patient as Fig. 24.11, after two Subcisions®.

Conclusions

Subcision® is a simple, effective (Figs. 24.11 and 24.12) and low cost surgical method for the treatment of advanced cellulite and some other skin conditions.

It is a precise surgical procedure for the treatment of severe cellulite, in which the septa that retain the skin are cut, resulting in redistribution of the traction and tension forces among the fat lobules, giving an immediate improvement to the skin relief.

Complications are rare and easily treated. The production of new connective tissue from the hematomas occurs in two to five weeks and normally persists for a considerable time in the correction of the treated defect. The results are technique dependent and are usually long-lasting [3].

REFERENCES

1. DS Orentreich, N Orentreich. Subcutaneous incisionless (subcision) surgery for the correction of depressed scars and wrinkles. Dermatol Surg 21:543–49, 1995.
2. DM Hexsel, R Mazzuco. Subcision: Uma alternativa cirurgica para a lipodistrofia ginoide ("celulite") e outras alteracoes do relevo corporal. An Bras Dermatol 72:27–32, 1997.
3. DM Hexsel, R Mazzuco. Subcision: a treatment for cellulite. Int J Dermatol 39:539–44, 2000.
4. Sultan Al-Khenaizan. Nokor needle marking: a simple method to maintain orientation during subcision Journal of Drugs in Dermatology 2007.
5. DM Hexsel, R Mazzuco, T Dal'Forno, CL Hexsel. Simple technique provides option for treating scars and other skin depressions. J Cosm Dermatol 17(1):35–41, 2004.
6. M Alam, N Omura, MS Kaminer. Subcision for acne scarring: technique and outcomes in 40 patients. Dermatol Surg 31(3):310–7, 2005.
7. P Luis-Montoya, P Pichardo-Velázquez, MT Hojyo-Tomoka, J Domínguez-Cherit. Evaluation of subcision as a treatment for cutaneous striae. J Drugs Dermatol 4(3):346–50, 2005.
8. A Karacalar, A Demir, L Yildiz. Subcision surgery for the correction of ear deformities. Aesthetic Plast Surg 28(4):239–44, 2004.
9. D Hexsel, M Soirefmann, CL Hexsel. Reduction of cellulite with Subcision. In: A Murad et al (eds). Body Rejuvanation. Taylor and Francis; 2009 (in press).
10. GL Vieira, PRS Rocha. Anestesia local. In: FP Fonseca, PRS Rocha. Cirurgia ambulatorial. Rio de Janeiro: Guanabara Koogan 1987: 49–71.
11. A Namias, B Kaplan. Tumescent anesthesia for dermatologic surgery. Cosmetic and noncosmetic procedures. Dermatol Surg 24(7):755–8, 1998.
12. McTH Calmont, B Leshin. Preoperative Evaluation of the Cutaneous Surgery Patient. In: GP Lask, RL Moy (eds). Principles and Techniques of Cutaneous Surgery. New York: McGraw-Hill; 1996: 101–12.
13. BB Hoffman, RJ Lefkowitz. Catecholamines, sympathomimetic drugs and adrenergic receptor antagonists. In: JG Hardman, LE Limbird, PB Mollinoff et al (eds). Goodman & Gilman's The Pharmacological Basis of Therapeutics. New York: McGraw-Hill; 1996: 199–248.

14. JL Fewkes. Antisepsis, anesthesia, hemostasis, and suture placement. In: KA Ardnt, PE Le Boit, JK Robinson, BU Wintroub (eds). Cutaneous Medicine and Surgery. Philadelphia: WB Saunders; 1996:128–138.

15. Vilhaça CM Neto. Anestesia –Parte 1. An Bras Dermatol 74(3):213–19, 1999.

16. D Hexsel, R Mazzuco, D Gobbato, CL Hexsel. Subcision. In: MP Kede, O Sabatovitch. Tratado de Medicina Estetica,1ª ed. Atheneu. Rio de Janeiro; 2003:350–359.

17. JK Robinson. Management of hematomas. In: JK Robinson, KA Ardnt, PE LeBoit, BU Wintroub (eds). Atlas of Cutaneous Surgery. Philadelphia: WB Saunders; 1996:73–77.

18. GH Sasaki. Comparison of results of wire subcision performed alone, with fills, and/or with adjacent surgical procedures. Aesthet Surg J 28(6):619–26, 2008.

19. K Balighi, RM Robati, H Moslehi et al. Subcision® in acne scar with and without subdermal implant: a clinical trial. J Eur Acad Dermatol Venereol 22(6):707–11, 2008.

25 Surgical Treatment: Liposuction, Liposculpture, and Lipoplasty
Gustavo Leibaschoff

- Liposuction is the name of the technique whereby fat is carried out through suction equipment (syringe or suction pump) without any idea about the harmonics of the body.
- Liposculpture is a technique for fat tissue extirpation through blunt 2–4 mm cannulae. Suction may be carried out with 20 or 60 cc syringes or suction pump (1 atm) with a tridimensional idea for recovery of the convexity and concavities of the shape of the body.
- We personally believe that the term "lipoplasty" is all-inclusive, and that the term "lipoplasty" involves all surgical, medical or rehabilitation therapeutic practices. It is sheer nonsense to assume that after-surgery procedures results are guaranteed. It is precisely the lack of comprehensive treatment that caused dissatisfaction in most patients who submitted to liposuction some years before.
- Liposculpture is a modeling of the contours, a real artistic job of architecture bound to restore the juvenile and harmonic forms of the face or body by working with the hypodermic fatty tissues.

Historical background

In 1921, the French surgeon Dujarrier tried to remove adipose tissue from the internal area of a dancer's knee by means of an obstetric curet. The limb was later amputated because of the ensuing infection [1]. In 1964, the German surgeon Schrudder tried to repeat the same operation using a different technique [2]. Thus, lipoexeresis was born, though physicians were unwilling to accept it because it frequently resulted in lymphorrhea and cutaneous unevenness. Some years later, in 1974, the Italian surgeon Arpad Fisher and his son Giorgio developed in Rome a new technique, called liposculpture, that included the use of blunt cannulae and a liposuction device [3]. In 1978, Drs. Meyer and Kesserling reported a liposuction technique that used a sharp cannula connected to a 0.5 atmosphere suction device.

But it was only in 1977 when the French surgeon Illouz [21,22] first submitted to an international cosmetic surgery conference a new technique of his own based on a cannula similar to Fisher's [23,24]. Tunnels were excavated at different adipose tissue levels after injecting a hypotonic solution [4]. However, it was the French physician Fournier who first coined the term "lipoplasty" for his "dry" fat suction technique (meaning that no previous hypotonic infiltration was applied) that enabled contour remodeling [5].

Since 1980, "liposculpture" and "lipoplasty" have become widespread around the world. Research papers were submitted to major cosmetic and plastic surgery journals and scientific conferences [6].

The development of liposculpture is not complete, however, without Dr. Jeffrey Klein's research work. He developed tumescent anesthesia and thus set a landmark in lipoplasty [7]. There is previous research on local anesthesia by the Russian physician Vinieschewky (1916), who studied hydraulic tissue preparation, and other works on local anesthesia applied to large volumes carried out in USA during the 1930s and 1950s. Dr. Klein's revolution allowed lipoplasty to be carried out on outpatients under local anesthesia entailing little blood loss.

In his attempts to reduce blood loss and post-surgical trauma, Dr. Pierre Fournier showed in 1985 that fat might be extracted through single-use syringes [5].

Dr. Michele Zocchi developed ultrasonic-assisted liposculpture and submitted his first reports on this technique in his papers on the selective cavitation effects of ultrasound for adipose tissue lyses [8] (Fig. 25.2–25.3). Later on, in 1992, a specific device was introduced. Carried out by competent professionals, this method enables the controlled extirpation of great amounts of adipose tissue and also allows skin retraction. Unfortunately, complications derived from irresponsible use of ultrasound devices have limited their use to experts only, with optimal results [9].

Dr. Michele Zocchi, from Italy, was a visionary man of science, a genuine researcher, and an insightful observer who noticed ultrasound advantages and their potential contribution to lipoplasty. Ultrasonic-assisted liposculpture carried out through devices such as solid titanium ultrasonic probes enables selective destruction of fatty cells with no damage to venous and lymphatic vessels or fibers [10,11].

Dr. Leibaschoff and Dr. Ciucci have carried out direct and radioisotope lymphographies that demonstrate conclusively this selective destruction (Fig. 25.4) [12], as well as Tazi and Schefflan's videofibroscopies.

In 1992, Dr. Giorgio Fischer (Italy) developed orthostatic liposculpture. He designed an orthostatic couch that lets the physician operate and control liposculpture while the patient is in standing position [3].

Almost simultaneously, Dr. Marco Gasparotti (Italy) reported his superficial liposculpture methodology, which enables better skin retraction and a smooth, homogeneous, cutaneous surface [13].

In 1993, Jeffrey Klein made still another contribution by using 2 mm micro-cannulae of various lengths in tumescent liposculpture. By working through multiple entry orifices, he achieved excellent results and the patient's recovery was very quick [14].

Now we have a new machine for internal ultrasonic-assisted liposculpture, the Vaser, the safest machine to work in ultrasonic lipoplasty, with all the advantages of the ultrasonic machine [16].

Vaser pulsed ultrasound is a recently built device, which utilizes ultrasound energy to emulsify the fat tissue.

The main differences with previous ultrasound technologies concerns safety issues.

Due to the excessive ultrasound energy delivered by first- and second-generation UAL devices a series of complications were

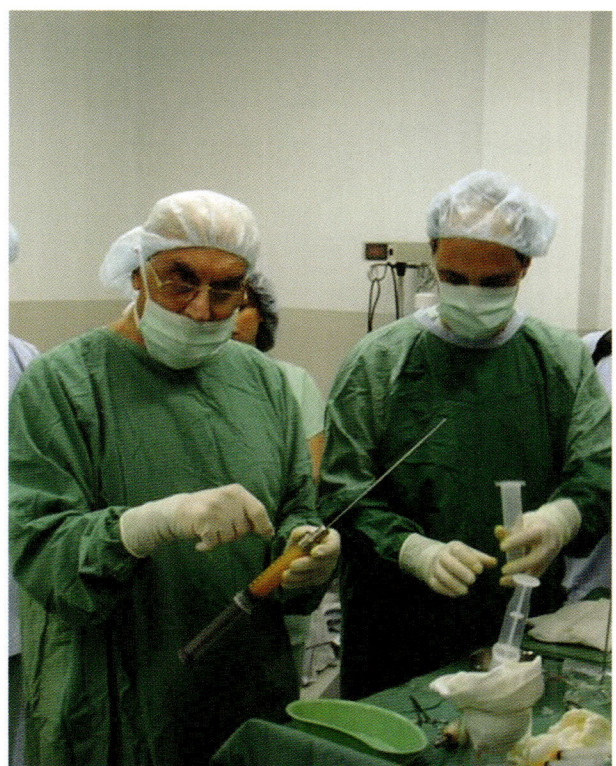

Figure 25.1 Fournier and the syringe, the basis of liposculpture.

(Fig. 25.5) the US market. The new device delivers nearly half the ultrasound energy in comparison with the older machines.

The shape and design of the new solid titanium probes increases efficiency of the system.

Superficial UAL allows (through minimal skin incisions) the utilization of two 2 mm solid titanium probes to fully undermine the subcutaneous tissue, thus allowing excellent skin retraction. Deeper planes are treated with two 9 mm or three 7 mm probes for faster emulsification. Grooved probes increase efficiency of the system. Three alarms control the system and prevent mistakes [20].

Lipoplasty has a threefold target: aesthetics, functionality, and restoration. But only surgeons properly trained in liposculpture may achieve this target. Lipoplasty is a surgical technique performed through mini-incisions. Thin tools a few millimeters in diameter are used under tumescent local anesthesia. Operations should be performed by surgeons who have experience in this field, under the control of anesthetists or cardiologists specialized in surgical monitoring.

Fournier said, "Liposculpture is the technique that uses disposable syringes to aspirate localized fat deposits and, if necessary, inject it where needed" [16] (Fig. 25.1).

We define Lipografting as the method consisting of the reinjection at different locations of the adipose tissue previously extracted through liposculpture and subsequently washed with physiologic solution to preserve adipocyte integrity [17].

Patient Selection

Liposculpture may be sometimes carried out under local anesthesia and as an ambulatory procedure, due to its characteristics as a less aggressive method. A wide variety of patients may be submitted to it. In each case, the following rules should be

described following UAL of 1995–2000 (seroma, mainly, but also burns, skin necrosis, and dysesthesia).

The initial enthusiasm for UAL decreased due to the complications rate and cost of equipment. In 2001 Vaser appeared on

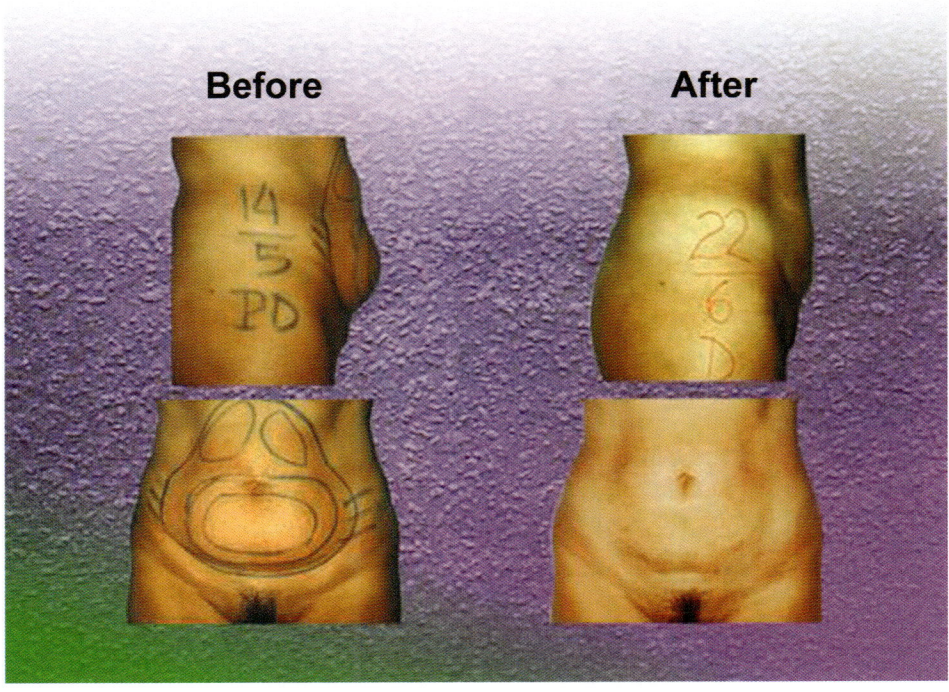

Figure 25.2 Before and after with ultrasound-assisted lipo (=1E, p. 215).

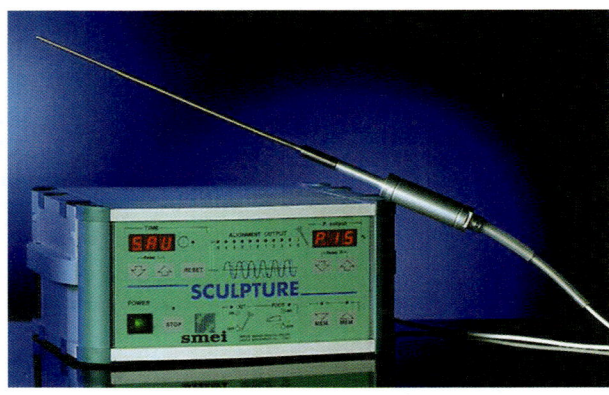

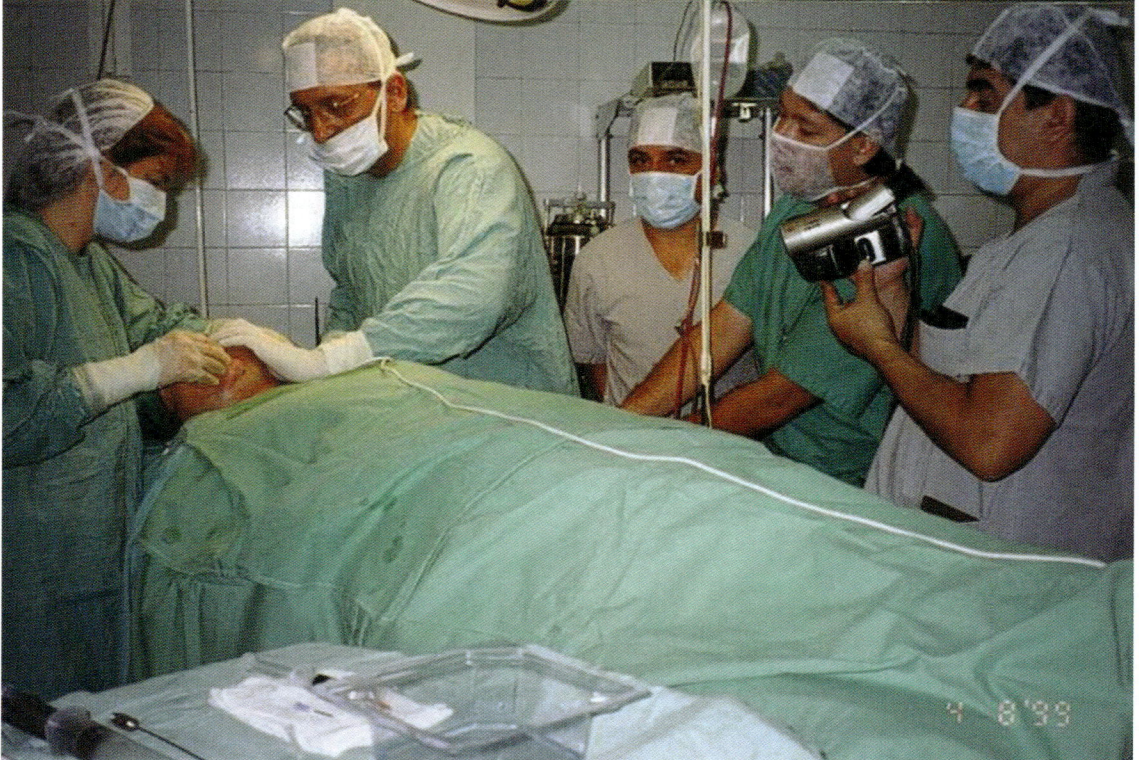

Figure 25.3 Dr Leibaschoff teaching about the use of Internal Ultrasound (first-generation of device of UAL) in the neck and face (=1E, p. 217).

observed in order to prevent future complications or the patient's disappointment:

- Liposculpture is a technique aimed at localized adiposity, but it is not a slimming technique. Hence, patient selection is essential, as well as the study of body contours and steatomeric areas.
- Use no more than 3000 cc of tumescent anesthesia solution.
- The safety of the lipoplasty with local anesthesia depend on the total amount of anesthetic drug (lidocaine); the dose and concentration are determined by kg of weight and this is the dosage each day.
- A maximum of three liters should be extracted.
- No more than 25% of the surface of the body.
- Mega-liposculpture should be avoided and have specific indications following the guides of the AACS and the research of P. Fournier [18,19].

- It is particularly indicated in patients showing good tropism and good cutaneous elasticity.
- The technique should not be applied to patients with a history of blood dyscrasia, renal, hepatic, cardiac affections, hypertension, diabetes, and those suspected of psychiatric disorders, as well as uninformed people.
- Technique should not be applied to patients with unreal expectations.

Pre-Surgical Visit

First of all, a long conversation should be had with the patient in order to understand the real motivation for the visit, how they were referred, their knowledge of the technique, and especially their expectations and fantasies about the results. It is very important to ascertain what they expect as a possible outcome of the operation. Then, the patient should be examined naked to detect

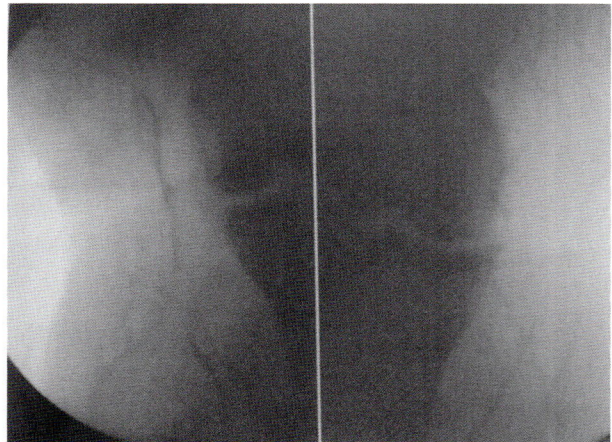

Figure 25.4 Lymphography in the inner knee.

examination areas and get a general impression of the body and its proportions, in order to assess possible outcomes according to body harmony.

The examination should be carried out with the patient in standing position and in different decubitus positions. In fact, we should remember that the fat tissue mass has its own mobility and changes according to different positions.

The patient should be required to contract different muscle groups in order to distinguish muscular flaccidity from "false *cullote de cheval*" (buttocks and saddleback), to differentiate abdomen anterior network dehiscence or flaccidity from swollen or dilated abdomen; thus defining the appropriate indications and techniques.

The history of previous treatments should be investigated, such as iontophoresis, electro-lipolysis, mesotherapy, and all methods that might have changed fatty tissue characteristics: drugs or other therapies, such as phosphatidilcholine, ozone therapy or masotherapy. We should examine skin quality and muscle group tonicity. Then we must provide our impression, suggest indications, and advise on possible risks.

It should be remembered that in many cases there is a gap between the fantasies of the patient and our real medical possibilities. This may lead to discontent, disappointment and complaints, and also legal proceedings. The patient should be

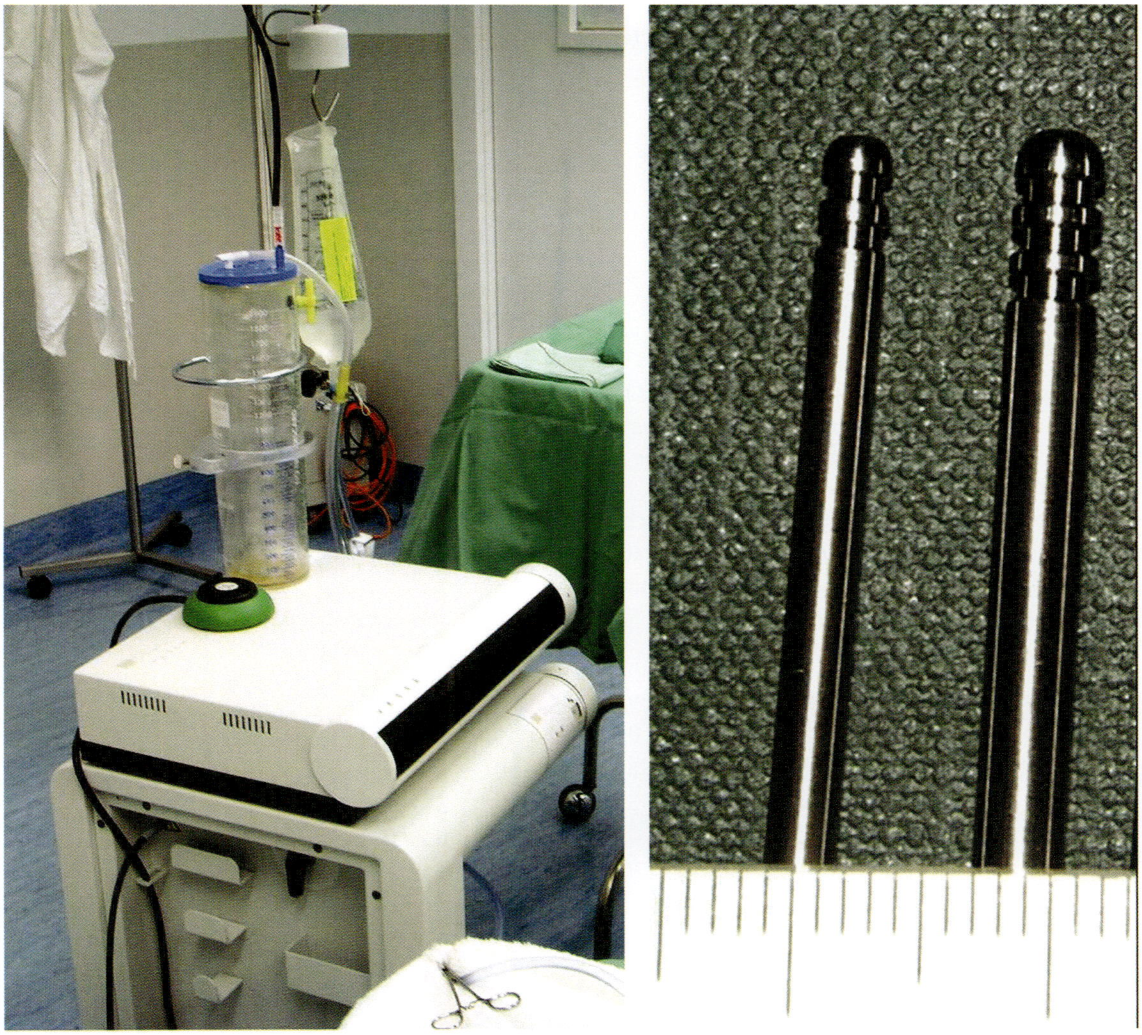

Figure 25.5 Vaser Grooved probes.

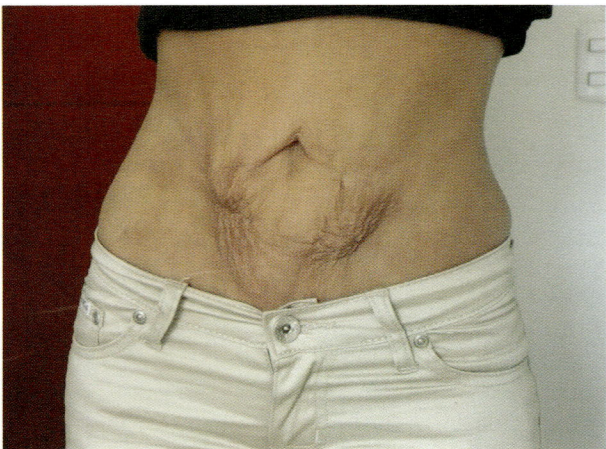

Figure 25.6 Very aggressive complication in liposculpture.

informed that immediate and later post-operative periods are not identical. Specific care for each period and possible limitations should be addressed.

In the event of a favorable decision, routine lab tests, proteingram (albumin content, lidocaine carrier), coagulation tests, cardiovascular surgical risk, and HIV tests should be required. Then, some other factors should be investigated: possible allergies to substances, especially to anesthetic drugs, skin disinfectants, history of keloids, and type of incision.

- Detailed Physical Exam
  - Abdomen: Hernias, Scars, Diastasis
  - Skin Alterations
  - Varicose Veins
  - Edema (lipoedema or lymphoedema
  - Retractions and Bumps
  - Flaccidity

Prescriptions
Aspirin and ibuprofen administration should be stopped at least seven days before the operation in order to avoid coagulation disorders. The use of all other unnecessary drugs should also be suspended a week prior to the operation.

Broad-spectrum antibiotics should be prescribed, such as ciprofloxacin 500 mg; 1 gr./day for five days after the operation. If necessary, an analgesic or non-steroidal anti-inflammatory (paracetamol) may also be prescribed.

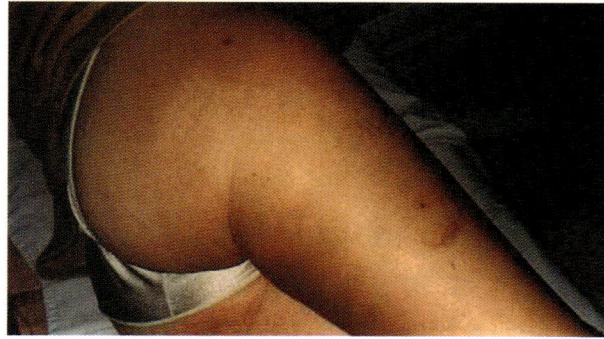

Figure 25.7 Post-op 48 hrs.

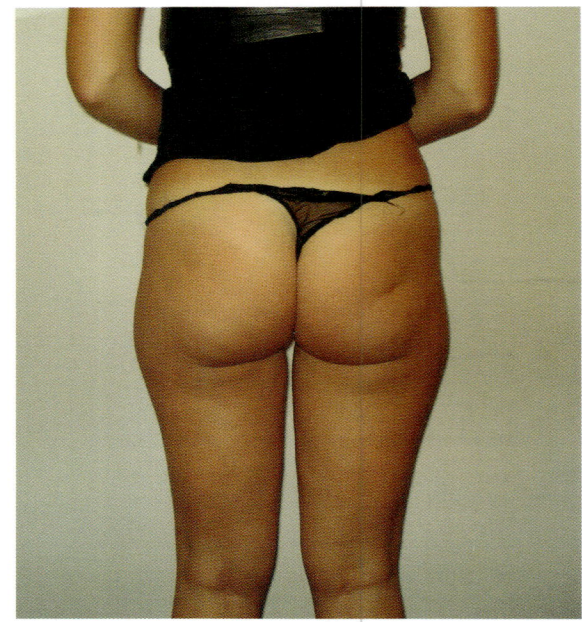

Figure 25.8 Take the pre-op photos without any marking. You can see the retraction in the right buttock and the localized obesity in the saddlebacks.

Exercise and sports should be stopped at least for two weeks, but the patient should walk every day after the lipo (after 48 hours, 1 mile a day in the first week); and also sun exposure of treated areas for approximately 15 days.

Care during immediate and later post-operative periods is very important.

When lipoplasty is finished, bimodal compression with absorbent pads is fundamental since it contributes to the patient's comfort and to a uniform skin and cellular subcutaneous tissue retraction. This is accompanied by an adequate compression and supporting binder. After 24 hours, pads are removed and replaced by a supporting non-compressive binder (hence allowing lymphatic precollector functioning). In the case of lower limb surgery, one week after the operation the patient should start wearing elasto-compressive hose (15 mm/Hg).

Immediate physical therapy consists in manual lymphatic drainage, 2 MHz external ultrasound, and magneto-therapy for one week. Then, subdermal therapy and carboxitherapy are introduced or continued.

The steps for a safe lipoplasty (lipo)

1. Take a picture before marking (Fig. 25.8).
2. Lipo starts with the marking (Fig. 25.9).
3. Lipo should be done in an operating room with all safety requirements including the presence of an anesthesiologist (Fig. 25.10).
4. Active and correct positioning of the patient for each area (Fig. 25.11).
5. Initiate the tumescent local anesthesia (Fig. 25.12).
6. Perform the tumescent local anesthesia in the area that is going to be done (Fig. 25.13).
   Formula of tumescent anesthesia solution: lidocaine 500 mg, 1 mg of adrenaline, 5 cc of bicarbonate in 1000 cc of saline solution.
7. After the end of the tumescent local anesthesia wait 20 minutes to start the lipo procedure, (Fig. 25.14).

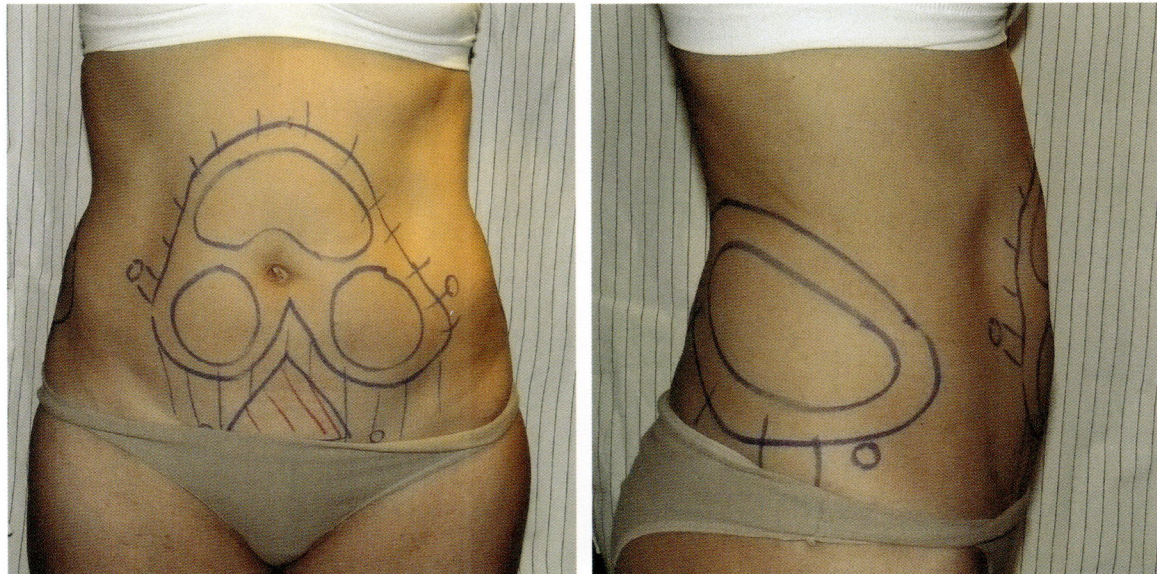

Figure 25.9 Liposculpture starts with the marking; good marking is made with two colors in standing-up position. The red areas are forbidden for liposuction; in the area with blue lines, the cannula pass without aspiration.

8. Starting the lipo procedure with a 2–3 mm diameter cannula and a syringe (Fig. 25.15).
   The basis of any lipo is the correct use of the syringe and the cannula. Afterward you will be proficient to be trained in assisted lipo (internal ultrasound, laserlypolisis).

9. Continue with lipo using syringe (Fig. 25.16).
   Notice that the left hand is always feeling the cannula movement and direction.

10. Next step a titanium cannula is used connected to a low-pressure aspirator (Fig. 25.17).

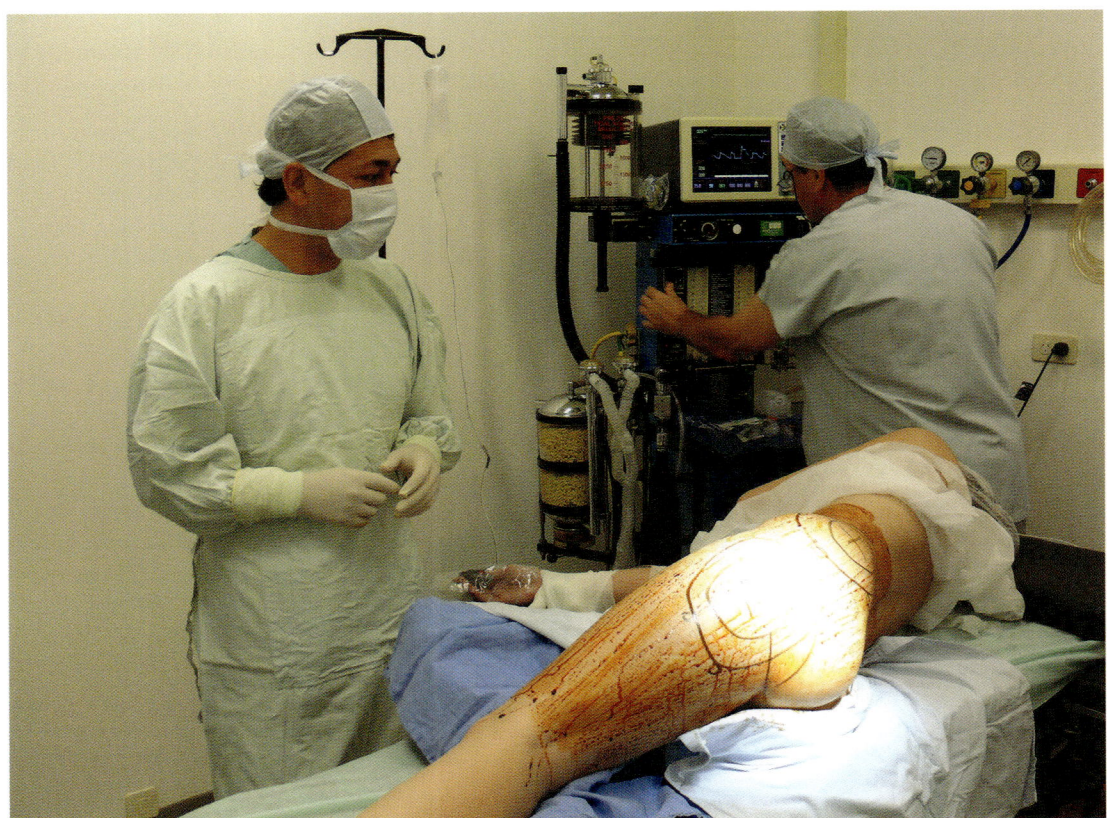

Figure 25.10 Liposculpture should be done in an operating room, with the presence of an anesthesiologist.

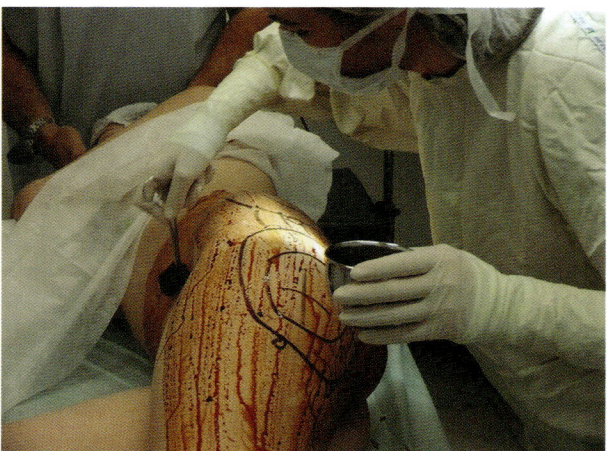

Figure 25.11 We work in aseptic conditions, with sterile draping and cleansing of the skin with iodopovinone.

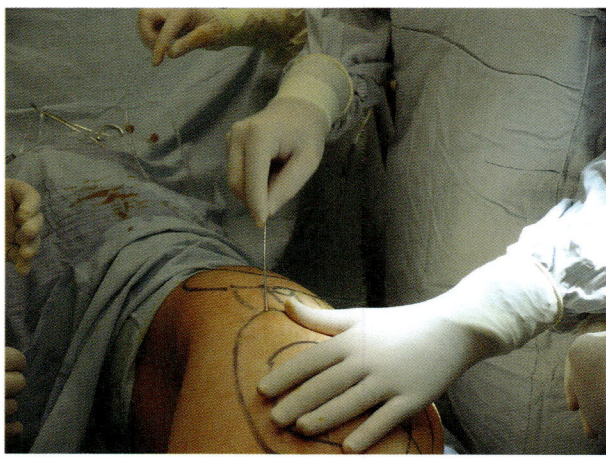

Figure 25.13 I introduce the local tumescent anesthesia through a small hole (2 mm) with an special blunt multiperforate cannula (2 mm).

During the aspiration, the assistant is helping with the skin stabilization.

11. **Post-operative scheme (Fig. 25.7)**

   Day 1: Relative rest in the bedroom. Start walking with bimodal elasto-compression (absorbent pads, compression and supporting binder).

   Day 2: The patient may start moving about. Wound healing. Light elasto-compression. Compression binder. Start with manual lymphatic drainage and external ultrasound. 2 MHZ and magnetotherapy showers are allowed, with caution in treated areas (Fig. 25.18).

   Days 3–7: The same as day 2.

   Day 15: Subdermal therapy starts, aimed at connective tissue restructuring.

   Day 21: Therapy may be associated with carboxitherapy.

Patients should be reminded that the best results may be observed only after some months (today we know that the first result will be at four months and the second at 14 months) (G.Sattler, Conference in the Annual Meeting of the American Academy of Cosmetic Surgery, January 2004).

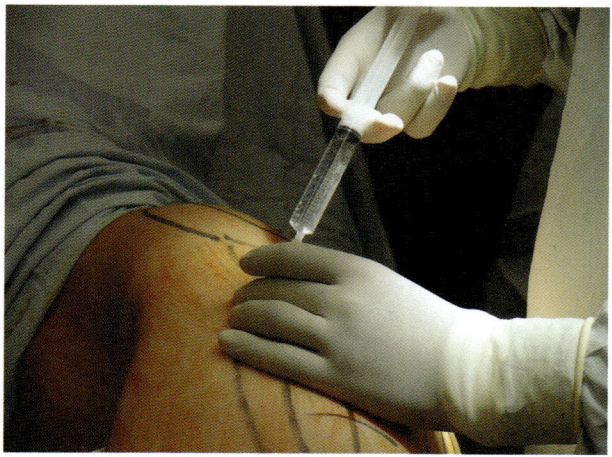

Figure 25.12 Local anesthesia for making the small holes (5 cc of local tumescent anesthesia).

Laserlypolisis

Advanced technique for the removal of localized excess of fatty tissue that can be used along or in combination with traditional liposuction to improve results.

History

1996/1998 First prototypes and early experimentation were done in Italy and Latin America during 1999. First patent was obtained.

1999/2000 Wide-scale trials were carried out in Brazil and Argentina.

By 2002 more than 2000 cases had been treated.

In the following years the method was further developed and perfected.

On October 31, 2006, Smartlipo™ obtained 510k approval from the American FDA and started marketing in the USA as well.

The technique uses the high peak power of the laser emission to rupture the membrane of the adipocytes. The effect is not only thermal but also thermomechanical, and the rapid and elevated absorption by the adipocyte membrane allows for creating an opening in the membrane itself with the spilling out of the cellular contents (Fig. 25.19).

The mix of the cell contents and the fluids from the tumescent anesthesia result in the production of an oily, low-viscosity aggregate which facilitates body modelling, and can be easily removed with low-pressure micro-pumps. (In my opinion it is important to always remove the emulsion with a 2 mm cannula and a 20 cc syringe.)

The first device was a Nd:YAG laser, at a 1064 nm wavelength, using 6 W power, 40 Hz frequency, 150 mj energy, and 100-microsecond pulse (Smartlipo™). This is the device which has more scientific papers about the use of Laserlypolisis. [25].

Many Nd:YAG devices were developed using different levels of power; nowadays there are devices using up to 30 W, increasing at the same time the efficacy of the technique as well as the complications. We need more research about the safety of these devices.

One of the great differences between Nd:YAG and diode laser is that the first is working with microsecond pulses and the diode in minisecond pulses [26].

Microscopic examination post-laserlypolisis [28].

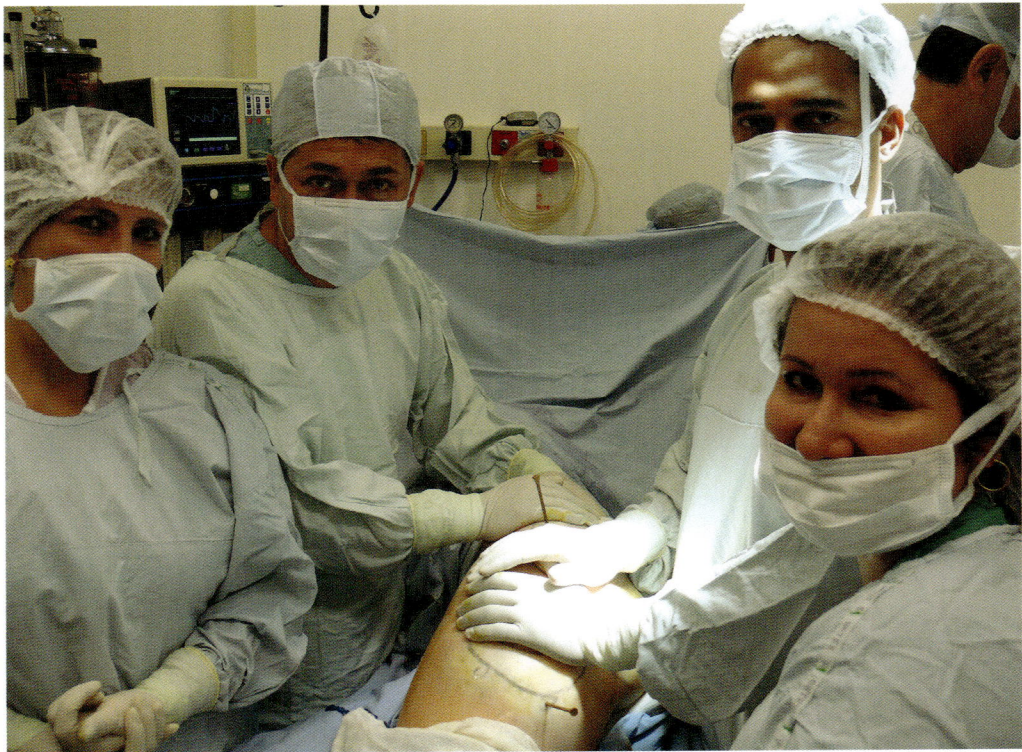

Figure 25.14 These photos were taken during a hands-on full-immersion training at the International Union of Lipoplasty.

The sections show varying degrees of subcutaneous cell tissue damage.

Laserlypolisis Indications
   Areas of moderate or potential flaccidity [27]
   Small or minimal areas of localized fat

Secondary liposuction
Difficult areas: face, neck, forearm, upper part of the stomach and knees.
In combination with traditional liposculpture to improve skin retraction and obtain an even and smoother skin surface.

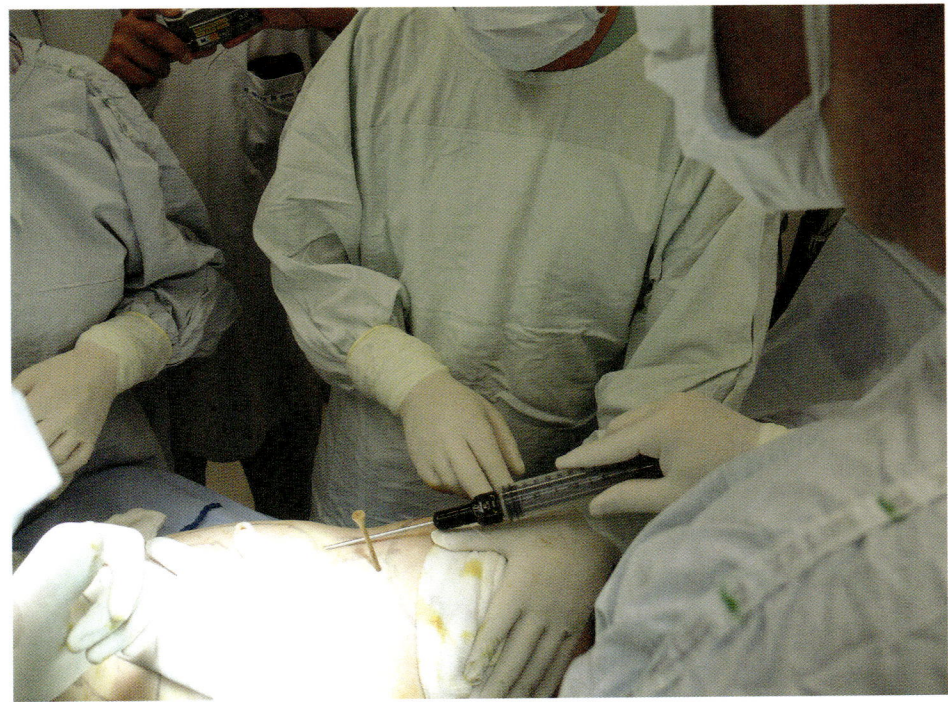

Figure 25.15 Start the liposculpture with syringe and blunt cannula.

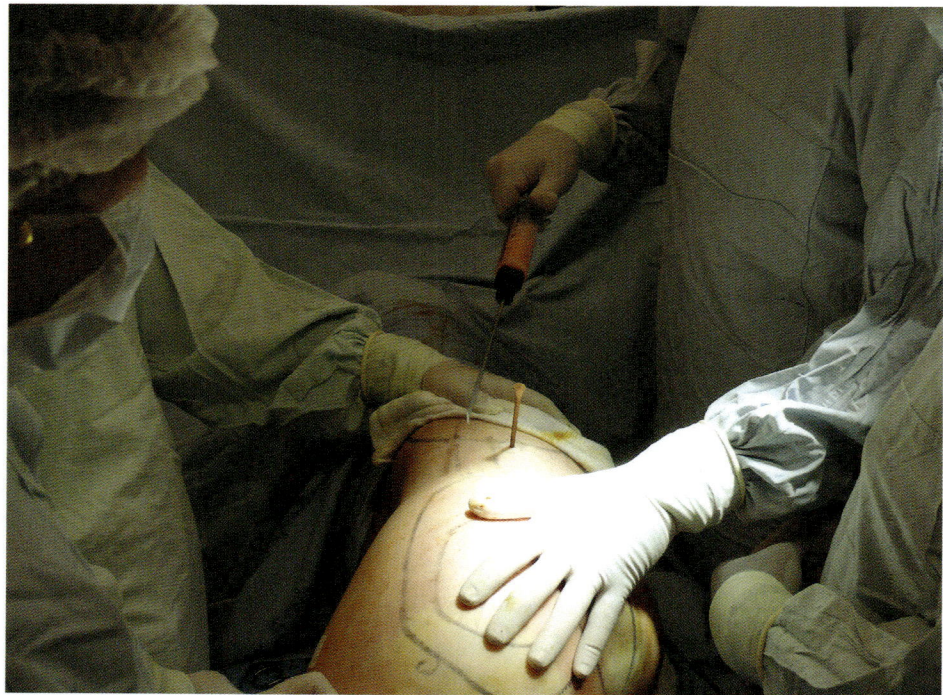

Figure 25.16 Continue the liposculpture with the syringe (look at the yellow fat inside).

Complications when using laserlypolisis have been reported but all those cases were related to the physician's lack of training and experience. There is a false belief that laserlypolisis is a non-surgical technique among professionals and patients.

When the complications rate increases the reputation of the method is damaged.

The key is to emphasize that you can't do the laserlypolisis procedure without experience and training in liposuction surgery.

Rules for a Safe Liposuction

1. Tumescent local anesthesia, respect the maximum doses
2. Assisted skin stabilization technique

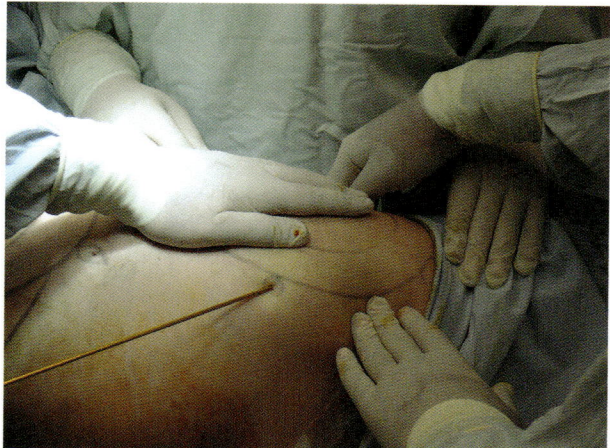

Figure 25.17 Use the cannula with aspiration and the hands working in the skin stabilization (to improve the result of the liposculpture).

3. Active positioning of the patient to allow the surgeon the procedure
4. Post-op open drainage
5. Take your time
6. Consider liposuction as a surgery; don't minimize the difficulty of the technique
7. DVT prevention in some cases
8. Keep the cannulas, probe or optical fiber always moving all the time to avoid burns
9. Pre-liposuction:

    The use of aesthetical medical procedures such carboxitherapy, endermologie, mesotherapy, etc. before the liposuction is an excellent way to improve the quality of the skin and subcutaneous tissues; that will maximize the efficacy of the liposuction.
10. Post-liposuction:

    After 24 hrs post-op the use of magnetotherapy, external ultrasound, lymphatic drainage and then after a week the use of endermologie and carboxitherapy will improve the skin retraction.

Facts in Determining a Safe Liposuction

Numbers of areas treated: Choose focal areas like hips and external thighs, upper and lower abdomen, internal thighs and internal knees, etc.

Volume of supranatant fat removed: Average less than 3000 cc.

Percent of body fat removed: No more than 25% of the body surface.

Dosage (mg/kg) of lidocaine: No more than 35 mg/kg per day.

Volume of intravascular fluid infused: It is useful to keep an IV open but it is not recommended to give more fluids.

Duration of surgical procedure: No more than 2 hours.

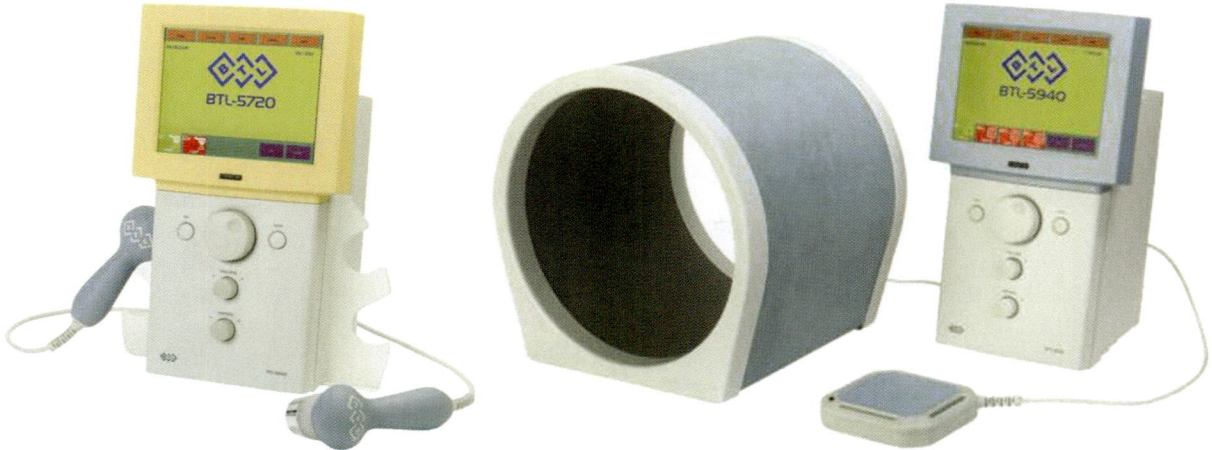

Figure 25.18 US 2 Mhz magnetotherapy.

Lipoplasty

From my point of view it's time to discuss the use and abuse of liposculpture.

In lipoplasty this principle is paraphrased by the statement, "excessive liposuction is unsafe and therefore unethical" (Fig. 25.6).

Statistics

Results after 20 years of performing 8500 liposculpture cases with local tumescent anesthesia:

Local Infection: 2

Post-operative focal subcutaneous panniculitis-like reaction: 0

Hematomas/seromas: 2

Allergic reaction to additional medication or adhesive tape: 20

Persistent post-operative edema: 5

Nausea associated to lidocaine : 10

Vasovagal reaction: 10

Excessive or persistent post-operative pain: 5

Post-operative fever: 2

Abnormally extended ecchymosed: 4

Unusual post-operative sleepiness/tiredness: 0

Permanent damage of sensitive nerves: 0

Cardiac arrhythmias requiring therapy: 0

Anemia: 0

Complications resulting in hospitalization: 0

Blood or fluid losses requiring transfusions: 0

Venous or fat embolism: 0

Hypovolemic shock: 0

Perforation of peritoneum or thorax: 0

Seizures: 0

Thrombophlebitis: 0

Toxic reactions to intravenous sedative or narcotic: 0

Death: 0

The sharing of experiences from other colleagues in meetings and congresses is very important but it is not enough. It is important to have also the skills that any surgical technique requires to maximize patient safety and results.

Cosmetic surgical procedures are facing a fast technological advance and safety concerns should be a priority for each of us. Physicians must have updated knowledge and skills prior to incorporating any new technique to their practices.

The International Union of Lipoplasty through its actions promotes, supports and encourages the learning process to achieve a safe and rational use of liposuction.

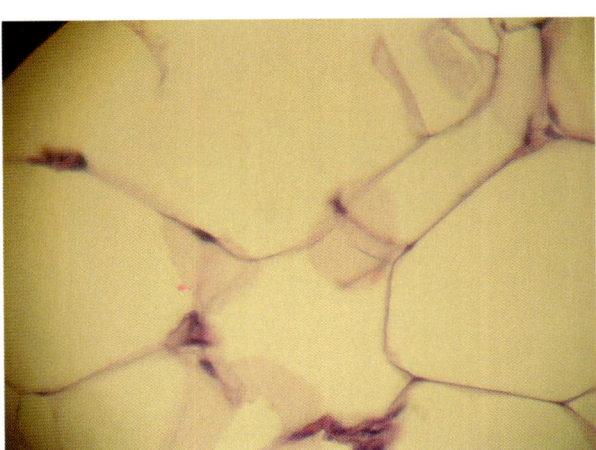 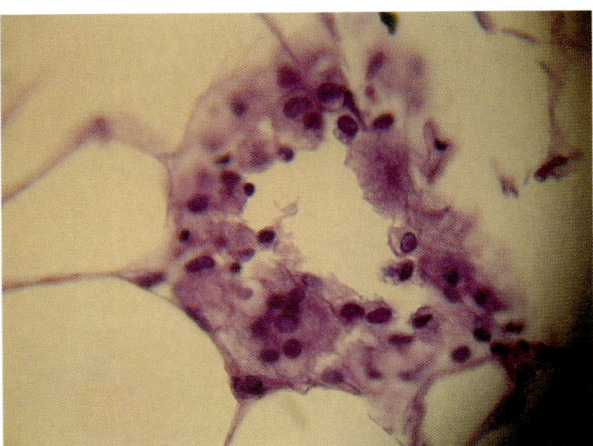

Figure 25.19 There is reversible (hydropic, balloon-like degeneration) and irreversible (fat necrosis with lipogranuloma formation in severe cases) cell damage.

REFERENCES

1. J Faivre. - Cirugie Esthetique 1992 Ed. Maloine - Pag 333.
2. J Faivre - Cirugie Esthetique 1992 Ed Maloine - Pag 333.
3. Fischer Giorgio. The evolution of Liposculture the american journal of cosmetic surgery 14 no 3:231–39, 1997.
4. YG Illouz. History and current concepts of lipoplasty. Clin Plast Surg 23:721, 1996.
5. PF Fournier. Liposculpturing: the syringe technique Paris: Arnette Blackwell; 1991.
6. M Gasparotti, LC, L Toledo. Superficial Liposculpture. New York, Springer-Verlag; 1993.
7. JA Klein. The tumescent technique for liposuction surgery. American Journal of Cosmetic Surgery 4:263, 1987.
8. ML Zocchi. Ultrasound-assisted lipoplasty: Technical refinements and clinical evaluations. Clin Plast Surg 23:575, 1996.
9. M Schefflin, H Tazi. Ultrasonic-assisted body contouring. Aesthetic Surgery Quarterly 16:117, 1996.
10. M Zocchi. Ultrasonic-assisted lipoplasty. Adv Plast Reconstr Surg 11:197, 1995.
11. G Leibaschoff. Ultrasonic liposculpture: in the treatment of liposclerosis/The american journal of cosmetic surgery 10 no.4:239–41, 1993.
12. G Leibaschoff, J Ferreira, JL Ciucci. Anatomic-radiologic comparison of the effects of liposculpture on the lymphatic system of the lower extremities. Amer J Cosm Surg 12:287–92, 1995.
13. M Gasparotti. Superficial liposuction yields superior results for most patients. Aesthet Surg J 17:64–66, 1997.
14. JA Klein. Tumescent technique for regional anesthesia permits lidocaine does of 35 mg/kg for liposuction. J Dermatol Surg Oncol 16:248, 1990.
15. W Cimino. Ultrasonic Surgery. Power quantification and efficiency optimization. Aesth Plast Surg 233–39, May – June 2001.
16. P Fournier. Liposculpture-ma technique Paris Arnette; 1989.
17. P Fournier. Facial recontouring with fat grafting. Dermatol Clin 8:523, 1989.
18. P Fournier. Therapeutic megalipoextraction or Megaliposculpture: Indication technique complications and results/The american journal of cosmetic surgery. 14 number 3:297–309, 1997.
19. V Sidor. Megalipoteraphy:problems and results the american journal of cosmetic surgery 14 number 3:241–49, 1997.
20. M Jewell, P Fodor, E Bolivar de Souza Pinto. Clinical application of Vaser assited Lipoplasty. Aesth Plast Surg 131–46, March April 2002.
21. YG Illouz. Remodelage Chirurgical de la silhouette par lypolise aspiration ou lipectomie sélective. Ann Chirurgical Plast Esthetique Paris 29(2):162–179, 1984.
22. YG Illouz. Body sculpturing by lipoplasty, Churchill Livingstone, 1989 – Nurbberger & Muller Classification; 33.
23. P Fournier. Liposculpture – Ma technique, Paris, Arnette Ed. 1989.
24. LS Toledo. Superficial Syringe Liposculpture for cellulite treatment – Plastic Surgery Symposium, Beverly Hills, California; 23–25th June 1990.
25. K Karen, R Geronemus. Laser lipolysis using a novel 1,064nm Nd:YAG laser. Dermatolo Surg 32:241–48, 2006.
26. A Goldman, G Blugerman, D Schavelzon et al. Laserlipolysis liposuction using Nd:YAG laser. Rev Soc Bras Cir Plast 17: 17–26, 2002.
27. AZD Badin, Lea Mara Moraes, Luciana Godek et al. Laserlipolysis: Flaccidity under control. Aesth Plast Surg 26:335–39, 2002.
28. G Leibaschoff et al. A double-blind, prospective, clinical, surgical, histopathological and ultrasound study comparing the effectiveness and safety of liposuction performed using Laserlipolysis and Internal Ultrasound Lipoplasty method, and assessing the evolution in patients. 25th Annual Meeting of the American Academy of Cosmetic Surgery, Phoenix Arizona, 2009.

26 Study Protocols in Cellulite
Débora Zechmeister do Prado, Amanda Stapenhorst, and Marie-Laurence Abella

Introduction

Before market launching, all drugs, cosmetics, nutraceuticals and devices must undergo to a series of clinical trials designed to evaluate their safety and efficacy according to the parameters of toxicity, potency, dose finding, and field conditions.

A research protocol is a document that contemplates the fundamental parameters of clinical trials, including ethical aspects and personnel responsibilities. The conduction of a clinical trial is set out in the protocol that represents the structured written plan of the study for helping the investigator organize his research with a logical, focused and efficient approach [1].

The latest research studies on cellulite have come out with new findings, about cellulite. However, regardless of the fact that cellulite is a widely discussed topic all over the world, there are still very few publications based on scientific research clinical trial protocols. Some of these studies fail to follow the international standards of good clinical practice and also miss some parameters for high level of evidence studies, such as randomization, control, blinding, definition of inclusion and exclusion criteria, outcomes and clinical parameters of safety and efficacy, besides the use of validated and well-established methods for evaluation of results.

This chapter is aimed at the fundamental aspects of clinical research as ethical standards and good clinical practices as well as specific parameters for clinical research in the field of cellulite.

History

Overall, the history of clinical research has some important landmarks. Among them are:

- In 1947, the Nuremberg Code created and defined ten points for the protection of research subjects; these included informed consent containing comprehensive information about the nature, purpose and risks of the trial, and the right to withdraw from the study at any time.
- The Declaration of Helsinki was created by the World Medical Association in 1964. It was designed to define ethical codes that would provide direction for all participants in medical research involving human subjects. Its principal amendments were done in Tokyo (1975), Venice (1983), Hong Kong (1989), Somerset West (1996) and Edinburgh (2000).
- The International Conference on Harmonisation of Technical Requirements for Registration of Pharmaceuticals for Human Use (ICH) took place at a meeting in April 1990 in Brussels. It represents the real concept of good clinical practices (GCP). The aim of ICH is to ensure that good quality, safe and effective drugs are developed and registered in the most efficient and cost-effective manner. These activities are pursued in the interest of the consumer and public health, to prevent unnecessary duplication of clinical trials in humans and to minimise the use of animal testing without compromising the regulatory obligations of safety and effectiveness.

Ethical Aspects

Study subjects must be treated with respect and not used only to obtain results. A research protocol should follow national and international laws and rules to protect the subjects [3]. To achieve greater harmonization in the interpretation, application and conduction of a study, all clinical studies should be carried out according to the Nuremberg Code, Helsinki Declaration and GCP/ICH Guidelines.

Protocol documents, such as the protocol itself, informed consent, declaration of a suitable facility, main investigator's resumé, trial budget, among others, must be sent to the Ethics Committee (EC) for approval [4] before beginning the study.

The EC is an independent body constituted of medical/scientific professionals and non-medical/non-scientific members, whose responsibility is to guarantee the protection of the rights, safety and well-being of human subjects involved in a trial and to provide public assurance of that protection. They review and provide opinion on the protocol, informed consent and other documents related to the research subjects [1]. The main ethical concern is whether the research will place the patients at undue risk, and whether the subjects will be fully informed about the nature of the study.

A scientific research protocol must provide informed consent. This is a document consisting of a written, signed and dated form in which each research subject voluntarily confirms his or her willingness to participate in a particular trial [3]. The informed consent should provide a clear, easy to understand explanation of all the important information about the study. It should be presented by a trained person and be confidential. After having been informed of all aspects of the trial, the subjects are free to decide whether they are going to participate [4].

The clinical trial can only begin after the EC approval. The research protocol should remain essentially unchanged except for minor details. If it becomes necessary to modify the protocol, a clear description of the rationale for the modification should be provided in a protocol amendment and communicated to the EC [5].

Clinical Trial Responsibilities

Clinical trials are developed and conducted by trained professionals working at different levels of responsibility.

Sponsor

The sponsor's responsibility is to implement and maintain quality assurance and a quality control system to ensure that trials are conducted according to protocols and data are generated, documented and reported in compliance with the protocol and the applicable regulatory requirements made by the EC. The sponsor is responsible for providing information about the product under investigation, if applicable. He/she is also responsible for designating qualified personnel who will be readily available to advise on trial-related medical questions or problems [6].

The clinical research associate (CRA) is the representative of the sponsor. According to the legislation, the purpose of the CRA is to verify that the rights and well-being of human subjects are protected, that all the trial data is accurate, complete and verifiable, and to check "in loco" if the trial is being conducted in compliance with the currently approved protocol/amendment.

Most trials are sponsored by the company manufacturer of the drug, cosmetic, nutraceutical or device, but in some cases, the study is investigator-initiated. In such cases, the main investigator assumes the sponsor's responsibilities.

Main or principal investigator
The main investigator must be qualified by education, training and experience to assume responsibility for the proper conduct of the trial. He/she should meet all the qualifications specified by the applicable regulatory requirement(s), and should provide evidence of such qualification through up-to-date curriculum vitae and/or other relevant documentation requested by the sponsor and the regulatory authorities. The investigator(s) should be familiar with the appropriate use of the investigational product or device [1].

Co-investigator
The co-investigator is the person who helps the main investigator follow the study. He/she is a physician who helps to include and evaluate the study subjects, deals with adverse events, takes responsibility over all medical procedures defined by the main investigator, clarifies all the medical questions asked by the research subjects, aids the CRA when necessary, among other responsibilities.

Clinical trial coordinator
The clinical trial coordinator is responsible for all operational actions regarding the study. It is her/his responsibility to help the main investigator to proceed in accordance with the study protocol, meeting all methodological and ethical demands to obtain reliable results guaranteeing the well-being of the research subjects.

Other clinical trial staff
A clinical trial involves a great number of people, each one with a different position such as research assistants, nurses, and secretaries. They must be trained and fully informed regarding the study to avoid mismatched information that could confuse the research subjects and compromise data accuracy. They should be warned about the ethical issues regarding clinical trials.

Study Protocol Structure
The protocol should provide an overview of the study, with an introduction, the reasons and objectives of the research, detailed methodology, and evaluation of outcomes. It must explain the study design (comparative, controlled, open-label, randomized, blind, etc.), the study population, the calculation of the sample size according to the main criteria of judgment, and how the data will be obtained [7]. Also, it must contain ethical aspects, management of possible adverse events and guarantees of the accuracy and quality of data. Other information essential to write a scientific research protocol is: title, identifying number and date, sponsor, main investigator's and other staff responsibilities including name,

address and telephone number of the investigator(s) responsible for conducting the trial. It should contain a statement that the trial will be conducted in compliance with the protocol and applicable regulatory and GCP/ICH requirements [2].

The title of the protocol should express the main purpose of the research. The title is usually the first part of the protocol to be read and therefore should transmit maximum information in fewer words. It should indicate the area of research, introduce the research question and specify the research method to be used [8].

Criteria of judgment must be precisely described: main criteria and secondary criteria. Formal sample size calculations are required for all clinical trials. These indicate how many study subjects are needed, as well as if the research ideas are correct, and if it is very likely that a statistically significant result will be obtained. It is important to give a limited description of the statistical methods used for the sample calculation.

The protocol should specify methods of allocation to treatment groups and blinding, in case of blind studies. In conducting a controlled trial, randomized allocation is the preferred means of assuring comparability of test groups and minimizing the possibility of selection bias. Blinding is an important factor in reducing or minimizing the risk of biased study outcomes. A trial where the treatment assignment is not known by the study participant because of the use of placebo or other methods of masking the intervention is referred to as a single blind study. When the investigator and staff who are involved in the treatment or clinical evaluation of the subjects and analysis of data are also unaware of the treatment assignments, the study is double blind [4].

The management of an adverse reaction should be specified in the protocol. An adverse reaction is defined as any medical occurrence in a patient or clinical investigation subject that does not necessarily have a causal relationship with the study treatment [1].

All the adverse events must be reported to the sponsor and according to the severity to the Ethics Committee and always according to the local regulation. The immediate report shall be followed by a detailed written explanation of the adverse event. In the exceptional case of reported deaths, all information must be provided by the investigator to the sponsor and the EC [5].

A serious adverse reaction is a medical occurrence that at any dose may result in death. It is an adverse, life-threatening adverse event that requires admission to hospital, resulting in permanent disability or in congenital anomaly/birth defect. All relevant information about suspected adverse reactions that are fatal or life-threatening must be reported as soon as possible to the Ethics Committee [3] always in accordance with local requirements.

Study Protocols in Cellulite
Evidence-based argumentation and a fundamental theory are essential to the development of a reliable cellulite research protocol. In such cases, all scientific requirements for a study protocol must be achieved, as explained above. However, despite differences in each cellulite study design regarding the objectives and nature of the investigational product, some specific requirements could be followed:

Inclusion and exclusion criteria

Some specific inclusion and exclusion criteria to select the research subjects should be included in any cellulite study:

Inclusion Criteria:

- The age range for cellulite studies is usually 18 to 45 years old, which is the period in a woman's life when cellulite could be present without interference of other associated conditions, such as flaccidity;
- Usually only female patients are included in a cellulite clinical trial, since women are most affected by this skin condition;
- Evaluation of the cellulite grade should be done to verify whether the subject presents the appropriate grade for the study;
- The range of BMI (Body Mass Index) should be defined, since weight influences cellulite. It is important to include subjects with normal weight/height ratio (BMI = Weight/Height^2) from19.0 to 24.9 kg.m^{-2} or overweight subjects, in some cases, with BMI from 25.0 to 29.9 kg.m^{-2}. As weight is an important factor (besides this), the subject must agree to maintain a stable weight throughout the duration of the study in order not to bias the results of the study (e.g. less than 2 kg of weight change are acceptable in most protocols);
- Subjects must have healthy skin in the area that will be measured;
- Subjects must agree not to use any slimming products or any other cellulite treatment during a determinate period preceding the study and during the study;
- Subjects must have a regular menstrual cycle, since hormonal changes are one of the causes of aggravated cellulite;
- The research subjects must want to take part in the study and be likely to follow the study procedures, and be available for the study visits according to the protocol.

Exclusion Criteria:

- Pregnant or lactating subjects or those who plan to get pregnant during the trial period;
- Subjects presenting varicose veins or history of phlebitis in the cellulite area or conditions such as psoriasis, eczema, erythema, edema, scars, wounds and other visible lesions, as these conditions could interfere with the evaluation of study results;
- Subjects with chronic diseases like diabetes, hypertension or undergoing oncological treatment that could interfere with the conduction of the study and evaluation of results;
- Subjects who have clotting disorders;
- Subjects who used some kind of cellulite-treatment in the last 30 days before the beginning of the study or those who underwent any kind of surgical procedure in the area of treatment, usually in the past three months before the study;
- Subjects using the following medications: analgesics, anti-inflammatory, antihistaminic, corticoids, diuretics, venotonics and those susceptible to hematomas or ecchymosis;
- Subjects receiving cosmetic, dermatological surgical or medical treatment likely to interfere with the study evaluations;
- Subjects making use of or who are planning to use and expose the area of treatment to the sun, artificial UV tanning or sunless tanning products;
- Subjects who have been on a slimming diet in the past three months before the study or who wish to do so during the study, as it could interfere in the study evaluations;
- Subjects who intend to start an intensive sport, because it could cause weight loss, probably reducing the cellulite grade during the study.

Clinical and cosmetic evaluation

The medical history of the research subject is the first thing to be done in the initial study visit. The patient should be questioned about the age of cellulite onset, history of disease, surgeries, presence of hormonal or vascular disease, the occasional or regular use of medicines or the use of any medicine that may contribute to increasing the deposit of fat. Questions should be asked about other aspects, such as: smoking, pregnancy, diet, physical exercise etc. [9].

The physical examination should be performed with the patient in a standing position and with muscles relaxed. Cellulite can be better observed with the application of the pinch test or muscle contraction. Overhead or tangential illumination of the patient facilitates visualization of cellulite. Palpation should always be performed to check the elasticity of the skin and subcutaneous tissue [9,10]. Evaluation of cellulite grade shall be performed, at all measurement times, by a very experienced person (specialist), the same person for the duration of the study and for all subjects, and always in the same condition of lighting. Validated scales, such as the Cellulite Severity Scale [14] are preferable in clinical trials. Localisation of the sites to be measured by instruments and how to locate these at the different evaluation visits must be completely reproducible.

Photographic images

Colour photographs of each cellulite area must be taken under normal conditions in the upright position with and without pinching (thigh and buttock on each side) according to a clearly defined procedure in the protocol.

The patients should stand at a predetermined distance and the pictures should be taken focusing on the area between the waist and the knees.

A digital camera with zoom should be used. The camera should be adjusted to a tripod, and the distance between the camera and the subject should be regulated according to the precision of the pictured area. The same camera should be used by the same operator for the duration of the study and the condition of lighting must be perfectly controlled.

There are a few photographic systems specifically designed to take standard pictures of cellulite patients, such as IntelliStudio and Vectra 3D from Canfield Scientific, Inc.

Methods evaluated

Cellulite should be evaluated using qualitative, semi-qualitative and quantitative methods. Recent studies investigating anti-cellulite treatments mostly used digital photography, visual scoring, circumferential thigh measurements, BMI and subjective assessments. Results of studies relating to anti-cellulite efficacy are provided in order to give an overview of investigative methods [11].

Measurement of the circumference of the thighs and buttocks should be performed, for all measurement times, in accordance with a procedure precisely defined in the protocol.

BMI is widely used by some authors. It is a quantitative method that uses the measure of weight and height to assess the degree of obesity [9].

The current scale for cellulite classification (grades 0 to III) [12,13] describes different grades of cellulite, but some aspects that affect the severity and morphology of cellulite should only be accessed by Hexsel, Dal'Forno & Hexsel Cellulite Severity Scale (CSS) [14]. CSS is a very useful semi-quantitative tool that addresses cellulite severity to 15 scores. Chapter 4 describes the CSS.

The two-dimensional ultrasound is a noninvasive method for evaluating variations and alterations of the subcutaneous fatty tissue, and with the assistance of Doppler, it evaluates the local circulation [9]. It is a useful method to evaluate the results of cellulite treatments on clinical trials. Choice of frequency of ultrasound is made according to the zone of interest. It is very interesting to evaluate the junction between hypodermis and dermis.

High-resolution magnetic resonance imaging measures the thickness of adipose tissue, but does not allow evaluation of the dermis or microcirculation. [9,15]. It is also an efficient but very costly method to evaluate cellulite in clinical trials.

Additional evaluation methods include a newly validated quality of life questionnaire (CelluQOL®) [16] that is very useful (see chapter 1), and also self-questionnaires, as secondary endpoints due to their subjectivity.

Conclusion

A well-planned and written research protocol is very important to prevent failure when collecting crucial information, as well as to check if the objectives of the study can be achieved and to plan precisely the research. A well-planned study design, reliable and accessible methodology and an experienced staff assure the quality of any clinical trial. It is easier to obtain EC approval when a well-written scientific protocol is presented, such as the sponsor agreement when the investigators initiated the studies.

Although cellulite is a great concern to many women, it has received little attention in the scientific world. The physiopathology of cellulite has not been well elucidated by the researchers, so studies in this area are a little scanty, and dissension and controversy are rife. New research protocols with new methods of evaluation are needed to develop studies in order to gain a better understanding of these skin conditions. They are important in obtaining new therapies and products.

REFERENCES

1. SB Hulley, TB Newman, SR Cummings. Getting Started: The Anatomy and Physiology of Clinical Research. In: SB Hulley, SR Cummings, WS Browner et al. Designing Clinical Research, 3rd ed. Lippincott USA; 2006: 97–106.
2. World Health Organization. Handbook for Good Clinical Research Practice (GCP): Guidance for Implementation, Geneva; 2002: 3–7.
3. LMP Silva, F Oliveira, C Miccioli. O processo de consentimento na pesquisa clínica: da elaboração à obtenção. Arq Bras Oftalmol 68(5):704–7, 2005.
4. EA Castilho, J Kalil. Ethics and medical research: principles, guidelines, and regulations. Rev Soc Bras Med Trop 38(4): 344–47, 2005.
5. ICH - Harmonised Tripartite Guideline for Good Clinical Practice. General Considerations for Clinical Trials, 4th ed; 1997: 1–13.
6. LM Friedman, CD Furberg, DL DeMets. Introduction to Clinical Trials. In: LM Friedman, CD Furberg, DL DeMets. Fundamentals of Clinical Trials, 3rd ed. Springer Verlag Pod; 1998: 1–12.
7. BF Luna. Seqüência Básica na Elaboração de Protocolos de Pesquisa. Arq Bras Cardiol 71(6):735–40, 1998.
8. KVS Soares, AA Castro. Projeto de Pesquisa para Ensaios Clínicos Randomizados. In: AA Atallah, NA Castro. Medicina Baseada em Evidências, São Paulo: Disciplina de Clínica Médica; 1998: 53–61.
9. D Hexsel, TO Dal'Forno, S Cignachi. Definition, Clinical Aspects, Associated Conditions, and Differential Diagnosis. In: MP Goldman, PA Bacci, G Leibaschoff, D Hexsel, F Angelini. Cellulite Pathophysiology and Treatment, New York: Taylor & Francis Group; 2006: 7–27.
10. MM Avram. Cellulite: a review of its physiology and treatment. J Cosmet Laser Ther 6:181–185, 2004.
11. S Bielfeldt, P Buttgereit, M Brandt et al. Non-invasive evaluation techniques to quantify the efficacy of cosmetic anti-cellulite products. Skin Research and Technology 1–11, 2008.
12. F Nürnberger, G Müller. So-called cellulite: an invented disease. J Dermatol Surg Oncol 4(3):221–9, 1978.
13. J Rao, KE Pabbo, MP Goldman. A Double-blind randomized trial testing the tolerability and efficacy of a novel topical agent with and without occlusion for the treatment of cellulite: a study and review of the literature. J Drugs Dermatol 3(4):417–25, 2004.
14. D Hexsel, T Dal'Forno, C Hexsel. A Validated Photonumeric Cellulite Severity Scale. J Eur Acad Dermatol Venereol 23(5): 523–8, 2009.
15. MP Goldman. Cellulite: A Review of Current Treatments. Cosmetic Dermatology 15(2):17–20, 2002.
16. D Hexsel, M Weber, ML Taborda, JF Souza. Preliminary results of the elaboration of a new instrument to evaluate quality of life in patients with cellulite - CelluQol®. Poster 1192, 67th Annual Meeting of the American Academy of Dermatology, San Francisco; 2009.

27 Digital Photography and Other Imaging Techniques in Cellulite

Ana Beatris Rossi, Alex Nkengne, and Christiane Bertin

Introduction

Cellulite is an aesthetic skin condition, characterized by a dimpled skin appearance in the lower legs, buttocks and abdomen. Based on the pathophysiology of cellulite, involving adipose tissue, dermis and vascular alterations, the evaluation of skin temperature and skin relief are good non-invasive methods to assess the level of cellulite. Skin temperature can be measured using either contact or infrared thermography. Digital photography and 3D imaging are two techniques that can document skin relief. Digital photography can also be used as an objective method to document and measure cellulite changes, demonstrate treatment efficacy and provide a barometer for patient/physician expectations and treatment planning.

This chapter describes some key elements for photographing cellulite, provides guidance on critically evaluating the cellulite photos, summarizes different equipment and storage options and presents some new imaging methods used in clinical research.

Digital Photography

Dermatologists have documented skin conditions with photography for over a century [1]. In the past decade digital photography has experienced a rapid rise in technological development (i.e. digital SLR—single lens reflex—cameras, increased resolution, better optics and processing, etc.) and a dramatic reduction in cost, providing physicians with access to powerful tools for acquisition, storage and manipulation of photographic images. Research has shown photography significantly improves patients' understanding about treatment progression [2]. Consequently, photography is the easiest and most effective way to communicate the benefits of treatment to patients, peers and the public.

Requirements to Perform Macro Photography

The minimum set up to document cellulite with photography should include a digital camera, light source, computer to store, analyze and display the images and possibly a color printer to share the images with the patient.

We identified four key elements in cellulite photography: photographer, camera, light source, and subject.

The photographer

The photographer is the conduit to obtaining a good photographic image of cellulite. Some of the responsibilities of the photographer are to ensure the correct positioning of the camera, light source and subject, uniform cellulite illumination and taking the photograph. Standardizing the setup and procedure are crucial to photographing and evaluating any change in cellulite due to treatment. The photographer must be patient, especially early on, and keep the subject calm to achieve a good quality work.

The camera

Current standard digital cameras available (point and shoot cameras: e.g. Canon Powershot, Sony Cybershot and Nikon Coolpix) have a resolution of over ten million pixels (i.e. 10 megapixels). Since Kaliyadan [2] has demonstrated that a resolution of four million pixels is enough in most dermatological usage, other criteria such as color balance and optical distortion should be used to compare digital cameras. Attention should also be paid when choosing a compression format that will not visibly alter the images during the storage process. Low quality jpg should be avoided. Details on types of digital storage and image formats are given in the third part of the chapter (Image Management).

Light source

In photography in general, and particularly photographing cellulite, light source positioning is crucial. Improperly positioned light can create shadows and artificially increase the perceived amount of cellulite. Fig. 27.1 provides examples of the same subject being illuminated by the same light source, placed in three different positions. We can observe that depending on the position of the light source, the light falls uniformly over the cellulite region or the shadows cast in the cellulite region artificially increases the apparent cellulite severity.

In order to obtain homogeneous lighting, a reflective panel can be used. In addition, a dark and opaque background provides greater control of the subject illumination. Most importantly, the positioning of the light source should be the same in all time-points for the same subject.

If the only lighting system used is the flash in the camera, this should be positioned at a distance that would allow taking a larger area, using a high-definition photo and after select and crop the area of interest.

Subject

The relative position of the subject to the camera enables the acquisition of the same field of view before and after cellulite treatment. The physician should have a standardized setup and imaging procedure to aid in correlating the before and after treatment images. For instance, to help maintain the same distance between the camera and patient, simple markings for the patient's feet and the camera tripod could be used. Further correlation between the two images could be accomplished using anatomical landmarks such as veins and scars. The "after treatment" image should be compared to the "before treatment" image immediately after acquisition to check for consistency and to be retaken if necessary.

The subject's stance determines the shape of the muscles. In most cases, it is recommended to photograph the subject in a relaxed, standing position. However, when taking photos of the gluteus area, asking the subject to contract the gluteus muscles helps making the cellulite more evident. Again, it's important to compare photos to achieve the same grade of muscle contraction in all time-points. A horizontal stabilizer bar can help reduce subject motion during the image acquisition. Fig. 27.2 illustrates the difference in cellulite perception between a relaxed posture and

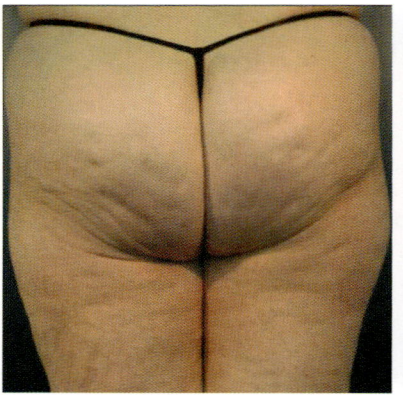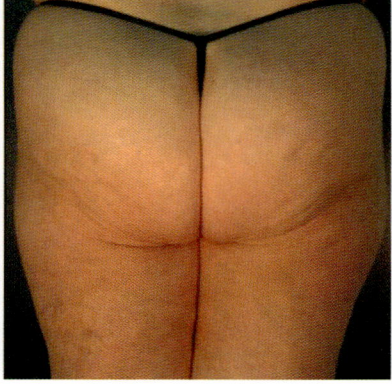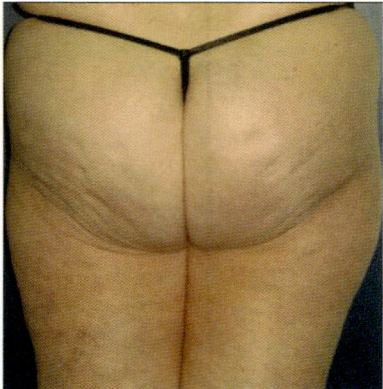

Figure 27.1 Different visual aspect of cellulite due to changes in light source positioning

contracting the gluteus muscles. The contracted muscles increase the perceived amount of cellulite on the subject.

Image Standardization

The primary treatments for cellulite are based on devices or cosmetics. For both types of treatments there is no strict control from health authorities, and no regulatory exigency to conducting randomized controlled clinical studies to demonstrate efficacy and safety. Many cellulite treatments use 'before and after' photos as promotion and demonstration of efficacy. The comparison of pictures acquired before and after treatment requires the use of an acquisition protocol standardizing the photography conditions in terms of the subject and camera positioning and illumination.

When observing before and after photos, it is important to determine if the 'improvement' is real and not due to not well-standardized photography acquisition. For instance the subject may have contracted her muscles in the "before" photo and relaxed in the "after" photo. One simple method to identify whether the muscles are contracted is to look at the curve of the gluteus fold. The curve is rounded when there is no contraction and tends to be closer to 90° when it is contracted. In addition, the shape of the shadow between the buttocks should be similar in the two photos (e.g. Fig. 27.3).

Ideally the subject should have a minimal amount of clothing on, as the difference in clothing or position of the clothes can distract attention and minimize/maximize differences when comparing images from before and after treatment.

To ensure good image standardization, the camera should be placed on a tripod and both distance from the subject to the tripod and the height (floor to camera) should be recorded for each subject. This ensures the same measurement parameter for the before and after photo.

OTHER IMAGING TECHNIQUES USED IN RESEARCH
Photographs of Pinched Thighs
Image acquisition

Manual palpation is one way to assess the severity of cellulite. The dimpled appearance of skin is accentuated when the skin is pinched. The skin can be pinched either with the hands or a device. Pinching the skin with the hands is a simple low-cost method. Since applying a consistent known pressure to the skin is difficult, using the hands to pinch the skin is not generally used as a research tool to measure cellulite (Fig. 27.4).

Another method is to use a device that can apply a known standardized pressure to the skin. One system proposed by Perin [3] and his team acquires macroscopic photographs of the external surface of the thigh being pinched with a consistent pressure (Fig. 27.5).

Their system exerts a tangential pressure of approximately 200 g/cm^2 on the surface of the skin. The tangential pressure depends on the positioning of the system on the thigh and a protocol is designed to enable consistent pressure across time-points. Perin and his colleagues evaluated the repositioning of the gripping system and have found it consistent in their experimental conditions (a deviation of 6 mm was observed on a surface of 160×100 mm).

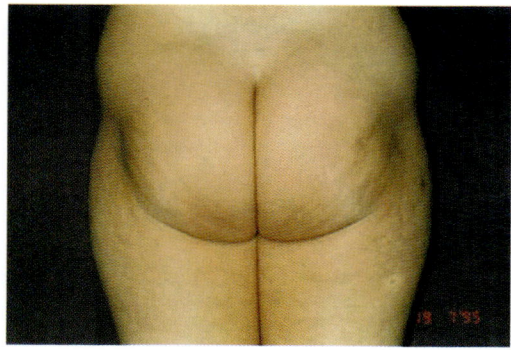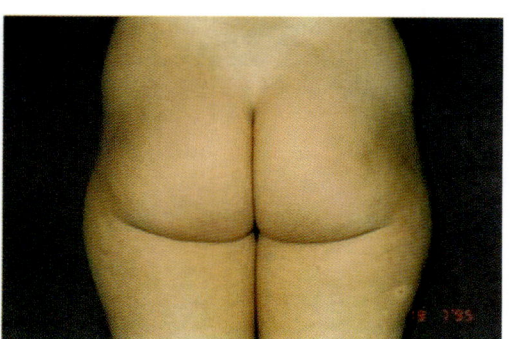

Figure 27.2 Subjects with gluteus contracted (left) and relaxed (right).

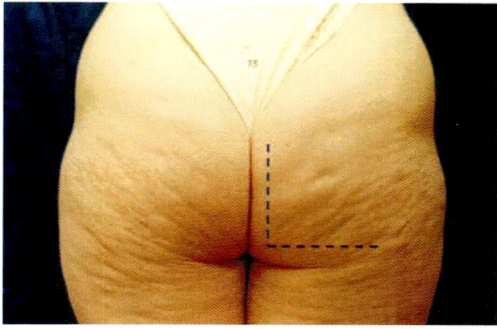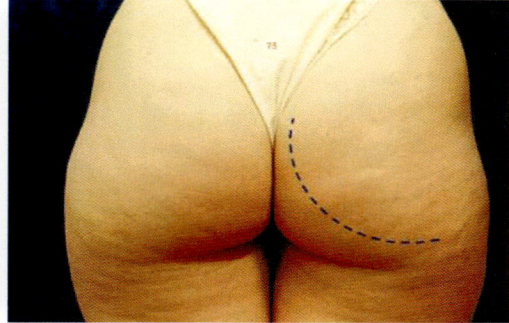

Figure 27.3 Differences between relaxed and contracted gluteus muscles. In the contracted photo (left), the intergluteus fold-tight angle is closer to 90°, whereas in the relaxed photo (right) the same line is rounded. Note the shape of the shadow is different and smaller in the contracted photo.

As for other digital photos, the standardization of subjects positioning and lighting enables to obtain comparable results across time-points. The subjects stand up in a controlled upright position, with their feet slightly open and they hold a horizontal bar for their body equilibrium. The camera is placed in front of the subjects' thigh, perpendicularly to the skin surface. The light source is placed to tangentially enlighten the skin surface below. This setup provides images with high dimple contrast, owing to the shadow they project (Fig. 27.6a).

Image analysis
Perin et al. proposed a seven-grade photonumerical scale to evaluate cellulite images of a pinched thigh. This scale was tested and validated demonstrating high level of repeatability and reproducibility. This method has the added benefit of providing the patient with meaningful figures.

The images can be analyzed to determine skin roughness (Fig. 27.6b). Briefly, the illuminant component of the image is extracted from the cellulite color images to provide information related to the distribution of light on the skin. The dimples appear lightened while the holes are shadowed. Profile lines are then extracted from the grey-level illuminant image and various roughness parameters such as the average roughness (Ra) and maximal amplitude (Rz) can be calculated.

We have investigated the correlation between roughness parameters (Ra, Rz) and the classical four points clinical grading of the cellulite [4] and found that the roughness parameters are correlated to the clinical score (see Fig. 27.7). Bertin et al. [5] also demonstrated that the method is sensitive enough to document changes related to the use of cosmetic products.

These two-dimensional regular images allow the documentation of cellulite and extraction of the roughness parameters. In order to assess the efficacy of a cosmetic or a device treatment, the standardization of the acquisition conditions is mandatory. The cellulite is even more visible when the thigh is pinched. This step also requires specific equipment that delivers a constant tangential pressure to the skin. When well standardized, this is a specific, reproducible and sensitive method to measure cellulite. However, the roughness parameters extracted from 2D images are based on light and shadow information and therefore represent an indirect measurement of the skin roughness.

Three-Dimensional Skin Surface Images
3D measurements can be performed to directly assess the skin surface texture and relief. Three digital imaging techniques have been progressively adapted for skin applications since the end the 90s [6]. They were first developed to measure skin wrinkles [7],

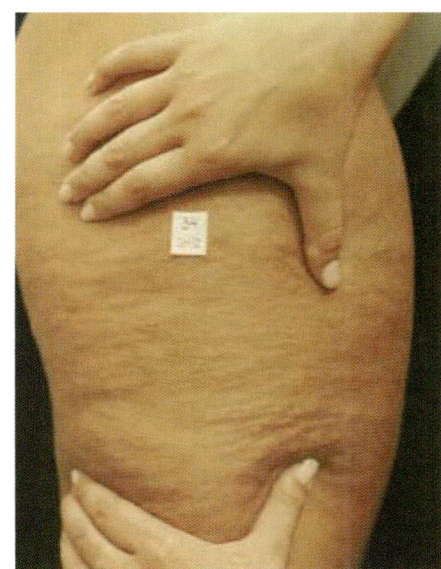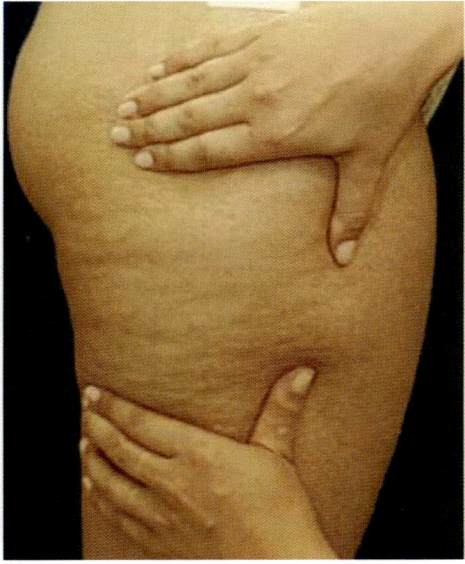

Figure 27.4 Pressure can accentuate the orange peel aspect of cellulite. The variation in hand pressure in the same subject provides different visual aspects.

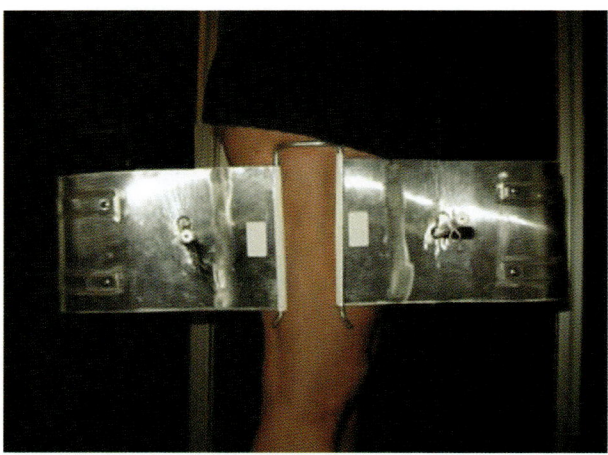

Figure 27.5 Pressure system developed by Perin et al.

and then extended to other applications such as facial shape or lips volume. A 3D device has successfully characterized cellulite levels *in vivo* [8].

Image acquisition

Suitable devices for 3D acquisition in a clinical center should be accurate, reproducible, noninvasive and affordable. There are three main techniques that currently meet these criteria. The techniques differ in how they scan the skin surface, but deliver similar 3D topographic surface maps. Each of the techniques has advantages and limitations (Table 27.1).

Laser scanning techniques. The cellulite area is scanned using a laser that is rasterized as a spot or stripe. The displacement of the laser is automatically controlled. The duration of the acquisition depends on the density of the cloud of points (spatial resolution) that is required. As an example, Smalls et al. [8] used a Cyberware Rapid 3D Digitizer (Cyberware, Inc., Monterrey, CA) to record 3D data of thigh cellulite. The scanner allowed them to collect a cloud of 256×512 pixel images (131,072 data points) in less than 40 seconds. The corresponding field of view was 402×170 mm and the spatial resolution of their acquisition was 0.5×0.38 mm. Today, faster devices such as the Konica Minolta VI-910 (Konica, Minolta Holding, Inc., Tokyo, Japan) enable the acquisition of 76,800 points in 0.3 seconds and 307,000 points in 2.5 seconds.

Structured light projection techniques. This method has been widely used to assess the skin roughness [7,9,10]. The principle is to project structured light patterns on the surface to be measured. The light pattern is distorted following the shape and the relief of the surface (Figs 27.8 and 27.9). By recording this deformation using a fast and high-resolution camera, the point's cloud is reconstructed using the triangulation principle. The Dermatop V3 (Breuckmann, Germany) are able to perform acquisition in less than 0.4 second for 1280×1024 points.

Stereophotographic techniques. Stereophotographic methods are inspired by the human perception of 3D information. Humans combine images from their two eyes to infer 3D information about the environment. Stereophotography applies the same principle to create 3D surfaces from two 2D images acquired using a regular camera. Consequently, the systems are usually made with one or two cameras that are able to acquire two images of the subject at different angles. Some systems also include a speckle texture light projector that enables a more precise recomposition of 3D data when the region of interest presents low contrast.

As for the previously described image methods, the acquisition of 3D images requires a well-standardized protocol as already described. While we prefer having the volunteers standing up (Fig. 27.9), Smalls asked them to sit on a flat surface with knees at a 90° angle [8]. This constraint is certainly linked with the long time their acquisition system requires (around 40 seconds).

Image analysis

The 3D image is a topographic surface composed with three main types of information: the overall shape, the waviness and the roughness.

We can use a few simple image-processing steps to separate the overall shape or curvature of the thigh and/or gluteus from the cellulite. The shape corresponds to the overall curvature of the region of interest (thigh or gluteus) and is not subject to variation related to the cellulite. Therefore, a low pass filter is applied on the image to remove this shape and to compensate the curvature of the image. After this step, a flattened surface containing only the waviness and the roughness of the skin is obtained. According to the sensitivity of the acquisition device, the roughness usually corresponds to the skin texture and is consequently removed with a high pass filter. Finally, only the waviness is analyzed since it is the

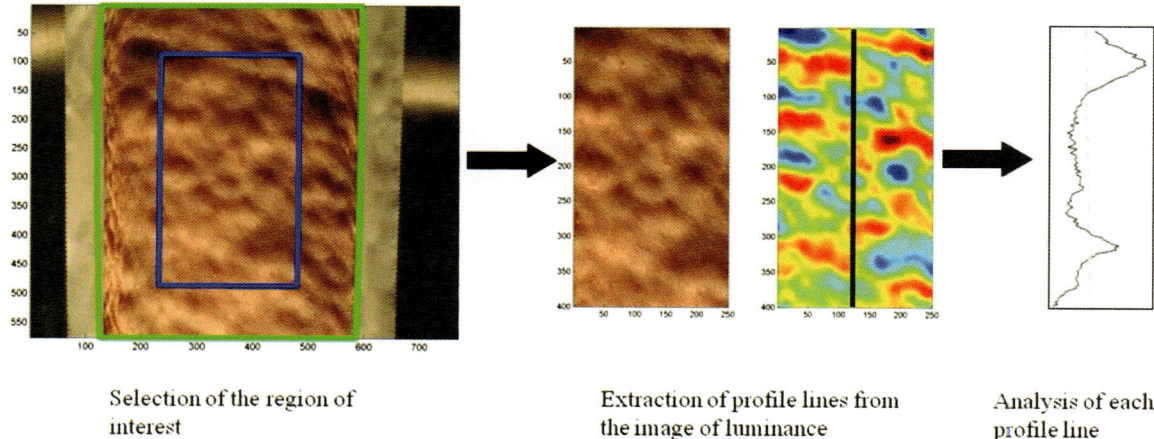

Selection of the region of interest

Extraction of profile lines from the image of luminance

Analysis of each profile line

Figure 27.6 Details of skin surface when pinched by the "pressure system" (a) and roughness parameters assessment (b).

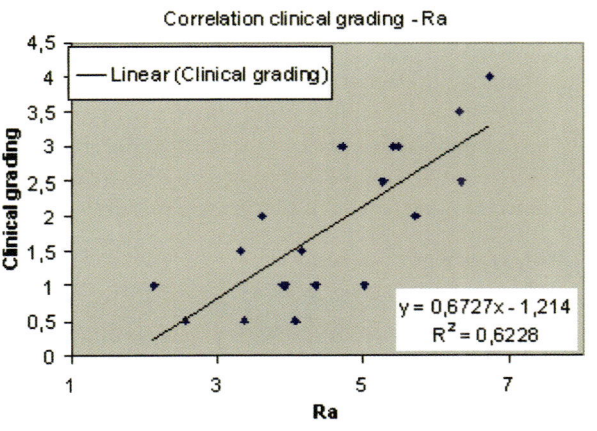
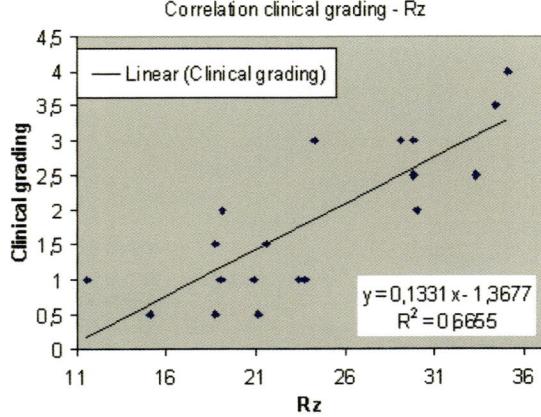

Figure 27.7 Correlation between the roughness parameters Ra, Rz and the clinical grading of the cellulite state using the four grades scale described by A. Rossi.

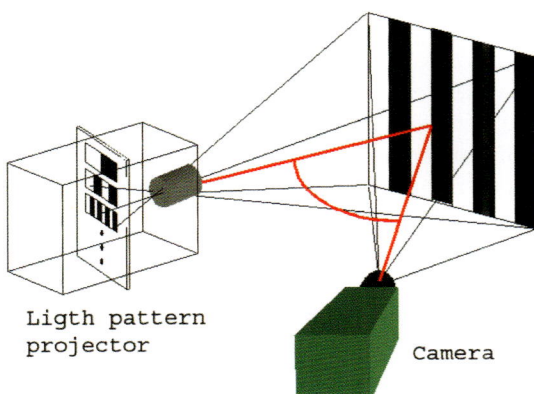

Ligth pattern projector   Camera

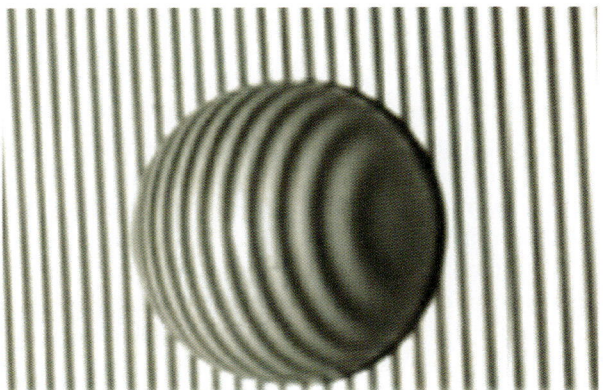

Figure 27.8 Principle of the structured light projection technique.

only component of the signal related to the dimpling of the skin caused by the orange peel aspect of cellulite (Fig. 27.10).

After having removed the body shape and the roughness of the skin, several parameters, such as the total dimple volume can be calculated to quantify the level of cellulite. Similarly to the line roughness parameters Ra, Rz, the surface roughness parameters such as mean roughness Sa and the maximum amplitude deviation Sz can be calculated directly from the surface data. The method based on the calculation of these parameters is sensitive and reproducible. Results from this method correlate well with the clinical grading of the cellulite (unpublished data).

Thermography

The measurement of the skin temperature has been used as a diagnostic tool for several diseases since the early 70s. The rationale is to measure the heat variations related to near surface blood flow in the hypodermal vascular network [11,12]. The heat changes are

Table 27.1 Comparison of three different 3D acquisition techniques. For each criteria, the best technology is rated with a triple "+"

Technology	Speed	Image quality	Cost
Laser scanning	+	++	++
Structured light	++	+++	+
Stereophotography	+++	+	+++

due to morphological modifications in adipocytes and blood flow in the different grades of cellulite [13]. Thermography indirectly evaluates blood flow through this vascular network. Two different thermal imaging techniques can assess skin temperature: contact thermography and infrared thermography.

Contact thermography

The first thermal images were obtained in the early seventies by taking pictures of encapsulated liquid crystals (ELC) plates. This method has been reported in the literature as the contact thermography. ELC plates are generally made by a set of flexible pillow detectors containing arrays of crystals which change color at a specific temperature [14]. Several types of crystals are distributed in a close space (pixel), each one sensitive to a specific temperature. Thus, the temperature is measured with an ordinal scale with a limited range. This system allows measuring temperatures with a seven-color scale ranging from 26.5 to 30.5°C. As an example, the Cell-meter RSW27S is a system made with a thermal plate and a camera for assessing cellulite on the thighs.

Image acquisition. The thermal plate is pressed against the desired body part using a metal frame. The color changes are recorded using a regular digital camera. The position of the camera, magnification and white balance are standardized to have reproducible pictures across time-points. An acquisition protocol is needed in order to acquire comparable pictures throughout all time-points. This protocol is usually close to those used for

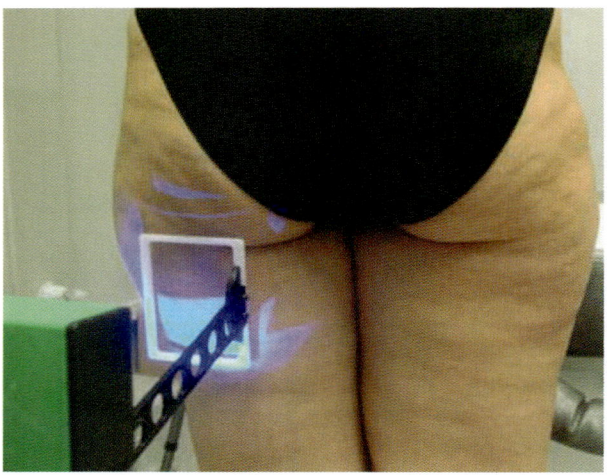

Figure 27.9 Acquisition of a 3D image using structured light projection techniques.

macrophotography. However, particular caution should be taken to handle thermal changes related to the physiological process. For example, the pictures should be taken at the same period of the day and menstrual cycle. The impact of physical activity, smoking, caffeine and emotional state should also be reduced to a minimum by keeping the patient in a controlled environment before image acquisition. Environmental factors influencing the body heat should also be controlled (room temperature and humidity).

Image analysis. The analysis of contact thermography images is sometimes qualitative [15]. Contact thermography images are generally compared to standard scale images. The two important thermal parameters for assessing cellulite severity are the overall temperature and its homogeneity. During the first stage of cellulite, adipocytes are small and well distributed resulting in a homogenous and hot skin. As the severity increases, irregular nodules appear and the skin temperature becomes more unbalanced and cold. Fig. 27.11 shows an example of thermal image

from two people, one without cellulite and the other with a severe grade of cellulite.

Contact thermography is an inexpensive and fast way to investigate the skin temperature and therefore evaluate the blood flow network. However, it requires direct contact with the skin, which can lead to interference in the measurement. Infrared thermography can be used to tackle this drawback.

Infrared Thermography

Infrared cameras are used to record infrared radiation emitted from the body. Infrared radiation is related to skin temperature. A higher skin temperature will emit more infrared radiation. Thermal cameras generally provide monochromatic images, where each pixel value corresponds to the temperature. The images are usually displayed using a color look-up-table (Lut) that goes from blue (cool points) to white (warm points). Infrared cameras can detect a wide range of temperature (from –20°C to 300°C) with a sensitivity of less than 0.02°C.

Image acquisition

The acquisition process requires the same positioning constraints as 2D macro photography, and the same standardization as for the contact thermography. The size of the thermal sensor is generally small (320 × 240 pixels), requiring careful selection of the distance between the subject and camera to maximize exposure to the area of interest. Due to the high sensitivity of the camera, physiological and environmental factors should be precisely monitored during the acquisition process. When recording skin cellulite images, it may be helpful to include thermal landmarks in the camera's field of view. As an example, the cellulite area to be examined could be delimited by small bandages (Fig. 27.11).

Image analysis

The images recorded using an infrared camera are processed automatically since the pixel values correspond to the real temperature (Fig. 27.11). The average temperature is calculated. The homogeneity of the skin temperature is obtained using parameters such as Ra and Rz or Sa and Sz.

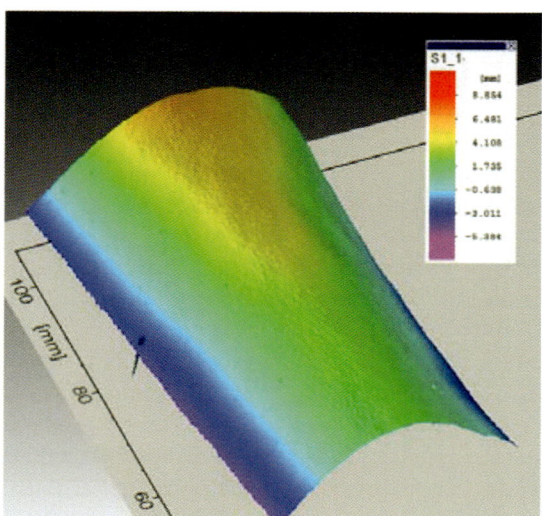
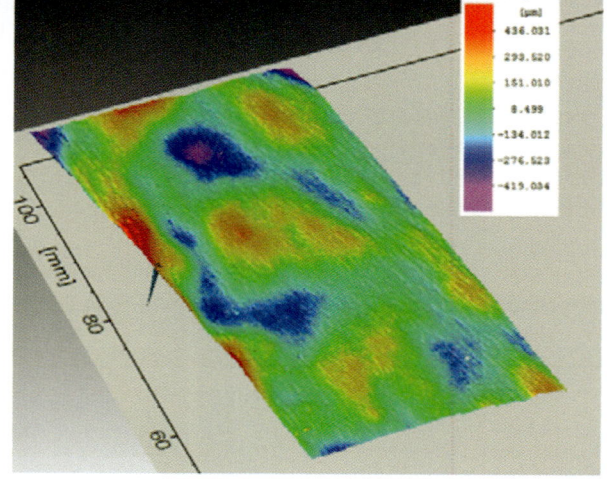

Figure 27.10 Example of 3D images before and after the removal of the waviness.

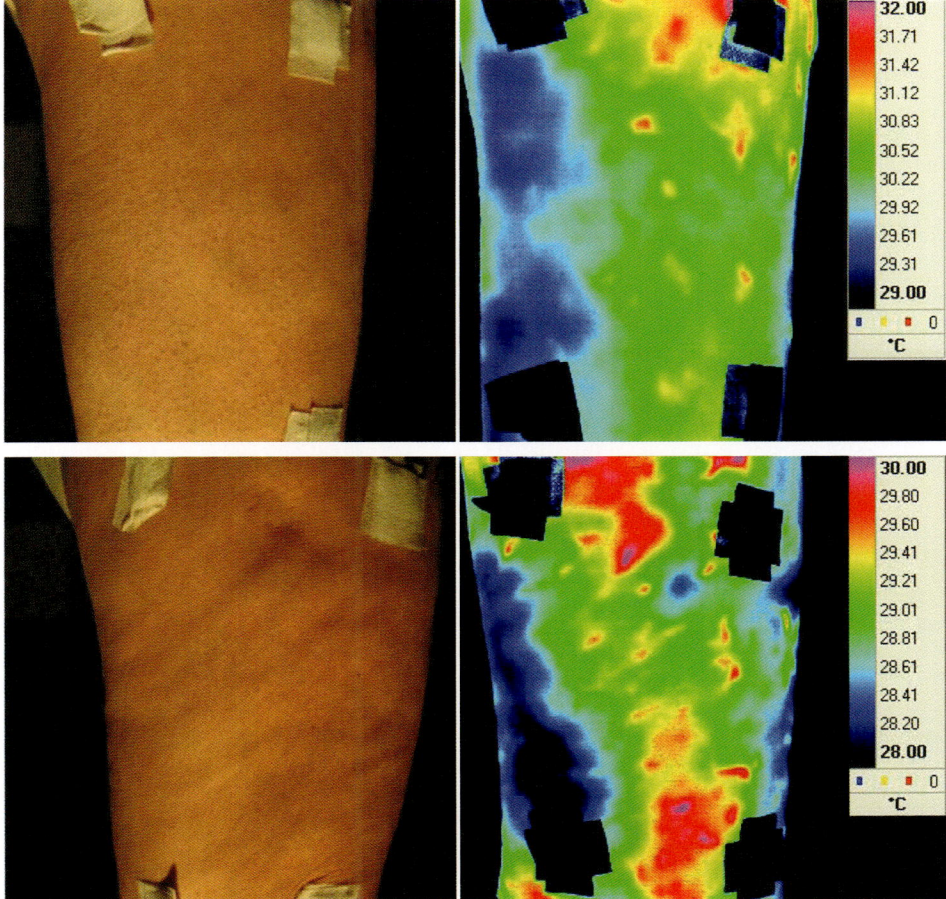

Figure 27.11 Contact thermography image from subjects without cellulite (top) and with cellulite (bottom).

Image Management

Apart from the image acquisition device (regular, 3D or infrared camera), a digital imaging system also includes a computer for image processing and visualization and a storage media. The computer to support a photographic system should have good power computation and enough random access memory (RAM). Most desktops and laptops currently available with 1 GB of RAM are powerful enough to process 2D and infrared images. More computation power (i.e. faster processor and more RAM) is needed for 3D images. A typical system for 3D image processing should have at least 2 GB of RAM. The system should also include a wide color corrected screen (e.g. 19 or 22 inch monitor) for viewing the images.

Finally, images should be digitally cataloged (i.e. easily saved, indexed and retrieved) based on the patients records. Several software packages are available to manage dermatological images (e.g. Dermapix®, Quantificare, France). The images should be saved on an external hard drive (over 1 terabyte) and backed up on a separate source. One potential solution is to use web-based image cataloging to archive medical images with respect with confidentiality requirements.

Acknowledgements

We would like to express our gratitude to Eotech (Marcoussis, France) for providing some of the illustrations used in this chapter, Aline Papillon for the support in the literature search, and Michael Cobb for the critical review of the content.

REFERENCES

1. D Ratner, C Thomas, D Bickers. The uses of digital photography in dermatology. Journal of American Academy of Dermatology. 41(5 Pt 1):749–56, 1999.
2. F Kaliyadan. Digital photography for patient counseling in dermatology—a study. Journal of European Academy of Dermatology and Venereology 22(11):1356–8, 2008.
3. F Perin, C Perrier, JC Pittet et al. Assessment of skin improvement treatment efficacy using the photograding of mechanically-accentuated macrorelief of thigh skin. International Journal of Cosmetic Science. 22(2):147–56, 2000.
4. AB Rossi, AL Vergnanini. Cellulite: a review. Journal of European Academy of Dermatology and Venereology 14(4):251–62, 2000.
5. C Bertin, H Zunino, J Pittet et al. A double-blind evaluation of the activity of an anti-cellulite product containing retinol, caffeine, and ruscogenine by a combination of several noninvasive methods. International Journal of Cosmetic Science 52(4):199–210, 2001.
6. S Jaspers, H Hopermann, G Sauermann et al. Rapid in vivo measurement of the topography of human skin by active image triangulation using a digital micromirror device. Skin Research and Technology. 5(3):195–207, 1999.

7. P Friedman, G Skover, G Payonk et al. 3D In-Vivo Optical Skin Imaging for Topographical Quantitative Assessment of Non-Ablative Laser Technology. Dermatologic Surgery 28(3):199–204, 2002.

8. L Smalls, C Lee, J Whitestone et al. Quantitative model of cellulite: three-dimensional skin surface topography, biophysical characterization, and relationship to human perception. International Journal of Cosmetic Science 27(4):253, 2005.

9. U Jacobi, M Chen, G Frankowski et al. In vivo determination of skin surface topography using an optical 3D device. Skin Research and Technology 10(4):207–14, 2004.

10. P Sandoz, D Marsaut, V Armbruster et al. Towards objective evaluation of the skin aspect: principles and instrumentation. Skin Research and Technology 10(4):263–70, 2004.

11. RB Barnes. Thermography of the Human Body Infrared-radiant energy provides new concepts and instrumentation for medical diagnosis. Science 140(3569):870–7, 1963.

12. S Bornmyr, H Svensson. Thermography and laser-Doppler flowmetry for monitoring changes in finger skin blood flow upon cigarette smoking. Clinical Physiology and Functional Imaging 11(2):135–41, 1991.

13. S Curri. Cellulite and fatty tissue microcirculation. Cosmetics and toiletries 108(4):51–8, 1993.

14. RA Sherman, AL Woerman, KW Karstetter. Comparative effectiveness of videothermography, contact thermography, and infrared beam thermography for scanning relative skin temperature. J Rehabil Res Dev 33(4):377–86, 1996.

15. C Kuhn, F Angehrn, O Sonnabend, A Voss. Impact of extracorporeal shock waves on the human skin with cellulite: A case study of an unique instance. Clinical Interventions in Aging. 3(1):201, 2008.

Index